HANDBOOK OF SYMPTOMS IN DOGS AND CATS

T0155191

Handbook of Symptoms in Dogs and Cats

Assessing Common Illnesses by Differential Diagnosis

Christian F. Schrey

Translated by Heidi Joeken

Dr. med. vet. Christian F. Schrey M.S., M.R.C.V.S.
Tierarztpraxis am Olivaer Platz Lietzenburger
Straße 107
10707 Berlin
www.vet-berlin.de

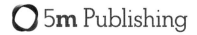

First published 2000

This edition published by 5m Publishing 2017

Authorised translation of the third German language edition, Christian
F. Schrey, Leitsymptome und Leitbefunde bei Hund und Katze

©2014 by Schattauer GmbH, Stuttgart/Germany

Copyright © Christian F. Schrey 2017

Heidi Joeken asserts her right to be known as the translator of this work

Published by
5M Publishing Ltd,
Benchmark House,
8 Smithy Wood Drive,
Sheffield, S35 1QN, UK
Tel: +44 (0) 1234 81 81 80
www.5mpublishing.com

A Catalogue record for this book is available from the British Library

ISBN 978-1-910455-72-2

Book layout by Servis Typesetting

Printed by Replika Press Pvt Ltd, India

Illustrations by Schattauer

Important note:

Medicine is an ever-changing science, so the contents of this publication, especially
recommendations concerning diagnostic and therapeutic procedures, can only give
an account of the knowledge at the time of publication. While utmost care has been
taken to ensure that all specifications regarding drug selection and dosage and treatment
options are accurate, readers are urged to review the production information sheet and
any relevant material supplied by the manufacturer, and, in case of doubt, to consult a
specialist. The publisher will appreciate being informed of possible inconsistences. The
ultimate responsibility for any diagnostic or therapeutic application lies with the reader.

No special reference is made to registered names, proprietary names trademarks,
etc. in this publication. The appearance of a name without designation as proprietary
does not imply that it is exempt from the relevant protective laws and regulations and
therefore free for general use.

Contents

To the three bright sparks
in my life, giving me perspective
Sabiene, Noona and Philipp

Foreword

This book arose out of frustration – as a new vet you may find yourself working on your own and feeling helpless when presented with a bleeding patient. There is no reference manual available that can help you quickly orientate yourself and find possible different diagnoses easily.

I hope that I can spare a lot of my colleagues this frustration and here welcome the 3rd edition. My thanks go to Mr Alexander Hüttig, Dr. Steven Kellner, Dr. Bärbel Löblich-Beardi, Dr. Meinhard Maurer, Prof. Dr. Roland Rudolph, Ms Antje Stolle-Malorny, Mr PD Dr. Günter Wilsdorf and Dr. Karl-Heinz Kirschstein for their altruistic and committed co-operation with this project.

My thanks also go to Schattauer Publishers, in particular to Mr Dipl.-Psych. Dr. med. Wulf Bertram but also to all members of staff who made the realisation of this project possible.

Berlin, February 2014.
Dr. med. vet. Christian F. Schrey

List of Abbreviations

αHBDH	Alpha-Hydroxybutyrate Dehydrogenase
ACTH	Adrenocorticotropic hormone
ADH	Antidiuretic hormone
Alb	Albumin
Amyl	Amylase
ANA	Antinuclear antibodies
ANP	Atrial Natriuretic Peptide
ANTU	Alpha Naphtylthiourea
AP	Alkaline Phosphatase
ARVC	Arrhythmogenic right ventricular Cardiomyopathy
ASD	Atrial Septal Defect
AV–Block	Atrioventricular Block
BAERA	Brain-auditory-evoked-response Audiometry
BE	Bacterial Examination
BG	Blood Glucose
BGA	Blood Gas Analysis
Bili	Bilirubin
BNP	Brain Natriuretic Peptide
BSR	Blood Sedimentation Rate
BW	Body weight
Ca	Calcium
CAV-1	Canines Adenovirus-1
CEA	Collie Eye Anomaly
CGH	Congenital Hypothyroidism
Chol	Cholesterol
CLAD	Canine Leucocyte Adhesion Deficiency
CN	Cranial nerve
CNS	Central Nervous System
CPSE	Canine Prostate-Specific Arginine Esterase
Crea	Creatinine
CRP	C-reactive Protein
CS	Cervical Spine
CSNS	Congenital stationary night blindness
CT	Computed tomography
DCMP	Dilated cardiomyopathy

DEA	Dog Erythrocyte Antigen
DEET	Diethyltoluamide
DIC	Disseminated intravasal coagulation (Consumptive coagulopathy)
Diff BC	Differential Blood Count
DM	Degenerative Myelopathy
ECG	Electrocardiogram
EEG	Electroencephalogram
EF	Episodic Falling
EIC	Exercise Induced Collapse
ELISA	Enzyme-linked immunosorbent assay
ENM	Hereditary Necrotising Myelopathy
EME	Eosinophilic meningoencephalitis
EMG	Electromyogram
Eos	Eosinophil granulocytes
Erys	Erythrocytes
FDP	Fibrin Degradation Products
FeLV	Feline Leukaemia virus
FIP	Feline infectious Peritonitis
FIV	Feline Immunodeficiency virus
FLUTD	Feline Lower Urinary Tract Disease
FORL	Feline Odontoclastic Resorptive Lesions
FUS	Feline Urological Syndrome (previously used term, now FLUTD)
GGT	Gamma-Glutamyl Transferase
Glob	Globulin
GME	Granulomatous meningoencephalitis
GnRH	Gonadotropin Releasing Hormone
GOT/AST	Glutamate Oxaloacetate Transaminase/Aspartate Aminotransferase
GPT/ALT	Glutamate-Pyruvate Transaminase/Alanine Aminotransferase
Hb	Haemoglobin
HCG	Human Chorionic Gonadotropin
HCMP	Hypertrophic cardiomyopathy
Hct	Haematocrit
HNPK	Hereditary Nasal Parakeratosis
IGF-1	Insulin-Like Growth Factor
IGS	Imerslund-Gräsbeck Syndrome
JEB	Junctional Epidermolysis Bullosa
K	Potassium

LDH	Lactate dehydrogenase
LE-Cells	Lupus erythematosus cells
Leuc	Leucocytes
LMN	Lower motor neuron
LS	Lumbar spine
Lympho	Lymphocytes
MCH	Mean corpuscular haemoglobin
MCHC	Mean corpuscular haemoglobin concentration
MCV	Mean corpuscular volume
Mg	Magnesium
Mono	Monocytes
MRT	Magnetic resonance tomography
N	Normal Finding
Na	Sodium
Neutro	Neutrophil granulocytes
NSAID	Non-steroidal anti-inflammatories
P	Phosphate
PDA	Patent ductus arteriosus
PNS	Peripheral nervous system
PT	Prothrombin Time
PTT/aPTT	(Activated) partial Thromboplastin Time
RI	Reticulocyte Index
SA-Block	Sinoatrial-Block
SARD	Sudden acute retinal detachment/Atrophy
SIADH	Syndrome of inappropriate ADH secretion
STH	Somatotropic Hormone
TBE	Tick borne encephalitis
TLI	Trypsin-like immunoreactivity
TP	Total Proteine
TRH	Thyrotropin-releasing Hormone
Trigl	Triglycerides
TSH	Thyroid Stimulating Hormone
UMN	Upper motor neuron
Urea	Urea
Vit	Vitamin
VSD	Ventricular Septal Defect
WPW	Wolff-Parkinson-White Syndrome

How to Use this Book

This book is a reference manual for the small animal vet in clinical practice offering differential diagnoses for common symptomatic presentations.

Principal symptoms and findings are individually listed and the differential diagnoses are in order of the most common and sorted into different species.

Principal Symptom/Finding

Definition	
Most Common Causes	
Dog	Cat
+++ Listing in decreasing order frequency	+++ Listing in decreasing order of frequency

Classification of the different causes

- Most common differential diagnoses in the dog and/or in the cat
- Rare differential diagnoses in the dog and/or in the cat

- (non–endemic pathogen in UK)

A suggestion of diagnostic approaches will follow each principal symptom with recommendations of tests in order of declining priority.

Diagnostic Approach

Principal Symptom

1. **Case History**

2. **General Examination**

3. **Blood Tests**

- First Choice Examination Parameters (Basic Diagnostics)
- Second Choice Examination Parameters (Further Diagnostics)

1 General Symptoms

Further Relevant Principal Symptoms

Obesity

Excess Weight, Adiposis

Common Causes	
Dog	Cat
+++ Overfeeding, Lack of Exercise, Neutering (esp bitch)	+++ Overfeeding, Lack of Exercise, Neutering (esp male cat)
++ Hypercortisolism (Cushing's Disease)	++ Glucocorticoid Long-Term Therapy
++ Glucocorticoid Long-Term Therapy	++ Arterial Hypertension
+ Hypothyroidism	

With Polyphagia

- Hypercortisolism (Cushing's Disease) [Dog]
- Glucocorticoid Long-Term Therapy

With Normophagia

- High caloric food
- Lack of Exercise
- Castration
- Hypothyroidism [Dog]

Diagnostic Approach

Obesity

1. **Case History**

2. **General Examination**

3. **Blood Tests**
- GPT, AP
- Glc
- Chol, Trigl [Dog]

4. **Function Test**

- T_3/T_4, fT_4 [Dog]
- TSH/TRH Stimulation test [Dog]
- Thyroglobulin Antibodies
- Adrenal Gland
  - Dexamethasone Suppression test ACTH
  - Stimulation test
  - Cortisol/Creatinine Ratio

Anaemia

Reduction in the number of erythrocytes and/or of haemoglobin and/or of the haematocrit with normal blood volume

Regenerative Anaemia:

- Haemolytic Anaemia
- Blood Loss Anaemia

Non-Regenerative Anaemia:

- Aplastic Anaemia/ Bone Marrow Failure
- Deficiency Anaemia

Common Causes	
Dog	**Cat**
Haemolytic Anaemia	
+++ Immunoreactive Causes	+++ FeLV/FIV
++ Toxic Causes	++ Haemobartonella felis
++ Infectious Causes	++ Toxic Causes
	++ Immunoreactive Causes
Blood Loss Anaemia	
++ Ruptured organ/blood vessel	+++ Ruptured organ/blood vessel
++ Bleeding tumour (esp splenic/intestinal tumour)	++ Bleeding tumour
	+ Bleeding fracture/haematoma
++ Bleeding ulcer	
++ Bleeding fracture/haematoma	
++ Coagulopathy	
Aplastic Anaemia	
++ Toxic Causes	++ Immunoreactive Causes
++ Leukaemia	++ Toxic Causes
++ Chronic Renal Failure	++ FeLV/FIV, Leukaemia
	++ Chronic Renal Failure

Haemolysis

Infectious Causes

- Viruses
  - FeLV/FIV [Cat]
  - FIP Coronavirus [Cat]
- Parasites/Rickettsia
  - Babesia sp. [Dog]
  - Haemobartonella sp. [Cat]
  - (Ehrlichia sp. [Dog])
  - (Hepatozoon sp. [Dog])
  - (Dirofilaria sp. [esp Dog])
  - (Cytauxzoon sp. [Cat])

- Bacteria
  - Leptospira sp. [Dog]

Immunoreactive Causes

- Autoimmune haemolysis
- Drug allergy
- Neonatal Isoerythrolysis [Cat]
- Blood transfusion incompatibility

Toxic Causes

- Water enema [Cat]
- Drugs
  - Antibiotics
  - NSAIDs (esp paracetamol)
  - Propylene glycol
  - Antiarrhythmics
  - Anticonvulsants
  - Cimetidine
  - Levamisole
  - Metronidazole
  - Griseofulvin
  - Phenothiazin
  - Methylene blue
  - Cytostatics
  - Vaccinations
  - Vitamin K
  - Benzocain
  - Methionin
- Onions/Garlic/Broccoli
- Snake venom
- Heavy metal Poisoning

Other Causes

- DIC
- Haemangiosarcoma
- Septicaemia/Endotoxaemia
- Lymphatic Leukaemia/ Lymphoma

- Splenic torsion
- V.cava Syndrome (Dirofilariosis)
- Microangiopathy
- Heat stroke
- Pyruvate kinase deficiency [Dog]
- Phosphofructokinase deficiency [Dog]
- Copper storage disease [Dog]
- Vasculitis
- Feline Porphyria [Cat]
- Hypophosphataemia

Blood Loss

Acute Blood Loss

- Traumatic organ or blood vessel rupture
- Bleeding tumour
- Coagulopathy
- Epistaxis
- Acute gastrointestinal haemorrhage
- Acute urinary tract haemorrhage
- Bleeding aneurysm

Chronic Blood Loss

  - Chronic gastrointestinal haemorrhage
  - Haemorrhagic gastroenteritis
  - Bleeding tumour
- Chronic urinary tract haemorrhage
- Hook worm infestation
- Bleeding tumour
- Ectoparasitic infestation
- Coagulopathy

- Iron deficiency (Cause + Effect)

Bone Marrow Failure

Infectious Causes

- Viruses
  - FeLV/FIV [Cat]
  - Parvovirus
- Rickettsia
  - (Ehrlichia sp. [Dog])
- Parasites
  - (Leishmania sp. [Dog])

Endocrine Causes

- Hypothyroidism [Dog]
- Hypocortisolism (Addison's Disease) [Dog]
- STH Deficiency

Toxic Causes

- Drugs
  - Fenbendazole
  - Synthetic Oestrogens
  - Azathioprine [Cat]
  - Phenylbutazone
  - Metamizol
  - Acetylsalicylic acid
  - Chloramphenicol
  - Primidon
  - Sulfonamide/Trimetoprim
  - Tetracyclines
  - Cytostatics
  - Arsenic derivates
  - Griseofulvin [esp Cat]
- Endogenous Oestrogens
- Sertoli Cell Tumour [esp Dog]
  - Ovarian cysts
  - Granulosa Cell Tumour
- Organophosphates
- Heavy metals
  - Lead
  - Aluminium
  - Cadmium
- Radiotherapy

Erythropoetin Deficiency

- Chronic Renal Failure

Bone Marrow Tumours

- Multiple Myeloma [Dog]
- Lymphatic Leukaemia
- Myeloid Leukaemia

Other Causes

- Myelofibrosis/Osteofibrosis
- Autoimmune Disease
- Vitamin B_{12}-/Folic Acid Deficiency
- Copper Deficiency

Diagnostic Approach

Obesity

1. **Case History**

2. **General Examination**

3. **Blood Tests**
   - Hct, RBC, WBC
   - Hb, MCH, MCV, MCHC

- Diff Blood Count
  - Blood parasites
  - Morphology of erythrocytes
- TP, Alb, Glob
- GPT, AP, Urea, Crea
- Reticulocytes
- Bili, LDH
- Na, K, Ca, P
- Glc, Chol

COAGULATION
- Bleeding time
- Prothrombin time (PT/Quick)
- (Activated) partial Thromboplastin time (PTT/ aPTT)
- Fibrin Degradation Product (FDP)
- Thrombocyte number

MICROBIAL SEROLOGY
- FeLV-/FIV Antigen [Cat]
- Babesia Antibody [Dog]
- Ehrlichia Antibody [Dog]
- Leptospira Antibody [Dog]

IMMUNOSEROLOGY
- Microscope Slide Agglutination Test
- Coombs Test

- ANA Test

FUNCTION TESTS
- T_4, fT_4
- TSH-/TRH Stimulation Test [Dog]
- Adrenal Gland Function Test [Dog]
  - Dexamethasone Suppression test
  - ACTH Stimulation Test
  - Cortisol/Creatinine Ratio

FURTHER SEROLOGY
- Serum iron
- Serum Vitamin B_{12}-/Folic acid
- Serum led

4. Urinalysis
- Urine dip stick
- Specific gravity
- Urine sediment

5. Faecal Examination
- Intestinal parasites Occult blood
- Parvovirus Antigen Test [Dog]

6. Further Tests
- Bone Marrow Biopsy
- X-Ray Study
- Ultrasound

Abdominal Pain

Acute or chronic pain in the abdomen with diffuse or localised pain on palpation, tense abdominal wall, hunched back, shallow breathing, pain vocalisation and a preference to take in pressure relieving positions (back or prone position)

Common Causes	
Dog	Cat
+++ Gastroenteritis	+++ Gastroenteritis
++ Ileus	++ Ileus
++ Gastric Dilation/Volvulus	++ Constipation
++ Constipation	++ Tumours
++ Pancreatitis	++ Renal/Urinary Tract Disease
++ Gastric/Duodenal Ulcer	
++ Tumours	++ Peritonitis
+ Renal/Urinary Tract Disease	+ Pancreatitis
	+ Gastric Ulcer
+ Organ Rupture	

Cranial Abdomen

Acute Causes

- Gastric Dilation/ Volvulus [Dog]
- Gastric Perforation
  - Trauma
  - Foreign Body
  - Ulcer
- Acute Pancreatitis [esp Dog]

Chronic Causes

- Gastritis/Duodenitis
- Gastric/Duodenal Ulcer
- Chronic Pancreatitis
- Hepatitis/Cholangitis
- Splenic Torsion
- Gastric Carcinoma
- Hepatic Abscess
- Hepatic Tumour
- Cholelithiasis
- Splenitis/Splenic tumour

Caudal Abdomen

Acute Causes

- Obstruction of the Urinary Tract

  - FLUTD [Cat]
  - Urolithiasis
  - Urinary Bladder/Urethral Tumour
- Acute Prostatic Disease [Dog]
  - Prostatitis, Prostatic Abscess
  - Prostatic Carcinoma
- Traumatic Vessel/Organ Rupture
  - Urinary Bladder Rupture
  - Uterine Rupture
- Feline Aortic Thrombosis [Cat]
- Referred Pain Spinal Column
- Testicular torsion/ Cryptorchism [Dog]
- Colonic Ulcer
- Dystocia

Chronic Causes

- Cystitis
- Endometritis
- Chronic Prostatic Disease [Dog]
  - Prostatic Hyperplasia
  - Prostatic Cyst

- Prostatic Carcinoma
- Paraprostatic Cyst
- Colitis
- Tumour
- Perianal Disease
  - Anal Gland Abscess
  - Perianal Fistula
  - Perianal Tumour
  - Perineal Hernia
  - Perianal Wound

Diffuse Abdominal Pain

Acute/Chronic Causes

- Mechanical Ileus (Intestinal obstruction)
  - Foreign Body
  - Tumour
  - Intestinal Parasites
  - Intussusception
  - Incarceration (Hernia)
  - Volvulus
  - Adhesions
- Paralytic Ileus (Enteral Motility Disorder)
  - Mesenterial Infarction
  - Infectious Enteritis
  - Toxic Enteritis
  - Gastric/Duodenal Ulcer
  - Gastropexy [Dog]
  - Intestinal Perforation
  - Dysautonomia [Cat]
  - Pyloric Stenosis
  - Postoperative Intestinal Paralysis
  - Peritonitis
  - Uraemia
  - Sepsis
  - Hypokalaemia
  - Hypothyroidism [Dog]
  - Hepatic Encephalopathy

- Diabetic Ketoacidosis
  - Pancreatitis
  - Meteorism
  - Vagus Paralysis
  - General Anaesthesia
  - Atropine
  - Butylscopolamine
- Peritonitis
  - FIP Coronavirus [Cat]
  - Septicaemia
  - Mechanical Ileus
  - Penetrating Wounds
  - Blunt Trauma
  - Intestinal Perforation
  - Ulcer Perforation
  - Organ Rupture (urine, bile, pancreatic enzymes)
  - Retroperitoneal abscess/ haematoma
  - Ruptured Prostatic Abscess [Dog]
  - Pancreatitis
  - Postoperative Complications
  - Tumours
- Constipation
- Gastroenteritis
- Pyometra
- Tumors
- Referred Pain
  - Spinal Column
  - Thorax/Pleura
  - Kidneys
  - Cranial/Caudal Abdomen
- Dystocia
- Occlusion of the mesenteric artery
- Portal Vein Thrombosis
- Intestinal Adhesions

Dorsal Abdomen

Acute Causes

- Acute Nephritis/
  Pyelonephritis

- Retroperitoneal abscess/
  haematoma
- Renal Calculi
- Hydronephrosis
- Renal Infarction

Diagnostic Approach

Abdominal Pain

1. Case History

2. General Examination

3. X-Ray Study
- Abdomen
- Thorax
- Gastrointestinal Contrast
  Medium Study
- Cystography
- Urography

4. Ultrasound Examination
- Abdomen

5. Blood Tests
- Hct, Ery, Leuc
- TP, Alb, Glob
- GPT, AP, Urea, Crea, Bili, BG
- Amylase, Lipase [Dog]
- Blood Sedimentation Rate (BSR)
- Diff BC
- Na, K, Ca
- TLI Test
- Bile Acids
- FIP Profile [Cat]
  - TP
  - Alb/Glob Ratio
  - Bili
  - GOT/AST
  - Serum Electrophoresis

MICROBIAL SEROLOGY
- FeLV-/FIV Antigen [Cat]

6. Urinalysis
- Urine dip stick
- Specific gravity
- Urine sediment
- Urinary output/volume

7. Endoscopy
- Gastro-/Duodenoscopy
  ± Biopsy
- Colonoscopy ± Biopsy

8. Further Tests
- Fluid Analysis of body cavity
  Effusions
- Neurological Examination Spinal
  Reflexes
  - Bicipital reflex (C6–C8)
  - Triceps reflex (C7–T1)
  - Patellar reflex (L4–L6)
  - Interdigital Pain
    reflex
    (C6–T1 and L6–S1)
  - Cutaneous trunci reflex
    (C7–T1)
  - Anal sphincter reflex (S1–S3)
  - Urinary bladder – can it be
    expressed?

Abdominal Distention

Enlarged Abdomen	
Common Causes	
Dog	Cat
+++ Abdominal effusion/Ascites	+++ Abdominal effusion
++ Hypercortisolism (Cushing's Disease)	++ Tumours
	++ Organ enlargement
++ Tumours	
++ Gastric dilation/volvulus	
++ Organ enlargement	

Organ Enlargement

Renomegaly

- Viral Nephritis
  - FeLV/FIV [Cat]
  - FIP Coronavirus [Cat]
- Bacterial Nephritis
  - Leptospira sp. [Dog]
- Toxic Nephritis
  - Ethylene glycol Poisoning
- Renal Congestion
  - Hydronephrosis (Urinary Tract Obstruction)
- Renal Tumours
  - Lymphosarcoma [esp Cat]
  - Sarcoma
  - Nephroblastoma
  - Adenocarcinoma
  - Renal Epithelial Carcinoma [Dog]
- Other Causes
  - Renal abscess
  - Renal haematoma
  - Renal cysts [Cat]
  - Compensatory Renal Hypertrophy
  - Tumour Metastasis

Splenomegaly

- Splenic Congestion
  - Right Sided Cardiac Failure
  - Splenic Torsion
  - Hepatic Cirrhosis
  - Sedation/General Anaesthesia
- Splenic Tumours
  - Haemangiosarcoma [esp Dog]
  - Lymphosarcoma
  - Mast Cell Tumour
  - Multiple Myeloma
  - Malignant Histiocytosis [St Bernard Dog]
  - Fibrosarcoma
- Parasitic Splenitis
  - Toxoplasma sp.
  - (Leishmania sp. [esp Dog])
  - (Dirofilaria sp. [esp Dog])
- Viral Splenitis

- FeLV/FIV [Cat]
- FIP Coronavirus [Cat]
- CAV-1 (Hepatitis c. c.) [Dog]
- Bacterial Splenitis
  - Brucella sp. [Dog]
  - Salmonella sp.
  - Mycobacterium sp.
  - Septicaemic Pathogens
- Rickettsial Splenitis
  - Haemobartonella sp. [Cat]
  - (Ehrlichia sp. [Dog])
- Immunoreactive Splenitis
  - Feline Hypereosinophilic Syndrome [Cat]
  - Lupus erythematosus
  - Immunohaemolytic Anaemia
- Other Causes
  - Splenic abscess/haematoma
  - Tumour Metastasis

Hepatomegaly

- Viral Hepatitis
  - CAV-1 (Hepatitis c. c.) [Dog]
  - FeLV/FIV [Cat]
  - FIP Coronavirus [Cat]
- Bacterial Hepatitis/Cholangitis
  - Salmonella sp.
  - E. coli
  - Staphylococcus sp.
  - Bacillus sp. [Dog]
  - Leptospira sp. [Dog]
- Parasitic Hepatitis/Cholangitis
  - Toxoplasma sp.
  - Capillaria sp.
  - (Leishmania sp. [esp Dog])
  - (Opisthorchis sp. [Cat])
- Immunoreactive Cholangitis

- Feline lymphocytic Cholangiohepatitis
- Metabolic Hepatosis
  - Feline Hepatic Lipidosis [Cat]
  - Glycogen Storage Disease
  - Copper Storage Disease [Dog]
  - Diabetes mellitus
  - Amyloidosis
  - Hypercortisolism (Cushing's Disease) [Dog]
  - Glucocorticoid Long Term Therapy
- Hepatic Congestion
  - Right Sided Cardiac Failure
  - Pericardial Disease
  - Cardiac Arrhythmias
  - Vena cava syndrome (Dirofilaria sp. [Dog])
  - Bile Duct Obstruction
  - Thrombosis
- Hepatic Tumours
  - Bile Duct Adenoma/
  - Carcinoma
  - Hepatocellular Adenoma/ Carcinoma
  - Lymphosarcoma
  - Haemangioendothelioma
  - Mast Cell Tumour
  - Tumour Metastasis
- Toxic Hepatosis

NSAID

- Paracetamol
- Phenylbutazone
- Naproxen
- Acetylsalicyl Acid
- Ibuprofen
- Indometacin

Anticonvulsants

- Phenobarbital
- Primidon
- Diazepam

Antibiotics

- Ampicillin
- Erythromycin
- Nitrofurantoin
- Tetracyclines

Inhalation Anaesthetics

- Halothan
- Methoxyflurane

Others

- Griseofulvin
- Procainamide
- Warfarin
- Haloperidol
- Phenothiazine
- Cimetidine
- Vitamin A
- Glucocorticoids
- Cytostatics
- Aflatoxines
- Household Agents
- Poisonous Plants
- Heavy metals
- Bile Duct Obstruction
  - Pancreatic Carcinoma
  - Acute Pancreatitis
  - Bile Duct Carcinoma
  - Cholelithiasis
  - Intestinal Tumour (Papillary tumour)
  - Enteral Foreign Body
- Other Causes
  - Hepatic Cysts
  - Biloma
  - Hepatic Abscess
  - Haematoma

Gastric/Intestinal Enlargement

- Gastric Overload (Polyphagia)
- Gastric Dilation/Volvulus [Dog]
- Intestinal Obstruction (Ileus)
- Constipation
- Meteorism

Uterine Enlargement

Pregnancy
Pyometra
- Hydrometra
- Mucometra
- Uterine tumours

Ovarian Enlargement

- Ovarian Cysts
- Ovarian Tumours
  - Granulosa Cell Tumour
  - Cystadenoma/-carcinoma [Dog]

Urinary Bladder Enlargement (Obstruction of the Urinary Tract)

- Urolithiasis
- FLUTD [Cat]
- Prostate Enlargement [Dog]
  - Prostatic Cysts
  - Prostatic Hyperplasia
  - Prostatitis/Prostatic Abscess
  - Prostatic Carcinoma
  - Paraprostatic Cyst
- Bladder/Urethral Tumours
  - Transitional Cell Carcinoma

- Leiomyoma/-sarcoma
- Fibroma
- Squamous Cell Carcinoma
- Polyp
- Papilloma
- Canine Transmissible Venereal Tumour [Dog]
- Neurological Causes
  - Sphincter Spasm (UMN Lesion)
  - Detrusor Atony (LMN Lesion)
  - Reflex Dyssynergia [Dog]
- Other Causes
  - Pelvic Fractures
  - Spinal disease
  - Abdominal tumours
  - Cystitis/Urethritis

Abdominal Effusion/ Ascites

Transudate

- Hypoalbuminaemia
  - Protein-losing enteropathy and nephropathy
  - Hepatic cirrhosis/ portosystemic shunt
  - Cachexia
  - Burns
- Tumours
- Obstruction of lymphatic vessels
- Hepatic cirrhosis

Modified Transudate

- Right Sided Cardiac Failure
- Pericardial Disease
- Tumours

Exudate

- Pus
  - Penetrating wounds
  - Ruptured Pyometra
  - Intestinal perforation
  - Ileus
  - Septicaemia/Ruptured abscess
  - Peritonitis
- Blood
  - Traumatic rupture of an organ or vessel
  - Coagulopathies
  - Splenic rupture/ haemangiosarcoma [Dog]
- Chyle
  - Obstruction of lymphatic vessels
  - Retroperitoneal haematoma
  - Lymphangiectasia [Dog]
  - Hepatic cirrhosis
  - Cardiac disease
  - Ileus
  - Acute pancreatitis
  - Tumours
- Pseudochylous Effusion
  - Tumours
  - Chronic inflammation
- Urine
  - Rupture of the bladder/ ureteral or urethral avulsion
- Bile
  - Rupture of the gall bladder
  - Hepatic rupture
- Other causes
  - Intestinal torsion/volvulus
  - Testicular torsion/ cryptorchism
  - Gastric/Intestinal rupture
  - Pancreatic rupture

– Acute Pancreatitis
– Tumours
– FIP [Cat]
– Diaphragmatic hernia
– Vena cava Syndrome
(Dirofilaria sp. [Dog])

Other Causes

• Weakness of the abdominal
muscles

– Hypercortisolism (Cushing's
Disease) [esp Dog]
• Pneumoperitoneum
– Penetrating Wounds
– Gastric/Intestinal
perforation
– Uterine perforation
• Obesity
• Umbilical hernia

Diagnostic Approach

Abdominal Distention

1. Case History

2. General Examination

3. X-Ray Study
• Abdomen
• Thorax

4. Ultrasound Examination
• Abdomen
• Heart (Doppler
Echocardiography)

5. Blood Tests
• Hct, Ery, Leuc
• TP, Alb, Glob
• GPT, AP, Urea, Crea, BG
• FIP Profile [Cat]
– TP
– Alb/Glob Ratio
– Bili
– GOT
– Serum electrophoresis
• Diff BC
• Amylase, Lipase [Dog]
• TLI Test

• Bile acids
• Bilirubin

COAGULATION
• Bleeding time
• Prothrombin time (PT/Quick)
• (Activated) partial
Thromboplastin time (PTT/aPTT)
• Fibrin degradation product (FDP)
• Thrombocyte number

MICROBIAL SEROLOGY
• FeLV-/FIV Antigen [Cat]
• Dirofilaria immitis Antigen [Dog]

FUNCTION TESTS
• Adrenal Gland function tests
[Dog]
• Dexamethasone Suppression test
• ACTH Stimulation test
• Cortisol/Creatinine Ratio

**6. Fluid Analysis of
Abdominal Effusion**
• Colour/Consistency/Smell
• Specific gravity

- Albumin/Globulin Ratio
- Rivalta Test [Cat]
- LDH, Bili, Crea, Amylase, Lipase
- Chol, Trigl
- Ether Clearance Test
- Cytology
- Bacterial culture

7. Urinalysis
- Urine dip stick
- Specific gravity
- Urine sediment

8. Further Tests
- Angiography
- Laparotomy

Bite and Scratch Wounds

Wound infection in humans, caused by dog and cat bites as well as scratches

Dog Bite Wounds	Cat Bite/Scratch Wounds

• Bacterial wound infection
  – Staphylococcus sp.
  – Streptococcus sp.
  – Clostridium sp.
  – Bacteroides sp.
  – Pasteurella sp.
• Viral wound infection
  – (Rabies Virus)
	• Rickettsial wound infection
	  – Bartonella (Rochalimaea) henselae
	  – Bacterial wound infection
	  – Afipia felis
	  – Pasteurella sp.
	  – Staphylococcus sp.
	  – Streptococcus sp.
	  – Clostridium sp.
	  – Bacteroides sp.
	• (Viral wound infection
	  – Rabies Virus)

Tendency to Bleed

Haemorrhagic Diathesis: Spontaneous haemorrhages in various locations

- Epistaxis (Nose bleed)
- Haemarthrosis (Joint bleed)
- Haemoptysis (Coughing blood)
- Haematuria
- Hyphema (Bleed into the anterior chamber of the eye)
- Haematoma
- Haematorrhoea (Gastrointestinal bleed)
- Haemorrhage into a body cavity

- Pulmonary haemorrhage
- Haematemesis (Vomiting blood)
- Petechiae/Ecchymoses (Mucous Membrane Haemorrhage)

Thrombocytopenia: Decreased thrombocyte number
Thrombocytopathy: Thrombocyte dysfunction (Adhesion dysfunction, Aggregation dysfunction, Storage pool Defects)
Coagulopathy: Plasmatic clotting disorder

Common Causes	
Dog	Cat
+++ Dicoumarol poisoning	+++ Leukaemia
++ DIC	++ DIC
++ Von Willebrand Disease	++ Hyperviscosity syndrome
++ Haemophilia A	++ Arterial Hypertension
+ Infectious Thrombocytopenia	+ Haemophilia A
+ Immunothrombocytopenia	+ Infectious Thrombocytopenia
+ Tumours	+ Immunothrombocytopenia

Thrombocytopenia

↓ Production of Thrombocytes (Bone marrow damage)

- Infectious Causes
  - FeLV/FIV [Cat]
  - FIP Coronavirus [Cat]
  - Parvovirus
  - (Ehrlichia sp. [Dog])
- Toxic Causes
  - Phenylbutazone
  - Metamizole
  - Chloramphenicol
  - Phenobarbital
  - Sulfonamides
  - Tetracyclines
  - Cytostatic
  - Radiation
  - Heavy metal poisoning
  - Oestrogen
- Immunoreactive Causes
  - Infection
  - Drugs (Gold, Cephalosporines, Oestrogens, Vaccines)
  - Autoimmune Diseases
- Bone Marrow Tumours
  - Multiple Myeloma
  - Lymphatic Leukaemia
  - Myeloid Leukaemia
- Other Causes
- Myelofibrosis/Osteofibrosis

↑ Consumption of Thromocytes

- DIC
  - Septicaemia/Endotoxaemia
  - Gastric Dilation/ Volvulus
  - Pyometra
  - Urinary Tract Infections
  - Haemorrhagic Enteritis
  - Splenic Torsion
  - Acute Pancreatitis

- Shock
- Heart Failure
- Liver Failure
- Haemolysis
- Snake Venom
- Heat Stroke
- Electrical Accident
- Burns
- FIP [Cat]
- Tumour Disease
- (Dirofilaria sp. [Dog])
- Immunoreactive Causes
  - Infection
  - Drugs
  - (Gold, Cephalosporines, Oestrogens, Vaccines)
  - Autoimmune Diseases
- Infectious Causes
  - FeLV/FIV [Cat]
  - FIP Coronavirus [Cat]
  - Parvovirus
  - Distemper Virus [Dog]
  - CAV-1 (Hepatitis c. c.) [Dog]
  - Canine Herpesvirus [Dog]
  - Leptospira sp. [Dog]
  - Salmonella sp.
  - Haemobartonella sp. [Cat]
  - Babesia sp. [Dog]
  - (Ehrlichia sp. [Dog])
  - (Histoplasma sp.)
- Splenomegaly
- Chronic Haemorrhage
- Thrombosis [esp Cat]

Thrombocytopathy

Congenital Causes

- Von Willebrand Disease [esp Dog]

- Chediak-Higashi Syndrome [Cat]
- Thrombasthenia (Glanzmann) [Dog]
- Platelet Aggregation Defect [Basset Hound/Pomeranian]
- Cyclic Neutropenia [Grey Collie]

Acquired Causes

- Drugs
  - NSAID (esp Acetylsalicylic acid)
  - Glucocorticoids
  - Antibiotics
  - Antihistamines
  - Dextrans
  - Local Anaesthetics
- Uraemia
- Hepatic Failure
- Acute Pancreatitis
- Bone Marrow Tumours
  - Multiple Myeloma
  - Lymphatic Leukaemia
  - Myeloid Leukaemia
- Hyperviscosity Syndrome
  - Multiple Myeloma
  - Lymphatic Leukaemia
  - FIP Coronavirus [Cat]
  - Lupus Erythematosus
  - Polycythaemia vera
  - Dehydration
  - (Leishmania sp. [esp Dog])
  - (Ehrlichia sp. [Dog])

Plasmatic Coagulopathy

Congenital Causes

- Factor VIII Deficiency (Haemophilia A) [male Dogs + Cats]

- Factor IX Deficiency
  (Haemophilia B) [male Dogs +
  Cats]
- Von Willebrand Disease [Dogs;
  rarely Cats]
- Factor VII Deficiency [Beagle]
- Factor X Deficiency [Cocker]
- Factor XI Deficiency [Dog]
- Factor XII Deficiency
  (Hagemann) [Cat]
- Vitamin K dependent
  Coagulopathy [Devon Rex Cats]

Acquired Causes

- Vitamin K Deficiency/
  Antagonism
  - Hepatic Failure
  - Malabsorption Syndrome
  - Obstructive Jaundice
  - Damage of the intestinal
    flora (Antibiotics)
  - Rodenticide Poisoning

- DIC
  - Septicaemiea/Endotoxaemia
  - Gastric Dilation/Volvulus
    [Dog]
  - Pyometra
  - Urinary Tract Infections
  - Haemorrhagic Enteritis
  - Splenic Torsion
  - Acute Pancreatitis
  - Shock
  - Heart Failure
  - Liver Failure
  - Haemolysis
  - Snake Venom
  - Heat Stroke
  - Electrical Accident
  - Burns
  - FIP Coronavirus [Cat]
  - Tumour Diseases
  - (Dirofilaria sp. [Dog])
- Other Causes
  - Heparin Treatment
  - Fibrinolytic Treatment

Diagnostic Approach

Tendency to Bleed

1. **Case History**

2. **General Examination**

3. **Blood Tests**
- Hct, Ery, Leuc, Hb
- Diff BC
- MCV, MCV, MCHC
- TP, Alb, Glob
- GPT, AP, Urea, Crea, BG
- FIP Profile [Cat]
  - TP
  - Alb/Glob Ratio

  - Bili
  - GOT/AST
  - Serum Electrophoresis
- Serum Electrophoresis

MICROBIAL SEROLOGY
- FeLV-/FIV Antigens [Cat]
- Babesia Antibodies [Dog]
- Ehrlichia Antibodies [Dog]
- Leptospira Antibodies [Dog]

COAGULATION
- Bleeding time

- Prothrombin time (PT/Quick)
- (Activated) partial Thromboplastin time (PTT/ aPTT)
- Thrombocyte Count
- Fibrin Degradation Product (FDP)
- Autoantibodies against Thrombocytes
- Von Willebrand Disease
- Determination of Factors II-XII

IMMUNOSEROLOGY
- Coombs Test
- ANA Test
- Microscope Slide Agglutination Test

FUNCTION TESTS
- T_4 [Cat]

4. Urinalysis
- Urine dip stick
- Specific gravity
- Urine sediment
- Bence-Jones Proteins

5. X-Ray Study
- Thorax
- Abdomen
- Skull/Tympanic Bulla

6. Further Tests
- Bone Marrow Biopsy/Cytology
- Blood Pressure Measure (indirect/direct)
- Ultrasound
- Liver biopsy

Pyrexia and Hyperthermia

Fever/Pyrexia: Increased body temperature (> 39.7°C) as a result of impaired hypothalamic thermoregulation
Hyperthermia: Increased body temperature (> 39.7°C) as a result of increased heat supply, increased heat generation or reduced heat emission

Common Causes	
Dog	Cat
+++ Infectious Diseases	+++ Infectious Diseases
++ Drug Fever	++ Drug Fever
++ Tumour Fever	++ Tumour Fever
++ Heat Stroke	++ Hyperthyroidism
++ Arthropathies	+ Haemophilia A

Pyrexia

Infectious Causes

- Viral Infections
  - FeLV/FIV [Cat]
  - FIP Coronavirus [Cat]
  - Cat Flu Syndrome [Cat]
  - Distemper Virus [Dog]
  - Parvovirus
  - CAV-1 (Hepatitis c. c.) [Dog]
- Bacterial Infections
  - Gram-positive and Gram-negative
  - Septicaemia/Endotoxaemia
  - Lyme Borrelia sp. [Dog]
  - Brucella sp. [Dog]
- Rickettsial Infections
  - Haemobartonella sp. [Cat]
  - (Ehrlichia sp. [Dog])
  - (Rickettsia sp. [Dog])
- Parasitic Infections
  - Toxoplasma sp.
  - Babesia sp. [esp Dog]
  - (Leishmania sp. [esp Dog])
  - (Cytauxzoon sp. [Cat])
  - (Hepatozoon sp. [Dog])
  - (Dirofilaria sp. [esp Dog])
  - Larva migrans
- Mycotic Systemic Infections
  - Cryptococcus sp. [Cat]
  - (Histoplasma sp.)
  - (Blastomyces sp.)
  - (Coccidioides sp.)

Immunoreactive Causes

- Polyarthritis
- Polymyositis
- Glomerulonephritis
- Allergy
- Lupus erythematosus
- Pemphigus Complex
- Immune Haemolytic Anaemia
- Immunothrombocytopenia
- Vasculitis

Drug Fever

- Tetracyclines
- Sulfonamides
- Penicillins
- Amphotericin B
- Antimon preparations
- Barbiturates
- Antihistamines
- Acetylsalicylic acid
- Paracetamol
- Procainamide
- Cytostatics
- Arsenic preparations
- Vaccines

Tumour Fever

- Solid Tumours
- Tumour metastasis
- Myeloproliferative Tumours

Other Causes

- Arthropathies
- Bacterial sources of infections Endocarditis
  - Abscess/dental abscess
- Blunt Trauma
- Recurrent infections due to Immunosuppression
- Arterial Thromboembolism
- Hypothalamic Diseases

Hyperthermia

↑ Heat Supply

- High Outdoor Temperature
- High Humidity

↑ Heat Generation

- Excitement
- Exercise
- Tachypnoea/Dyspnoea

- Seizures
- Hyperthyroidism [Cat]
- Malignant Hyperthermia (Anaesthesia)
- Phaeochromocytoma

↓ Heat Emission

- Heat Stroke
- Obesity

Diagnostic Approach

Pyrexia and Hyperthermia

1. **Case History**

2. **General Examination**

3. **Oropharyngeal Examination**

4. **Blood Tests**
- Hct, Ery, Leuc
- GPT, AP, Urea, Crea, Bili, BG
- FIP Profile [Cat]
  - TP
  - Alb/Glob Ratio
  - Bili
  - GOT/AST
  - Serum electrophoresis
- Thrombocytes
- Diff BC
- TP, Alb, Glob
- Amylase, Lipase [Dog]
- TLI Test
- Bile Acids

MICROBIAL SEROLOGY
- FeLV-/FIV Antigen [Cat]
- Toxoplasma Antibodies

- Lyme Borrelia Antibodies [Dog]
- Dirofilaria Antigen [Dog]
- Leishmania Antibodies [Dog]

IMMUNE SEROLOGY
- ANA Test
- Coombs Test

FUNCTION TESTS
- T_4, fT_4 [Cat]

5. **X-Ray Study**
- Abdomen
- Thorax
- Skull
- (Tympanic bulla + teeth)
- Contrast medium study of the gastrointestinal tract

6. **Urinalysis**
- Urine dip stick
- Specific gravity
- Urine sediment

7. **Ultrasound**
- Abdomen ± biopsy
- Heart

8. Further Tests
- Lymph node biopsy/cytology
- Peritoneal lavage/cytology
- Blood culture (BE)
- Tracheobronchial lavage/cytology/BE
- Bone Marrow biopsy/cytology
- Arthrocentesis/Synovial analysis
- Spinal tap/analysis
- Laparotomy

Hypothermia

Reduction of the internal body temperature
Reduction of the external body temperature

Common Causes		
Dog		Cat
+++ Sedation/Anaesthesia		+++ Sedation/Anaesthesia
++ Circulatory shock		++ Circulatory shock
++ Lack of Exercise		++ Lack of Exercise
++ Neonate		++ Neonate
++ Hypothyroidism		++ Feline Aortic Thrombosis

↓ Internal Body Temperature

↓ Heat Production

- Sedation/Anaesthesia
- Circulatory Shock
- Hypothyroidism [Dog]
- Lack of Exercise as a result of systemic disease
- Hypothalamic disease
- Bradycardic cardiac arrhythmias
- Hypoglycaemia
- Cachexia
- Immature Thermoregulation (Neonates/Premature litters)

↑ Heat Loss

- Exposure to the cold

- Small animals/Neonates
- Lack of exercise as a result of trauma/paralysis
- Burns

↓ External Body Temperature

Shock

- Hypovolaemic Shock
- Cardiogenic Shock
- Neurogenic Shock
- Poisoning

Vascular Thrombosis

- Feline aortic thrombosis [Cat]
- Arterial thrombosis

Diagnostic Approach

Hypothermia

1. **Case History**

2. **General Examination**

3. **Blood Tests**
- Hct, Erys, Leuc, Hb
- TP, Alb, Glob
- GPT, AP, Urea, Crea, BG
- Na, K, Ca
- Diff BC
- Blood Gas Analysis (BGA)
- Thrombocytes
- Serum electrophoresis

MICROBIAL SEROLOGY
- FeLV-/FIV Antigen [Cat]

FUNCTION TESTS
- T_4, fT_4
- TSH-/TRH Stimulation Test [Dog]

4. **Urinalysis**
- Urinary output/volume
- Urine dip stick
- Specific gravity
- Urine sediment

5. **X-Ray Study**
- Thorax
- Abdomen

6. **Ultrasound**
- Heart (Doppler Echocardiography)
- Abdomen

7. **Further Tests**
- Measure of the femoral pulse [Cat]
- Neurological Examination
- Electrocardiogram (ECG)
- Blood Pressure (indirect/direct)

Icterus/Jaundice

Yellow discolouration of the skin and mucous membranes due to accumulation of bilirubin

Common Causes	
Dog	Cat
Prehepatic Icterus	
+++ Toxic Haemolysis	+++ FeLV/FIV
++ Immunoreactive Haemolysis	++ Haemobartonella felis
++ DIC	++ Toxic Haemolysis
++ Neonate	++ Immunoreactive Haemolysis
Hepatocellular Icterus	
++ Hepatotoxins	+++ Feline hepatic lipidosis

Common Causes	
Dog	Cat
++ Liver tumours	+++ Feline Cholangiohepatitis
++ Right Sided Heart Failure	++ Hepatotoxins
	++ Liver tumours
	+ Right Sided Heart Failure
Posthepatic Icterus	
++ Obstructive Tumours	++ Obstructive Tumours

Prehepatic Icterus

Infectious Causes

- Leptospira sp. [Dog]
- FeLV/FIV [Cat]
- Haemobartonella sp. [Cat]
- Babesia sp. [esp Dog]
- (Ehrlichia sp. [Dog])
- (Dirofilaria sp. [Vena cava Syndrome] [Dog])
- (Hepatozoon sp. [Dog])

Immunoreactive Causes

- Drug Allergy
  - Penicillins
  - Cephalosporins
  - Sulfonamides
  - Phenylbutazone
  - Propylthiouracil
  - Levamisol
  - Paracetamol
- Autoimmune haemolysis
- Neonatal Isoerythrolysis [Cat]
- Blood transfusion incompatability

Toxic

- Drugs

  - NSAID (esp Paracetamol, Ibuprofen)
  - Antiarrhythmics
  - Anticonvulsants
  - Cimetidine
  - Levamisol
  - Metronidazole
  - Griseofulvin
  - Phenothiazin
  - Methylene blue
  - Vitamin K
  - Benzocain
  - Methionin
- Water enema [Cat]
- Onions
- Snake venom
- Heavy metal poisoning

Other Causes

- Haemorrhage
  - Trauma
  - Tumours
  - Rodenticide Poisoning
  - DIC

Hepatocellular Icterus

Infectious Causes

- Viral Hepatitis

- CAV-1 (Hepatitis c. c.) [Dog]
- FeLV/FIV [Cat]
- FIP Coronavirus [Cat]
- Bacterial Hepatitis/Cholangitis
  - Salmonella sp.
  - E. coli
  - Staphylococcus sp.
  - Bacillus sp. [Dog]
  - Leptospira sp. [Dog]
- Parasitic Hepatitis/Cholangitis
  - Toxoplasma sp.
  - Capillaria sp.
  - (Leishmania sp. [esp Dog])
  - (Opisthorchis sp. [Cat])

Toxic Causes (Hepatotoxins)

- Antibiotics
  - Ampicillin
  - Erythromycin
  - Nitrofurantoin
  - Tetracyclines
- Antimycotics
  - Griseofulvin
  - Ketoconazole
- NSAID
  - Paracetamol
  - Phenylbutazone
  - Naproxen
  - Acetylsalicylic acid
  - Ibuprofen
  - Ketoprofen
  - Indometacin
- Inhalation Anaesthetics
  - Halothan
  - Methoxyfluran
- Anticonvulsants
  - Phenobarbital
  - Primidon
  - Diazepam
- Glucocorticoids
- Cytostatics
- Other drugs
  - Procainamide
  - Warfarin
  - Haloperidol
  - Phenothiazide
  - Cimetidine
  - Vitamin A
- Household Agents
- Other poisons
  - Aflatoxines
  - Poisonous Plants

Hepatic Tumours

- Primary tumours
  - Bile Duct adenoma/carcinoma
  - Hepatocellular adenoma/carcinoma
  - Lymphosarcoma [esp Cat]
  - Haemangioendothelioma
- Tumour Metastasis
  - Mammary carcinoma
  - Mast cell tumour
  - Lymphosarcoma [esp Cat]

Other Causes

- Lymphocytic Cholangiohepatitis [esp Cat]
- Liver abscess
- Feline hepatic lipidosis [Cat]
- Diabetes mellitus
- Hyperthyroidism [Cat]
- Hypercortisolism (Cushing's Disease) [Dog]
- Pancreatitis
- Right sided heart failure
- Cholelithiasis (Gall stones)
- Hepatic cysts

- Hepatic cirrhosis
- Amyloidosis
- Glycogen storage disease
- Copper storage disease [Dog]

Posthepatic Icterus

Bile Duct Obstruction

- Choledocholithiasis (Bile duct stones)

- Bile Duct adenoma/carcinoma
- Acute Pancreatitis
- Pancreatic tumours
- Cholangitis/Cholecystitis
- Diaphragmatic hernia
- Small intestinal tumour (Papillary tumour)

Diagnostic Approach

Icterus/Jaundice

1. **Case History**

2. **General Examination**

3. **Blood Tests**
- Hct, Ery, Leuc
- Hb, MCH, MCV, MCHC
- Diff BC
  - Blood parasites
  - Erythrocyte morphology
- TP, Alb, Glob
- GPT, AP, Urea, Crea, BG
- Bili, Chol, LDH
- FIP Profile [Cat]
  - TP
  - Alb/Glob Ratio
  - Bili
  - GOT
  - Serum electrophoresis
- Reticulocytes
- Na, K, Ca, P

COAGULATION
- Bleeding time
- Prothrombin time (PT/Quick)
- (Activated) partial Thromboplastin time (PTT/ aPTT)

- Fibrin Degradation products (FDP)
- Thrombocte number

MICROBIAL SEROLOGY
- FeLV-/FIV Antigen [Cat]
- Babesia Antibodies [Dog]
- Ehrlichia Antibodies [Dog]
- CAV-1 Antibodies [Dog]
- Leptospira Antibodies [Dog]
- Leishmania Antibodies [Dog]
- Dirofilaria Antibodies [Dog]
- Toxoplasma Antibodies

IMMUNOSEROLOGY
- Coombs Test
- ANA Test
- Microscope slide Agglutination test

FUNCTION TESTS
- Adrenal Gland [Dog]
  - Dexamethasone Suppression test
  - ACTH Stimulation test
  - Cortisol/Creatinine Ratio

FURTHER SEROLOGY
- Blood typing [Cat]

4. Urinalysis
- Urine dip stick
- Specific gravity
- Urine sediment

5. X-Ray Study
- Abdomen

- Thorax

6. Ultrasound
- Abdomen ± Liver biopsy
- Heart (Doppler Echocardiography)

7. Further Tests
- Bone Marrow Biopsy/Cytology

Infections, recurrent

Common manifestations of recurrent infections: Skin infections, urinary tract infections, respiratory tract infections, gastrointestinal infections rarer

Common Causes	
Dog	Cat
+++ Treatment failure	+++ Treatment failure
++ Bacterial focus of infection	++ FeLV/FIV
++ Diabetes mellitus	++ Bacterial focus of infection
++ Tumour disease	++ Diabetes mellitus
	++ Tumour disease

Persistent Infection

- Treatment failure
- Bacterial resistency
- Acute relapses of latent infections (Herpes virus)
- Bacterial focus of infection (endocarditis, abscess)

Immunodeficiency

Primary Immunodeficiency

- X-chromosomal combined immunodeficiency [Basset]

- Cyclic neutropenia [Grey Collie]
- Thymal hypoplasia
- IgA deficiency [German Shepherd Dog, Beagle, Shar-Pei]
- IgM deficiency [Doberman]
- C_3 deficiency [Brittany Spaniel]
- Chediak-Higashi Syndrome [Persian Cat]
- Mucopolysaccharidosis [Siamese Cat, European Shorthair Cat]

- Leucocyte adhesion deficiency [Irish Setter]

Secondary Immunodeficiency

- Malnourishment
- Viral Immunosuppression
  - FeLV/FIV [Cat]
  - Canine distemper virus [Dog]
  - Parvovirus
- Drug-induced immune suppression
  - Glucocorticoids
  - Cytostatics
  - Oestrogens
- Associated microbes
  Bacteria
  - Listeria sp. [Dog]
  - Pseudomonas sp.
  - Staphylococcus sp.
  - Nocardia sp.

Rickettsia
- (Ehrlichia sp. [Dog])

Fungi
- Microsporum sp.
- Trichophyton sp.
- Aspergillus sp.
- Candida sp.
- Cryptococcus sp.

Parasites
- Demodex sp.
- Toxoplasma sp.
- Pneumocystis sp.
- Other causes
  - Splenectomy
  - Bone marrow damage
  - Malignant tumours
  - Diabetes mellitus
  - Hyperoestrogenism
  - Liver cirrhosis
  - Chronic renal failure

Diagnostic Approach

Infections, recurrent

1. Case History

2. General Examination

3. Blood Tests

- Hct, Ery, Leuc
- Diff BC
- TP, Alb, Glob
- GPT, AP, Urea, Crea, BG
- Serum electrophoresis
- Immunoelectrophoresis

MICROBIAL SEROLOGY

- FeLV-/FIV Antigen [Cat]
- Toxoplasma Antibodies

- Ehrlichia Antibodies [Dog]
- Aspergillus Antibodies [Dog]

4. Urinalysis

- Urine dip stick
- Specific gravity
- Urine sediment

5. X-Ray Study

- Thorax
- Abdomen

6. Ultrasound

- Abdomen
- Heart

Further Tests
- Canine distemper antigen
  (Conjunctival smear) [Dog]
- Lymph node biopsy/cytology
- Blood culture
- Bone marrow biopsy/cytology

Performance Insufficiency

Performance dependent exhaustion and muscle weakness

Common Causes	
Dog	Cat
+++ Congestive heart failure	+++ Congestive heart failure
++ Respiratory Tract Disease	++ Respiratory Tract Disease
++ Metabolic Causes	++ Metabolic Causes
++ Neuromuscular Causes	++ Neuromuscular Causes

Cardiovascular Causes

Congenital Heart Disease

- Patent ductus arteriosus (PDA)
- (Sub-)Aortic stenosis
- Stenosis of the pulmonary artery
- Atrial Septal Defect (ASD)
- Ventricular Septal Defect (VSD)
- Valval dysplasia
- Tetralogy of Fallot
- Patent right aortic arch (Right sided aorta)
- Endocardial fibroelastosis
- Ebstein anomaly
- Transposition of the large vessels
- Anomalous pulmonary venous connection

Myocardial Disease

- Primary Cardiomyopathy

- Dilated cardiomyopathy
- Hypertrophic cardiomyopathy [esp Cat]
- Restrictive cardiomyopathy

Secondary Cardiomyopathy

- Metabolic causes
  - Hyperthyroidism [Cat]
  - Hypothyroidism [Dog]
  - Hypo-/Hyperkalaemia
  - Hypo-/Hypercalcaemia
  - Diabetes mellitus
  - Hypercortisolism (Cushing's Disease) [Dog]
  - Uraemia
  - Renal hypertension
  - Glycogen storage disease
- Alimentary Causes
  - Taurine deficiency [esp Cat]
  - Carnitine deficiency [esp Dog]
- Viral myocarditis

- Parvovirus
- Canine Distemper Virus [Dog]
- Herpesvirus
• Bacterial endocarditis/ myocarditis
  - Aerobes/Anaerobes
  - Lyme Borreliosis sp. [Dog]
  - Endotoxaemia
• Mycotic myocarditis
  - Cryptococcus sp. [Cat]
• Parasitic myocarditis
  - Toxoplasma sp.
  - (Hepatozoon sp. [Dog])
  - (Trypanosoma sp. [Dog])
  - Immunoreactive myocarditis
  - Polyarteritis nodosa
  - Lupus erythematosus
• Toxic myocarditis/ myocardosis
  - Doxorubicin
  - Heavy metals
• Traumatic myocarditis
  - Contusion
  - Atrial rupture

Valvular Heart Disease

• Mitral Valve Disease
  - Dysplasia
  - Endocarditis
  - Fibrosis
  - Functional dilation of the valvular annulus
• Valvular Pulmonary Stenosis Dysplasia
• Tricuspid Valve Disease
  - Dysplasia
  - Endocarditis
  - Fibrosis

  - Functional dilation of the valvular annulus
• Valvular Aortic stenosis Dysplasia
• Rupture of the Papillary Muscle

Cardiac/Pericardial tumours

• Haemangiosarcoma [esp Dog]
• Right sided atrial myxoma [Dog]
• Heart base tumour (Chemodectoma) [Dog]
Tumour metastasis
• Thyroid carcinoma
• Mesothelioma
• Cysts

Pericardial Disease (Pericardial Effusion) Modified Transudate

• Congestive heart failure
• Uraemia
• Hypoalbuminaemia
• Cardiac arrhythmias
• Pericardiodiaphragmatic hernia

Exudate

• Tumours
• Pericarditis
  - Canine Distemper Virus [Dog]
  - FIP Coronavirus [Cat]
  - Leptospira sp. [Dog]
  - Actinomyces sp.
  - Nocardia sp.
  - Mycobacterium sp.
  - Toxoplasma sp.
  - Pasteurella sp.

- Streptococcus spp.
- Staphylococcus spp.
- E. coli
- Cryptococcus sp. [Cat]

Blood

- Atrial rupture
- Haemangiosarcoma [Dog]
- Coagulopathies
- Foreign bodies

Arterial Thromboembolism

- Feline Aortic thromboembolism
  - Hypertrophic cardiomyopathy
  - Restrictive cardiomyopathy
  - Dilated cardiomyopathy
- Bottom hung window syndrome [Cat]
- Pulmonary thromboembolism
  - (Dirofilaria sp. [esp Dog])
  - (Angiostrongylus sp. [Dog])
  - Hypercortisolism (Cushing's Disease) [Dog]
  - DIC
  - Cardiomyopathy
  - Protein-losing nephropathy
  - Acute Pancreatitis
  - Septicaemia/Endotoxaemia
  - Immune haemolytic Anaemia
  - Bone trauma/surgery
  - Hyperviscosity syndrome

Pleural/ Mediastinal Causes

Thoracic effusion Transudate

- Congestive heart failure (Right sided heart failure)

- Hypoalbuminaemia

Modified Transudate

- Congestive heart failure
- Tumours
- Diaphragmatic hernia
- Pancreatitis
- Autoimmune Diseases
- Hepatic cirrhosis

Exudate

- FIP Coronavirus [Cat]
- Tumours
- Pyothorax
  - Actinomyces sp.
  - Nocardia sp.
  - Pasteurella sp.
  - Bacteroides sp.
  - Fusobacterium sp.
  - Pneumonia
  - Foreign body perforation
  - Oesophageal perforation
  - Tumour necrosis
  - Thoracocentesis
- Diaphragmatic hernia
- Lung lobe torsion

Blood

- Lung lobe torsion
- Trauma
- Coagulopathy
- Tumours

Chyle

- Congestive heart failure
- Tumours
- Trauma
- Lymphangiectasia [Dog]
- Diaphragmatic hernia

- Lung lobe torsion
- (Dirofilaria sp. [esp Dog])

Pneumothorax

- Traumatic Causes
  - Road traffic accident
  - Window fall [esp Cat]
  - Thoracic penetration
  - Thoracocentesis
  - Pressure ventilation
  - Oesophageal penetration
  - Tracheal penetration
  - Perforating rib fracture
  - Lung contusion/ Pleural rupture
- Spontaneous Causes
  - Pneumonia
  - Bullous emphysema
  - Larva migrans
  - Mycotic Granulomata
  - Pulmonary tumours
  - Pulmonary abscesses
  - Pulmonary cyst
  - Foreign bodies

Mediastinal Tumours

- Lymphadenopathy
- Lymphosarcoma [esp Cat]
- Heart base tumour (Chemodectoma) [Dog]
- Thyroid carcinoma
- Thymoma
- Mediastinal cysts
- Mesothelioma

Diaphragmatic Elevation

- Diaphragmatic rupture
- Gastric dilation/volvulus [Dog]
- Hepatomegaly
- Diaphragmatic paralysis
- Intraabdominal tumour
- Marked abdominal effusion

Pulmonary Causes

Pulmonary Oedema

↑ **Hydrostatic pressure**
- Left Sided Heart Failure
  - Dilated cardiomyopathy
  - Hypertrophic cardiomyopathy
  - Restrictive cardiomyopathy
  - Mitral valve disease
  - (Sub)Aortic stenosis
  - Ventricular septal defect
  - Patent ductus arteriosus (PDA)
- Overinfusion (esp Dextranes, full blood)
- Anaphylaxis
- Hyperthyroidism [Cat]
- Hypertension [esp Cat]
- Cardiac arrhythmias
- Rupture of the papillary muscle

↓ **Hydrostatic pressure**
- Hypoalbuminaemia + overinfusion

↑ **Permeability**
- Pneumonia
- Aspiration pneumonia/Smoke inhalation/irritant gases
- Uraemia
- Endotoxins
- DIC
- Lung contusion
- Seizures
- Acute Pancreatitis
- Traumatic brain injury
- Anaphylaxis

- Drowning
- Electrical shock
- Snake venom
- O_2 Poisoning

Pneumonia

- Viral Pneumonia
  - Canine Distemper Virus [Dog]
  - CAV-1 (Hepatitis c. c.) [Dog]
  - Cat Flu [Cat]
  - FIP Coronavirus [Cat]
  - FeLV/FIV [Cat]
  - Kennel cough [Dog]
- Bacterial Pneumonia
  - Bordetella sp.
  - E. coli
  - Klebsiella sp.
  - Pseudomonas sp.
  - Pasteurella sp.
  - Staphylococcus sp.
  - Streptococcus sp.
  - Mycoplasma sp.
  - Mycobacterium spp.
  - Chlamydia sp.
- Immunoreactive Pneumonia
  - Atopy/Inhalation Allergy
  - Bacterial/Fungal/Parasitic Allergy
  - Drug Allergy
  - Lupus Erythematosus
- Aspiration pneumonia
  - Megaoesophagus
  - Drug/Contrast Medium administration
  - Force Feeding
- Rickettsial Pneumonia
  - (Ehrlichia sp. [Dog])
  - (Rickettsia sp. [Dog])

- Parasitic Pneumonia
  - Toxoplasma sp.
  - Pneumocystis sp.
  - Capillaria sp.
  - Filaroides sp.
  - Aelurostrongylus sp. [Cat]
  - (Crenosoma sp. [Dog])
  - (Angiostrongylus sp. [Dog])
  - (Dirofilaria sp. [esp Dog])
  - (Paragonimus sp.)
  - Larva migrans
- Mycotic Pneumonia
  - Cryptococcus sp. [Cat]
  - (Histoplasma sp.)
  - (Blastomyces sp.)
  - (Coccidioides sp.)
  - Facultative pathogenic fungi
- Toxic Pneumonia
- Smoke inhalation/Irritant gases
- Uraemia
- Other causes
  - IgA deficiency
  - Dyskinesia of the cilicated epithelium
  - Foreign Bodies

Pulmonary Tumours

- Tumour metastases
  - Thyroid Carcinoma
  - Mammary Carcinoma
  - Haemangiosarcoma
  - Squamous Cell Carcinoma
  - Transitional Cell Carcinoma
  - Melanoma
  - Lymphosarcoma
  - Malignant Histiocytosis [Bernese Mountain Dog]
- Primary Tumours

- Adenocarcinoma
- Squamous Cell Carcinoma

Other Causes

- Pulmonary Haemorrhage
  - Pulmonary Contusion
  - Lung Lobe Torsion
  - Foreign Body
  - Coagulopathies
  - Pneumonia
  - Pulmonary Abscess
  - Pulmonary Tumours
- Atelectasis
- Emphysema
- Pulmonary Fibrosis

Metabolic Causes

Endocrine Diseases

- Hypothyroidism [Dog]
- Hypercortisolism (Cushing's Disease) [Dog]
- Diabetes mellitus
- Hyperthyroidism [Cat]
- Hypocortisolism (Addison's Disease) [Dog]

Electrolyte Disturbances

- Hyperkalaemia
- Hypokalaemia
- Hypercalcaemia
- Hypocalcaemia
- Hypernatraemia

Neuromuscular Causes

Polyneuropathy

- Infectious Causes
  - FeLV/FIV [Cat]
  - Toxoplasma sp.

- Neospora sp. [Dog]
- Immunoreactive Causes
  - Lupus erythematosus
- Metabolic Causes
  - Diabetes mellitus
  - Hypercortisolism (Cushing's Disease) [esp Dog]
  - Hypothyroidism [Dog]
- Toxic Causes
  - Organophosphate Poisoning (chronic)
  - Lead Poisoning
  - Cytostatics
  - Lindane
  - Botulism toxin
  - Tick toxin (Tick paralysis)
- Congenital Causes
  - Axonopathy
  - Demyelinisation Diseases
  - Lysosomal Storage Disease
  - Spinal Muscular Atrophy
- Other Causes
  - Nerve Root Compression Syndrome
  - Feline Dysautonomia [Cat]
  - Polyneuritis/ Polyradiculoneuritis [Dog]

Junctionopathy (Neuromuscular Junction)

- Myasthenia gravis
  - acquired
  - congenital

Polymyopathy

- Infectious Causes
  - Toxoplasma sp.
  - Neospora sp. [Dog]
  - Lyme Borreliosis sp. [Dog]
  - Leptospira sp. [Dog]

- Immunoreactive Causes
  - Lupus Erythematosus
  - Eosinophilic Myositis [Dog]
- Metabolic Causes
  - Hypokalaemia [esp Cat]
  - Hypercortisolism (Cushing's Disease) [esp Dog]
  - Hypothyroidism [Dog]
  - Hypoglycaemia
  - Vit E-/Selenium Deficiency
- Congenital Causes
  - Muscular Dystrophy

  - Dermatomyositis [Collie]
  - Glycogen Storage Disease

Other Causes

- Anaemia
- Infectious Diseases
- Organ Failure
- Bone/Joint Diseases
- Spinal Diseases
- Tumour Diseases
- Psychogenic Causes
- Age
- Drug Side Effects

Diagnostic Approach

Performance Insufficiency

1. **Case History**

2. **General Examination**

3. **Neurological Examination**

4. **Orthopaedic Examination**

5. **X-Ray Study**
- Thorax
- Abdomen

6. **ECG**

7. **Ultrasound**
- Heart (Doppler Echocardiography)
- Abdomen

8. **Blood Tests**
- Hct, Ery, Leuc, Hb
- Na, K, Ca, P
- TP, Alb, Glob
- GPT, AP, Urea, Crea
- BG, CK

- Diff BC
- FIP Profile [Cat]
- α HBDH
- Troponin
- ANP

MICROBIAL SEROLOGY
- FeLV-/FIV Antigen [Cat]
- Toxoplasma Antibodies
- Dirofilaria Antigen [Dog]
- Lyme-Borreliosis Antibodies [Dog]
- Ehrlichia Antibodies [Dog]

IMMUNOSEROLOGY
- ANA Test
- Autoantibodies against Acetyl-choline Receptors (Myasthenia gravis detection)

FUNCTION TESTS
- Adrenal Gland Function Tests [Dog]

- – Dexamethasone Suppression test
- – ACTH Stimulation test
- – Cortisol/Creatinine Ratio
- T_4, fT_4
TSH-/TRH Stimulation test [Dog]
- Thyroglobulin Antibodies

FURTHER TESTS
- Tensilon Test (Myasthenia gravis Test) [Dog]

9. Urinalysis
- Urine dip stick
- Specific gravity
- Urine sediment

10. Further Tests
- Non-selective Angiography
- Electromyogram (EMG)
- Muscle Biopsy
- Body Cavity Fluid Analysis

Lymph Node Enlargement, Peripheral

Lymphadenopathy: Swelling of the palpable peripheral lymph nodes:
Lnn. parotidei
Lnn. mandibulares
Lnn. retropharyngei laterales
Lnn. cervicales superficiales
Lnn. axillares
Lnn. inguinales superficiales
Lnn. poplitei

Common Causes

Dog	Cat
+++ Tumour metastasis (esp lymphatic leukaemia)	++ Infectious Diseases
++ Infectious Diseases	++ Tumour metastasis
++ Autoimmune Diseases	++ Autoimmune Diseases

Generalised Lymphadenopathy

Infectious Causes

- Parasitic Infections
  - Demodex sp.
  - Sarcoptes sp.
  - Toxoplasma sp.
  - Babesia sp. [esp Dog]
  - (Leishmania sp. [esp Dog])
- Rickettsial Infections
  - (Ehrlichia sp. [Dog])
  - (Rickettsia sp. [Dog])
- Mycotic Infections
  - Cryptococcus sp. [Cat]
  - Sporothrix sp. [Cat]
  - (Histoplasma sp.)
  - (Blastomyces sp.)
- Viral Infections

– FeLV/FIV [Cat]
FIP Coronavirus [Cat]
- Bacterial Infections

Immunoreactive Causes

- Feline hypereosinophilic syndrome [Cat]
- Lupus erythematosus
- Rheumatoid Arthritis
- Allergy

Tumorous Causes

- Lymphatic Leukaemia
- Tumour metastasis

Localised Lymphadenopathy

- Infection of the localised drainage region (abscess)
- Tumour metastasis of the local drainage region

Diagnostic Approach

Lymphadenopathy, Peripheral

1. **Case History**

2. **General Examination**

3. **Lymph Node Biopsy**
- Cytology
- Leishmania amastigote
- Tumour cytology
- Bacterial/Fungal/Protozoal Culture

4. **X-Ray Study**
- Thorax
- Abdomen
- Spine

5. **Blood Tests**
- Hct, Ery, Leuc
- Diff BC (+ Cytology)
- TP, Alb, Glob
- Serum electrophoresis
- GPT, AP, Urea, Crea, BG
- FIP Profile [Cat]
    – TP
    – Alb/Glob Ratio
    – Bili/GOT
    – Serum electrophoresis

MICROBIAL SEROLOGY
- FeLV-/FIV Antigen [Cat]
- Toxoplasma Antibodies
- Ehrlichia Antibodies [Dog]
- Leishmania Antibodies [Dog]
- Brucella Antibodies [Dog]
- Lyme Borreliosis Antibodies [Dog]
- Canine Herpes virus Antibodies [Dog]

IMMUNOSEROLOGY
- ANA Test
- Rheumatoid factor

6. **Urinalysis**
- Urine dip stick
- Specific gravity
- Urine sediment
- Bence-Jones Proteins

7. **Further Tests**
- Bone marrow biopsy/cytology
- Ultrasound
- Arthrocentesis/Synovial analysis

Oedema, subcutaneous

Extravascular collection of fluid in subcutaneous tissues

Common Causes	
Dog	Cat
++ Lymphoedema	++ Lymphoedema
+ Congestive heart failure	+ Congestive heart failure

Localised Oedema

↑ Hydrostatic Pressure

- Venous Thrombosis
- Tumours (esp Mammary)
- Arteriovenous Anastomosis

Disturbance of the Localised Permeability

- Trauma
- Surgical procedure
- Burns
- Cellulitis/Abscess
- Tumours
- Insect bite/sting
- Vaccine reaction
- Snake Venom
- Lymphangitis
- Lymphangioma/-sarcoma

Generalised Oedema

↑ Hydrostatic Pressure

- Right Sided Heart Failure
- Biventricular Congestive Heart Failure
- Right atrial/Vena cava Obstruction
  - (Dirofilaria sp. [esp Dog])

  - (Angiostrongylus sp. [Dog])
  - Tumours
  - Thrombosis
- Overinfusion in case of Oliguria/Anuria
- Hypoalbuminaemia

↓ Oncostatic Pressure (Hypoalbuminaemia)

- Hepatic cirrhosis/portocaval Shunt
- Exsudative body cavity effusion
- Cachexia/Marasmus
- Protein-losing enteropathy
- Protein-losing nephropathy
- Burns

Permeability Disturbances

- Septicaemia/Endotoxaemia
- Vasculitis
  - FIP Coronavirus [Cat]
  - Canine Coronavirus [Dog]
  - Septicaemia/Endotoxaemia
  - Polyarteritis nodosa
  - Allergy
  - Lupus erythematosus

- Rheumatoid Arthritis
- Uraemia
- Tumours
- (Ehrlichia sp. [Dog])
- (Rickettsia sp. [Dog])
* Trauma
* Burns
* Snake Venom

Lymphoedema

* Lymphostasis/Lymphatic obstruction

- Trauma
- Infiltrating Tumours
- Lymphangioma/-sarcoma
- Lack of exercise
* Congenital aplasia of lymphatic vessels

Myxoedema

* Hypothyroidism [Dog]

Diagnostic Approach

Oedema, subcutaneous

1. **Case History**

2. **General Examination**

3. **X-Ray Study**
* Thorax
* Abdomen

4. **Blood Tests**
* Hct, Ery, Leuc
* TP, Alb, Glob
* GPT, AP, Urea, Crea, BG
* Diff BC
* FIP Profile [Cat]
  - TP
  - Alb/Glob Ratio

- Bili
- GOT
- Serum electrophoresis

MICROBIAL SEROLOGY
* FeLV-/FIV Antigen [Cat]
* Dirofilaria Antigen [Dog]

Ultrasound
* Heart (Doppler Echocardiography)
* Abdomen

Further Tests
* Lymphangiography
* Faecal Examination

Sleep Disturbances

Insomnia: Sleeplessness/Nocturnal Unrest
Hypersomnia: Lethargy/Excessive Sleep/Somnolence
Sleep attacks: Bouts of periodically recurring sleeping episodes
Syncope: Spontaneous, reversible and short acting loss of consciousness

Coma: Deep unconsciousness with resistance to external stimuli
Narcolepsy: Transient sleep attack (can be aroused)
Cataplexy: Sudden and severe loss of muscle tone

Insomnia

- Congestive Heart Failure
- Arterial Hypertension [esp Cat]
- Respiratory Disease
- Painfulness
- Pruritus
- Hyperthyroidism [Cat]
- Drugs
  - Aminophylline
  - Caffeine
  - Amphetamines
  - Vitamin C
  - Glucocorticoids
- Central nervous Disease
- Seizures

Sleep Attacks

- Narcolepsy
- Cataplexy
- Syncope
- Seizures

Hypersomnia

- Systemic Disease
- Chronic Renal Failure
- Hypothyroidism [Dog]
- Central nervous Disease
- Electrolye Imbalance
- Coma
- Shock
- Drugs
  - Sedatives/Anaesthetics
  - Anticonvulsants
  - Antihistamines

Diagnostic Approach

Sleep Disturbances

1. Case History

2. General Examination

3. Neurological Examination

4. X-Ray Study
- Thorax
- Abdomen

5. Blood Tests
- Hct, Ery, Leuc, Hb
- TP, Alb, Glob
- GPT, AP, Urea, Crea, BG
- Na, K, Ca
- Diff BC

MICROBIAL SEROLOGY
- FeLV-/FIV Antigen [Cat]

FUNCTION TESTS
- T_4, fT_4
- TSH-/TRH Stimulation test [Dog]
- T_3 Suppression test [Cat]

6. Urinalysis	• Urine dip stick
• Urinary output/ volume	• Specific gravity
	• Urine sediment

Mucous Membrane Colour, abnormal

Alteration of the physiological mucous membrane colour (pink)

Pallor

Shock

- Hypovolaemic Shock
- Anaphylactic Shock
- (Septic/Endotoxic Shock)
- Cardiogenic Shock
- Neurogenic Shock

Anaemia

- Haemolytic Anaemia
- Blood Loss/Anaemia
- Aplastic Anaemia/Bone marrow failure
- Nutritional Anaemia

Red

Ocular Disease

- Conjunctivitis/Keratitis
- Uveitis
- Glaucoma

Other Causes

- Excitement
- Septicaemia
- Polycythaemia
- CO Intoxication

Yellow

Icterus/Jaundice

- Prehepatic Icterus
- Hepatocellular Icterus
- Posthepatic Icterus

Blue

Cyanosis

- Central Cyanosis
  - Heart Disease
  - Respiratory Disease
  - Pulmonary Disease
  - Other Diseases
- Peripheral Cyanosis
- Venous Thrombosis

Shock

Life-threatening circulatory failure with hypoperfusion and hypoxic cellular damage as a result of hypoxia

Clinical Shock Symptoms:
Pale mucous membranes (*not* with septic shock, *not* in decompensated shock)
Weak pulse (hypotension)
Delayed capillary refill time
Tachycardia Tachypnoea
Hypothermia (Hyperthermia with septic shock)
Low peripheral body temperature
Oliguria
Thirst

Hypovolaemic Shock

Blood Loss

- Traumatic Organ/ Blood Vessel Rupture
- Epistaxis
- Coagulopathy
- Bleeding Ulcer
- Bleeding Tumour
- Gastrointestinal haemorrhage
- Bleeding Urinary Tract

Plasma Loss

- Extensive Burns
- Extensive Wounds
- Protein-Losing Enteropathy (esp Parvovirosis)
- Protein-Losing Nephropathy
- Chronic fistula
- Effusion into body cavity

Fluid Loss

- Vomitus
- Diarrhoea
- Diuretics
- Fever
- Effusion into body cavity

Septic/Endotoxic Shock

Bacteriaemia

- E. coli
- Staphylococcus sp.
- Salmonella spp.
- Pseudomonas sp.

Risk Factors

- Abscesses
- Urinary Tract Infection
- Bile Duct Infection
- Pneumonia
- Peritonitis
- Pyometra
- Haemorrhagic Gastroenteritis
- Gastric Dilation/Volvulus [Dog]
- Ileus
- Surgery
- Immunosuppression
- Hypercortisolism (Cushing's Disease) [Dog]
- Tumour Disease
- Venous Catheter
- Diabetes mellitus

Anaphylactic Shock

- Drugs
  - Penicillins
  - Cephalosporins
  - Sulfonamides
  - Local anaesthetics
  - Dextranes
  - Organ extracts
  - Vaccines
  - Iodine Preparations
  - Vitamin K1 (i.v.)
  - Radiographic Contrast Medium
  - Hyposensitisation antigens
  - Blood Transfusion
- Insect /Snake Venoms
- Toxic Plants

Cardiogenic Shock

Congenital Heart Disease

- Patent ductus arteriosus (PDA)
- (Sub)Aortic Stenosis
- Pulmonary Stenosis
- Atrial Septal Defect (ASD)
- Ventricular Septal Defect (VSD)
- Valve dysplasia
- Tetralogy of Fallot
- Endocardial Fibroelastosis

Myocardial Disease

Primary Cardiomyopathy

- Dilated Cardiomyopathy
- Hypertrophic Cardiomyopathy [esp Cat]
- Restrictive Cardiomyopathy
- Secondary Cardiomyopathy
- Metabolic Causes
  - Hyperthyroidism [Cat]
  - Hypothyroidism [Dog]
  - Hypo-/Hyperkalaemia
  - Hypo-/Hypercalcaemia
  - Diabetes mellitus
  - Hypercortisolism (Cushing's Disease) [Dog]
  - Uraemia
  - Renal Hypertension
  - Glycogen Storage Disease
- Alimentary Causes
  - Taurine Deficiency [esp Cat]
  - Carnitine Deficiency [esp Dog]
- Viral Myocarditis
  - Parvovirus
  - Distemper Virus [Dog]
  - Herpes Virus
- Bacterial Endo-/Myocarditis
  - Aerobics/Anaerobics
  - Lyme Borrelia sp. [Dog]
  - Endotoxaemia
- Mycotic Myocarditis
  - Cryptococcus sp. [Cat]
- Parasitic Myocarditis
  - Toxoplasma sp.
  - (Hepatozoon sp. [Dog])
  - (Trypanosoma sp. [Dog])
- Immunoreactive Myocarditis
  - Polyarteritis nodosa
  - Lupus erythematosus
- Toxic Myocarditis/ Myocardosis
  - Doxorubicin
  - Heavy metals
- Traumatic Myocarditis
  - Contusion
  - Atrial Rupture

Heart Valve Disease

- Mitral Valve Insufficiency
  - Dysplasia

- Endocarditis
- Fibrosis
- Functional dilation of the annular ring
- Valvular Stenosis of the Pulmonary Artery
- Tricuspid Valve Insufficiency
  - Dysplasia
  - Endocarditis
  - Fibrosis
  - Functional dilation of the annular ring
- Valvular Aortic Stenosis
- Papillary Muscle Rupture

Pericardial Disease

- Viral Pericarditis
  - FIP Coronavirus [Cat]
- Bacterial Pericarditis
  - Streptococcus sp.

- Staphylococcus sp.
- E. coli
- Pasteurella sp.
- Mycobacterium sp.
- Actinomyces sp.
- Nocardia sp.
- Mycotic Pericarditis
  - Cryptococcus sp.
- Parasitic Pericarditis
  - Toxoplasma sp.
- Traumatic Pericarditis/ Pericardial Rupture
- Pericardial Tumours
  - Haemangiosarcoma
  - Heart Base Tumour (Chemodectoma)
  - Thyroid Carcinoma
  - Mesothelioma
  - Lymphosarcoma
  - Tumour Metastasis

Diagnostic Approach

Shock

1. Case History

2. General Examination

3. ECG

4. Blood Tests
- Hct, Ery, Leuc, Hb
- Na, K, Ca, P
- TP, Alb, Glob
- GPT, AP, Urea, Crea, BG
- Diff BC

5. X-Ray Study
- Thorax
- Abdomen

6. Ultrasound
- Heart (Doppler Echocardiography)
- Abdomen

7. Urinalysis
- Urinary output/volume
- Urine dip stick
- Specific gravity
- Urine sediment

2 Cardiovascular Principal Symptoms

Further Relevant Principal Symptoms

Cardiac/Respiratory Arrest

Absent respiration, pulse and heart sounds (asystole, ventricular fibrillation, electromechanical dissociation)

Common Causes		
Dog		Cat
+++	Trauma	+++ Trauma
++	Anaesthetic Incident	++ Anaesthetic Incident
++	Respiratory Tract Obstruction	++ Respiratory Tract Obstruction
++	Congestive Heart Failure	++ Congestive Heart Failure
++	Cardiac Arrhythmias	++ Cardiac Arrhythmias

Primary Cardiac Causes

Heart Disease

- Dilated Cardiomyopathy
- Hypertrophic Cardiomyopathy [esp Cat]
- Heart Tumours/Thrombosis
- Pericardial Effusion
- Congenital Heart Disease
- Valvular Heart Disease
- Infectious Myocarditis
- Toxic Myocarditis/ Myocardosis
- Atrial Rupture
- Rupture of the Papillary Muscle

Cardiac Arrhythmias

- Heart Disease
- Acidosis/Alkalosis
- Hyper-/Hypokalaemia
- Hypocalcaemia
- Hypomagnesaemia
- Hypovolaemia
- Septicaemia/Endotoxaemia
- Hypoxia
- Anaemia
- Anaesthetic Incident
- Trauma
- Electrical Shock
- Hypothermia

Primary Respiratory Causes

Respiratory Tract Obstruction

- Foreign body
- Blocked endotracheal tube
- Trauma
- Glottal oedema
- Tumours
- Tracheal collapse
- Recurrent laryngeal nerve paralysis [large dog breeds]

Pulmonary Disease

- Pneumonia
- Pulmonary Tumours
- Pulmonary Oedema
- Pulmonary haemorrhage
- Anaphylaxis
- Pulmonary thromboembolism
- Atelectasis
- Emphysema

Thoracic Disease

- Pneumothorax
- Pleural Effusion
- Diaphragmatic hernia/rupture
- Mediastinal Tumours
- Diaphragmatic Paralysis

Primary Neurological Causes

Cerebral Disease

- Traumatic brain injury
- Brain tumours
- Cerebral oedema
- Encephalitis
- Cerebral haemorrhage/abscess

Cervical Spine Disease

- Trauma/Vertebral fracture or luxation
- Haematoma/Abscess
- Disc prolapse
- Fibrocartilaginous Embolism
- Tumours

Diagnostic Approach

Cardiac/Respiratory Arrest

(following successful reanimation and intensive care monitoring)

1. ECG

2. Case History

3. General Examination

4. X-Ray Study
- Thorax
- Abdomen
- Skull
- Cervical Spine

5. Blood Tests
- Hct, Ery, Leuc, Hb
- Na, K, Ca, P, Mg
- TP, Alb, Glob
- GPT, AP, Urea, Crea, BG

- Blood gas analysis (BGA)
- Blood Sedimentation Rate (BSR)
- Diff BC

MICROBIAL SEROLOGY
- FeLV-/FIV Antigen [Cat]

6. Urinalysis
- Urinary output/volume
- Urine dip stick
- Specific gravity
- Urine sediment

7. Ultrasound
- Analysis of body cavity fluid

Heart Murmurs

Heart sound audible during auscultation caused by turbulence, noticeable either between the 1st and 2nd heart beat (systolic murmur), between the 2nd and 1st heart beat (diastolic murmur) or continuously (machinery murmur)

Common Causes	
Dog	Cat
+++ Mitral valve insufficiency	+++ Hypertrophic Cardiomyopathy
++ Dilated Cardiomyopathy	++ Restrictive Cardiomyopathy
++ Fever/Anaemia	++ Arterial Hypertension
++ Congenital heart disease	++ Cor pulmonale
+ Cor pulmonale	++ Fever/Anaemia
	++ Congenital heart disease

Systolic Murmur

Left Cranial
(2nd–4th Intercostal Space)

- (Sub)Aortic Stenosis
  - Dysplasia (congenital)
- Pulmonary Stenosis
  - Dysplasia (congenital)
  - Aelurostrongylus sp. [Cat]
  - (Dirofilaria sp. [esp Dog])
  - Angiostrongylus sp. [Dog]
- Other Causes
  - Physiological ejection phase murmur [puppies]
  - Anaemia/Hypoxia
  - Fever
  - Hyperthyroidism [Cat]
  - Hypertrophic Cardiomyopathy [esp Cat]
  - Pregnancy
  - III. degree AV block
- Tetralogy of Fallot
  - 1. Pulmonary Stenosis
  - 2. Ventricular Septal Defect
  - 3. Right ventricular Hypertrophy
  - 4. Overriding Aorta

Left Caudal
(5th–6th Intercostal Space)

- Mitral valve insufficiency
  - Endocarditis
  - Fibrosis
  - Dysplasia (congenital)
  - Functional dilation of the valvular anulus

Right Cranial
(2nd–4th Intercostal Space)

- (Sub)Aortic Stenosis
- Ventricular Septal Defect

Right Caudal
(5th–6th Intercostal Space)

- Tricuspid valve insufficiency
  - Endocarditis
  - Fibrosis
  - Dysplasia (congenital)
  - Functional dilation of the valvular anulus

Diastolic Murmur

Left Cranial
(2nd–4th Intercostal Space)

- Aortic valve insufficiency

- Bacterial endocarditis
- Fibrosis
- Functional dilation of the valvular anulus
- Pulmonary valve insufficiency
  - Bacterial endocarditis
  - Aelurostrongylus sp. [Cat]
  - (Dirofilaria sp. [esp Dog])
  - Angiostrongylus sp. [Dog]
- Other causes
  - Atrial Tumours
  - Anaemia
  - Ventricular Septal Defect
  - Atrial Septal Defect

Left Caudal
(5th–6th Intercostal Space)

- Mitral valve stenosis

Right Caudal
(5th–6th Intercostal space)

- Tricuspid valve stenosis

Continuous Murmur
(Machinery Murmur)
Left Cranial
(2nd–4th Intercostal Space)

- Patent ductus arteriosus (Left-Right Shunt)

Other Sounds

- Pericardial Sounds
  - Pericarditis
  - Pericardial Tumours
  - Pericardial Rupture
- Respiratory Sounds
- Thoracic Rubbing Sounds
- Extrathoracic Sounds

Diagnostic Approach

Heart Murmurs

1. **Case History**

2. **General Examination**

3. **X-Ray Study**
- Thorax
- Abdomen

4. **ECG**

5. **Ultrasound**
- Heart (Doppler-Echocardiography)
- Abdomen

6. **Blood Tests**
- Hct, Ery, Leuc, Hb
- TP, Alb, Glob
- GPT, AP, Urea, Crea, BG
- Na, K, Ca, Mg
- Diff BC
- Blood Gas Analysis (BGA)
- α HBDH
- Troponin
- ANP

MICROBIAL SEROLOGY
- FeLV-/FIV Antigen [Cat]

- Dirofilaria Antigen [Dog]

FUNCTION TESTS
- T_4, fT_4 [Cat]
- T_3 Suppression Test [Cat]

7. Urinalysis
- Urinary output/volume
- Urine dip stick

- Specific gravity

8. Further Tests
- Examination of the ocular fundus
- Blood Pressure Measurement (indirect/direct)
- Non-selective angiocardiography
- Analysis of body cavity fluid

Cardiac Arrhythmias

Physiological Heart Rate:
Dog: 70–160/min Sinus rhythm or respiratory sinus arrhythmia
    (puppies–220/min)
Cat: 160–240/min Sinus rhythm

Common Causes	
Dog	Cat
+++ Mitral valve insufficiency	+++ Hypertrophic Cardiomyopathy
++ Dilated Cardiomyopathy	
++ Congenital Heart Disease	++ Renal Failure
	++ Hyperthyroidism
++ General Illness	++ Hyper-/Hypokalaemia
+ Drugs (Digoxin intoxication)	++ General Illness

Slow and Regular

Sinus Bradycardia

- – Regular sinus rhythm
- Physiological
  - – Exercise
  - – Sleep
- Sick Sinus Syndrome
- Vagal tone
  - – Endotracheal tube
  - – Cardiac catheter
  - – Cerebral Pressure
  - – Oropharyngeal Disease
  - – Abdominal Pain

  - – Peritonitis
  - – Pancreatitis
  - – Vomitus
  - – Gastric ulcer
  - – Carotid Sinus Pressure
  - – Compression of the eyeball
  - – Tumours (neck, mediastinum)
- Electrolyte imbalances
  - – Hyperkalaemia
  - – Hypocalcaemia
- Drugs
  - – Digitalis glycosides

- Beta blockers
- Calcium antagonists
- Cimetidine
- Xylazine
- Acepromazine
- Halothan
• Other Causes
- Myocarditis
- Endocarditis
- Cardiomyopathy
- Heart Tumours
- Congenital Heart Defect
- Hypothyroidism [Dog]
- Uraemia
- Muscarine Poisoning

Sinus Arrest/III. Degree Sinoatrial Block

- Missing P Waves
- Escape rhythm
• Same causes as Sinus bradycardia

II. Degree Atrioventricular Block (Mobitz Type II)

- P Waves without subsequent QRS-T complexes
- Conduction of only every second, third or fourth atrial impulse
• Vagal Tone
• Hyperthyroidism [Cat]
• Electrolyte Imbalances
- Hyperkalaemia
- Hypocalcaemia
• Drugs
- Digitalis glycoside
- Beta blockers
- Calcium antagonists

- Xylazine
- Lidocaine
• Other Causes
- Myocarditis
- Cardiomyopathy
- Heart tumours
- AV-Node fibrosis
- Aortic stenosis
- Ventricular septal defect
- Muscarine Poisoning

III. Degree AV-Block

- P- and QRS-T complexes are unconnected
- Dissociation between atrial and ventricular activity
• Same causes as II. Degree AV-Block

Slow and Irregular

II. Degree SA Block

- Periodic or intermittent absence of P-QRS-T complexes
• Same causes as Sinus bradycardia

II. Degree AV Block (Mobitz Type I)

- Progressively prolonged PQ Interval until absence of QRS complex occurs (Wenckebach Phenomenon) with intermittent absence of one or more QRS-T complexes
• Same causes as II. Degree AV Block

Absolute Arrhythmia

- – Atrial fibrillation/flutters
- Same causes as atrial flutters/ fibrillation

Fast and Regular

Sinus Tachycardia

- – Regular sinus rhythm
- Physiological
  - – Exertion
  - – Vegetative
- Drugs
  - – Atropine
  - – Adrenalin
  - – Ephedrine
  - – Theophylline
  - – Ketamine
  - – Cocaine/Amphetamines
  - – Caffeine/Nicotine
  - – Alcohol
- Other Causes
  - – Hyperthyroidism [Cat]
  - – Fever
  - – Respiratory Disease
  - – Congestive Heart Failure
  - – Anaemia
  - – Hypovolaemia
  - – Acidosis
  - – Phaeochromocytoma

Atrial Tachycardia/AV Node Tachycardia

- – Three or more supraventricular extrasystoles
- Same causes as in supraventricular extrasystoles

Ventricular Tachycardia

- – Ventricular extrasystoles often in rapid succession or Bigeminy-/Trigeminy Rhythms
- Same causes as in ventricular extrasytoles

Ventricular Pre-excitation (Wolff-Parkinson-White Syndrome)

- – Premature ventricular excitation from the SA node via the Kent Bundle (among others) (Re-entry Mechanism)
- – Reduced PQ Interval
- – Widened delta Waves (between P- and R-Rise) and QRS complexes
- Congenital Defect
- Other Causes
  - – Ventricular septal defect
  - – Mitral valve fibrosis
  - – Hypertrophic cardiomyopathy [Cat]
  - – Hyperthyroidism [Cat]
  - – Myocarditis
  - – Endocarditis

Fast and Irregular

Atrial Fibrillation/Flutters

- – Highly frequent atrial fibrillations
- – Absent P Waves
- – Coarse or fine flutter waves
- – Normal QRS-T shape
- Same causes as in supraventricular extrasystoles

Ventricular Fibrillation

- Highly frequent ventricular contractions/fibrillations
- Chaotic, bizarrely shaped ventricular complexes (Torsade de pointes)
- Often arises out of R-on-T Phenomenon
• Same causes as in ventricular extrasystoles

Supraventricular Extrasystoles

- Highly frequent atrial contractions
- Distorted and premature P Waves
- Normal QRS-T complexes
- Not fully compensated rest
• Physiological
  - vegetative
• Sick Sinus syndrome
• Electrolyte Imbalances
  - Hypo-/Hyperkalaemia
• Drugs
  - Digoxin intoxication
  - Narcotics
• Other Causes
  - Valvular heart disease
  - Cardiomyopathy
  - Atrial tumours/thrombi
  - Patent ductus arteriosus
  - Hyperthyroidism [Cat]

Ventricular Extrasystole

- Premature ventricular excitation with electrical discharge from within the ventricular muscle
- Deformed ventricular complexes
- P Waves disconnected from QRS-T Complexes
- Complete compensatory pause
- Often arises out of R-on-T Phenomenon
• Physiological
  - vegetative
• Electrolyte Imbalance
  - Hypo-/Hyperkalaemia
• Drugs
  - Digitalis glycosides
  - Adrenalin
  - Narcotics
  - Antiarrhythmics
  - Theophylline
• Other Causes
  - Aortic stenosis
  - Myocarditis
  - Cardiomyopathy
  - Heart Tumours
  - Septicaemia/Endotoxaemia
  - Gastric Dilation/ volvulus [Dog]
  - Pyometra
  - Prostatic cysts [Dog]
  - Pancreatitis
  - Anaemia
  - Hypoxia
  - Uraemia
  - Fever
  - Acidosis
  - Seizures
  - Electrical Shock

Diagnostic Approach

Cardiac Arrhythmias

1. **Case History**

2. **General Examination**

3. **ECG**

4. **X-Ray Study**
- Thorax
- Abdomen

5. **Ultrasound**
- Heart (Doppler Echocardiography)

6. **Blood Tests**
- Hct, Ery, Leuc, Hb
- TP, Alb, Glob
- GPT, AP, Urea, Crea, BG
- Na, K, Ca, Mg
- Diff BC
- Blood Gas Analysis (BGA)
- α HBDH
- Troponin
- ANP

MICROBIAL SEROLOGY
- FeLV-/FIV Antigen [Cat]

FUNCTION TESTS
- T_4, fT_4 [Cat]
- T_3 Suppression Test [Cat]

FURTHER SEROLOGY
- Serum Digitalis Levels (Therapeutic control)

7. **Urinalysis**
- Urinary output/volume
- Urine dip stick
- Specific gravity

8. **Further Tests**
- Examination of the ocular fundus
- Blood Pressure Measure (indirect/direct)
- Non-selective angiocardiography
- Analysis of body cavity fluid

Heart Sounds, Pathological

1. **Heart Sound:** Beginning of the systole (closure of mitral and tricuspid valve)
2. **Heart Sound:** Beginning of the diastole (closure of aortic and pulmonary valve)
3. **Heart Sound:** Fast Ventricular filling phase
4. **Heart Sound:** Atrial contraction

1. Heart Sound

Loud
- Sympathetic tone
- Hyperthyroidism [Cat]

- Mitral valve prolapse

Quiet
- Pericardial effusion
- Thoracic effusion

- Pneumothorax
- Pulmonary emphysema
- Obesity
- Shock
- Mitral valve insufficiency
- Left bundle branch block

Split

- Ventricular extrasystoles
- Left–right Shunt
- Right bundle branch block

2. Heart Sound

Loud

- Sympathetic tone
- Arterial hypertension [esp Cat]

Quiet

- Hypotension
- Shock
- Left sided heart failure

Split

- Physiological in large dog breeds
- Pulmonary stenosis
- (Dirofilaria sp. [esp Dog])
- Mitral valve insufficiency
- Ventricular septal defect

- Atrial septal defects
- Ventricular extrasystoles
- Right bundle branch block

3. Heart Sound

- Anaemia
- Pregnancy
- Hyperthyroidism [Cat]
- Mitral valve insufficiency
- Tricuspid valve insufficiency
- Hypertrophic cardiomyopathy [esp Cat]
- Left–right Shunt

4. Heart Sound

- Pulmonary hypertension
- Pulmonary stenosis
- Arterial hypertension [esp Cat]
- Aortic stenosis
- Hypertrophic cardiomyopathy [esp Cat]
- Papillary muscle rupture
- III. Degree AV Block
- Anaemia
- Hyperthyroidism [Cat]

Midsystolic Clicks

- Mitral valve prolapse
- Pericardial adhesions

Diagnostic Approach

Heart Sounds, Pathological

1. **Case History**

2. **General Examination**

3. **ECG**

4. **X-Ray Study**
   - Thorax

- Abdomen

5. Ultrasound
- Heart (Doppler Echocardiography)

6. Blood Tests
- Hct, Ery, Leuc, Hb
- TP, Alb, Glob
- GPT, AP, Urea, Crea, BG
- Na, K, Ca, Mg
- Diff BC
- Blood Gas Analysis (BGA)
- α HBDH
- Troponin
- ANP

MICROBIAL SEROLOGY
- FeLV-/FIV Antigen [Cat]
- Dirofilaria Antigen [Dog]

FUNCTION TESTS
- T_4, fT_4 [Cat]
- T_3 Suppression Test [Cat]

FURTHER SEROLOGY
- Serum Digitalis Level

7. Urinalysis
- Urinary output/volume
- Urine dip stick
- Specific gravity

8. Further Tests
- Examination of the ocular fundus
- Blood pressure measure (indirect/direct)
- Non-selective angiocardiography
- Analysis of body cavity fluid

Cardiomegaly

Enlargement of the heart

Common Causes	
Dog	**Cat**
+++ Mitral valve insufficiency	+++ Hypertrophic cardiomyopathy
++ Dilated cardiomyopathy	++ Restrictive cardiomyopathy
++ (Sub)Aortic stenosis	++ Mitral valve insufficiency
++ Cor pulmonale	++ Arterial hypertension
++ Pulmonary stenosis	– Renal Failure
++ Ventricular septal defect	– Hyperthyroidism
++ Patent ductus arteriosus	++ Cor pulmonale
++ Atrial tumours	++ Atrial thrombosis
++ Pericardial effusion	

Left Atrium

- Mitral valve insufficiency
- Cardiomyopathy

- Dilated cardiomyopathy
- Hypertrophic cardiomyopathy [esp Cat]

- Restrictive cardiomyopathy
- Atrial tumours
  - Haemangiosarcoma [esp Dog]
  - Tumour metastasis
- Atrial thrombosis
- Left–right Shunt
  - Ventricular septal defect (VSD)
  - Atrial septal defect (ASD) (Shunt reversal)
  - Persistent ductus arteriosus (PDA)
- Right–left Shunt
  - Tetralogy of Fallot
  - Transposition of the large vessels
- Endocardial fibroelastosis

Left Ventricle

- Mitral valve insufficiency
- Cardiomyopathy
  - Dilated Cardiomyopathy
  - Hypertrophic cardiomyopathy [esp Cat]
  - Restrictive cardiomyopathy
- (Sub)Aortic stenosis [Dog]
- Patent ductus arteriosus (PDA)
- Arterial hypertension [esp Cat]
- Myocarditis

Right Atrium

- Atrial septal defect (Left-right Shunt)
- Tricuspid valve insufficiency
- Atrial tumours
  - Haemangiosarcoma [Dog]
  - Myxoma [Dog]
  - Tumour metastasis

- Atrial thrombosis with right ventricular enlargement
  - Cor pulmonale
  - Pulmonary stenosis
  - Tetralogy of Fallot
  - Left sided heart failure
  - Mitral valve stenosis
  - (Dirofilaria sp. [esp Dog])
- Tricuspid valve stenosis
- Ebstein Anomaly (Tricuspid valve displacement into the right ventricle)

Right Atrium

- Left–right Shunt
  - Ventricular septal defect (VSD)
  - Atrial septal defect (ASD)
  - Persistent Ductus arteriosus (PDA)
- Tricuspidvalve insufficiency
- Pulmonary stenosis
- Cor pulmonale
- Tetralogy of Fallot
  - Pulmonary stenosis
  - Ventricular septal defect
  - Overriding aorta
  - Right ventricular hypertrophy
- Ebstein Anomaly (Tricuspid valve displacement into the right ventricle)

Pulmonary Segment

- Pulmonary stenosis
- Cor pulmonale
  - Pulmonary/ Respiratory tract disease
  - (Dirofilaria sp. [esp Dog])

- – (Angiostrongylus sp [Dog])
- Thromboembolism of the pulmonary artery
- Left-right Shunt
  - – Ventricular septal defect (VSD)
  - – Atrial septal defect (ASD) (Shunt reversal)
  - – Patent ductus arteriosus (PDA)

  With dilation of the pulmonary veins
  - – Left sided heart failure
  - – Mitral valve stenosis
- Tetralogy of Fallot
  - – Pulmonary stenosis
  - – Overriding aorta
  - – Right ventricular hypertrophy
- Erroneous outlet of pulmonary veins into the Vena cava

Aorta

- (Sub)Aortic stenosis

- Patent ductus arteriosus (PDA)
- Arterial hypertension [esp Cat]
- Tetralogy of Fallot
  - – Pulmonary stenosis
  - – Ventricular septal defect
  - – Overriding aorta
  - – Right ventricular hypertrophy
- Persistent right aortic arch (Right aorta)
- Aortic aneurysm
- Aneurysm of Sinus valsalvae
- Connective tissue disease
  - – Ehlers-Danlos syndrome
  - – Osteogenesis imperfecta

Spherical Heart

- Pericardial effusion
  - – Atrial rupture
  - – Pericarditis
  - – Congestive heart failure
  - – Pericardial tumours
  - – Renal failure

Diagnostic Approach

Cardiomegaly

1. **Case History**

2. **General Examination**

3. **X-Ray Study**
- Thorax
- Abdomen

4. **ECG**

5. **Ultrasound**
- Heart (Doppler Echocardiography)

6. **Blood Tests**
- Hct, Ery, Leuc, Hb
- TP, Alb, Glob
- GPT, AP, Urea, Crea, BG
- Na, K, Ca, Mg
- Diff BC
- Blood Gas Analysis (BGA)
- α HBDH
- Troponin
- ANP

MICROBIAL SEROLOGY
- FeLV-/FIV Antigen [Cat]
- Dirofilaria Antigen [Dog]

FUNCTION TESTS
- T_4, fT_4 [Cat]
- T_3 Suppression Test [Cat]

FURTHER SEROLOGY
- Serum Digitalis level (Therapeutic control)

7. Urinalysis
- Urine dip stick

- Specific gravity
- Urinary output/ volume

8. Further Tests
- Faecal Examination
- Examination of the ocular fundus
- Blood pressure measure (indirect/ direct)
- Non-selective angiocardiography
- Analysis of body cavity fluid

Hypertension, Arterial

Increased Blood Pressure
Normal values (direct measurement):
Dog: 130–170 mmHg (Systole) 70–90 mmHg (Diastole)
Cat: 150–200 mmHg (Systole) 85–100 mmHg (Diastole)

Common Causes	
Dog	Cat
+++ Renal Failure	+++ Renal Failure
++ Diabetes mellitus	++ Hyperthyroidism
++ Hypercortisolism (Cushing's Disease)	++ Diabetes mellitus

Causes

- Idiopathic
- Chronic renal failure
- Hypercortisolism (Cushing's Disease) [Dog]
- Diabetes mellitus
- Hyperthyroidism [Cat]
- Central nervous Disease
- Hyperaldosteronism [Dog]
- Phaeochromocytoma

Diagnostic Approach

Hypertension, Arterial

1. Case History

2. General Examination

3. ECG

4. X-Ray Study
- Abdomen
- Thorax
- Excretory urography

5. Ultrasound
- Abdomen (kidneys, adrenal glands)
- Heart (Doppler Echocardiography)

6. Blood Tests
- Hct, Ery, Leuc, Hb
- TP, Alb, Glob
- GPT, AP, Urea, Crea, BG
- Na, K, Ca, P
- FIP Profile [Cat]
  - TP
  - Alb/Glob Ratio
  - Bili
  - GOT
  - Serum electrophoresis
- Diff BC
- α HBDH
- Troponin
- ANP

MICROBIAL SEROLOGY
- FeLV-/FIV Antigen [Cat]

FUNCTION TESTS
- T_4, fT_4
- T_3 Suppression Test [Cat]
- Adrenal gland function tests [Dog]
  - Dexamethasone Suppression test
  - ACTH Stimulation test
  - Cortisol/Creatinine Ratio
- Serum Aldosterone [Dog]

7. Urinalysis
- Urinary output/ volume
- Urine dip stick
- Specific gravity
- Urine sediment
  - Bacteria
  - Erys, Leuc
  - Epithelial cells
  - Urinary casts
  - Urinary crystals
  - Tumour cytology
- Bacterial culture (Cystocentesis)

8. Further Tests
- Examination of the ocular background
- Blood Pressure measure (indirect/direct)
- Renal biopsy

Pulse Alterations

Changes in the pulse quality

Absent Femoral Pulse

- Feline aortic thromboembolism [Cat]
- Thromboembolism of the femoral artery
- Cardiac Arrest
  - Asystole
  - Atrial Fibrillation
  - Electromechanical dissociation

Weak Pulse

- Arterial hypotension
- High diastolic blood pressure with low systolic blood pressure
- Hypovolaemia
- Mitral valve insufficiency
- (Sub)Aortic stenosis
- Cardiomyopathies
- Pericardial effusion
- Aortic thromboembolism [Cat]

Strong Pulse

- Exercise/Excitement
- Fever
- Anaemia
- Hyperthyroidism [Cat]
- Patent ductus arteriosus
- Aortic valve insufficiency

Pulse Deficit

- Cardiac Arrhythmias
  - Supraventricular extrasystoles
  - Ventricular extrasystoles

Jugular Venous Pressure

- Pulmonary stenosis
- Cor pulmonale
- (Dirofilaria sp. [esp Dog])
- Tricuspid valve insufficiency
- Cardiomyopathies
- Pericardial effusion
- Heart tumours
- Atrial thrombosis
- III. Degree AV Block

Diagnostic Approach

Pulse Alterations

1. **Case History**

2. **General Examination**

3. **X-Ray Study**

- Thorax
- Abdomen

4. **ECG**

5. Ultrasound
- Heart (Doppler-Echocardiography)
- Abdomen

6. Blood Tests
- Hct, Ery, Leuc, Hb
- TP, Alb, Glob
- GPT, AP, Urea, Crea, BG
- Na, K, Ca, Mg
- Diff BC
- Blood Gas Analysis (BGA)
- α HBDH
- Troponin
- ANP

MICROBIAL SEROLOGY
- FeLV-/FIV Antigen [Cat]

- Dirofilaria Antigen [Dog]

FUNCTION TESTS
- T_4, fT_4 [Cat]
- T_3 Suppression Test [Cat]

FURTHER SEROLOGY
- Serum Digitalis Level

7. Urinalysis
- Urinary output/volume
- Urine dip stick
- Specific gravity

8. Further Tests
- Angiography
- Examination of the ocular fundus
- Blood Pressure Measure (indirect/direct)

Syncope

Spontaneous, reversible and brief unconsciousness

Common Causes	
Dog	Cat
+++ Valvular Heart Disease	+++ Hypertrophic Cardiomyopathy
++ Dilated Cardiomyopathy	++ Valvular Heart Disease
++ Congenital Heart Disease	++ Pericardial Disease
+ Pericardial Disease	++ Hyperthyroidism
+ Neurological Causes	+ Neurological Causes

Cardiovascular Causes

Congenital Heart Disease

- Patent ductus arteriosus (PDA)
- (Sub)Aortic stenosis
- Stenosis of the pulmonary artery

- Atrial septal defect (ASD)
- Ventricular septal defect (VSD)
- Valve dysplasia
- Tetralogy of Fallot
- Endocardial fibroelastosis
- Ebstein Anomaly

- Erroneous outlet of pulmonary veins into the Vena cava

Myocardial Disease

Primary Cardiomyopathy
- Dilated cardiomyopathy
- Hypertrophic cardiomyopathy [esp Cat]
- Restrictive cardiomyopathy

Secondary Cardiomyopathy
- Metabolic Causes
  - Hyperthyroidism [Cat]
  - Hypothyroidism [Dog]
  - Hypo-/Hyperkalaemia
  - Hypo-/Hypercalcaemia
  - Diabetes mellitus
  - Hypercortisolism (Cushing's Disease) [Dog]
  - Uraemia
  - Renal hypertension
  - Glycogen storage disease
- Alimentary Causes
  - Taurine deficiency [esp Cat]
  - Carnitine deficiency [esp Dog]
- Viral Myocarditis
  - Parvovirus
  - Canine distemper virus [Dog]
  - Herpes virus
- Bacterial Endo-/Myocarditis
  - Aerobics/Anaerobics
  - Lyme Borreliosis sp. [Dog]
  - Endotoxaemia
- Mycotic Myocarditis
  - Cryptococcus sp. [esp Cat]
- Parasitic Myocarditis
  - Toxoplasma sp.
  - (Hepatozoon sp. [Dog])

- (Trypanosoma sp. [Dog])
- Immunoreactive Myocarditis
  - Polyarteritis nodosa
  - Lupus erythematosus
- Toxic Myocarditis/Myocardosis
  - Doxorubicin
  - Heavy metals
- Traumatic Myocarditis
  - Contusion
  - Atrial Rupture

Valvular Heart Disease

- Mitral valve insufficiency
  - Dysplasia
  - Endocarditis
  - Fibrosis
  - Functional dilation of the valvular anulus
- Valvular pulmonary stenosis
  - Dysplasia
- Tricuspid valve insufficiency
  - Dysplasia
  - Endocarditis
  - Fibrosis
  - Functional dilation of the valvular anulus
- Valvular Aortic stenosis
  - Dysplasia
- Papillary muscle rupture

Heart/Pericardial Tumours

- Haemangiosarcoma [esp Dog]
- Heart base tumour (Chemodectoma) [Dog]
- Myxoma [Dog]
- Thyroid carcinoma
- Mesothelioma
- Lymphosarcoma
- Cysts

Pericardial Disease (Pericardial Effusion)

Modified Transudate
- Congestive Heart Failure
- Uraemia
- Hypoalbuminaemia
- Cardiac arrhythmias
- Pericardio-diaphragmatic hernia

Exudate
- Tumours
- Pericarditis
  - Canine Distemper virus [Dog]
  - FIP Coronavirus [Cat]
  - Leptospira sp. [Dog]
  - Actinomyces sp.
  - Nocardia sp.
  - Mycobacterium sp.
  - Toxoplasma sp.
  - Pasteurella sp.
  - Streptococcus spp.
  - Staphylococcus spp.
  - E. coli
  - Cryptococcus sp. [esp Cat]

Blood
- Atrial rupture
- Haemangiosarcoma [esp Dog]
- Foreign body
- Coagulopathy

Arterial Thromboembolism

- Feline Aortic thromboembolism
  - Hypertrophic cardiomyopathy
  - Restrictive cardiomyopathy
  - (Dilated cardiomyopathy)
  - Pulmonary thromboembolism
    - (Dirofilaria sp. [esp Dog])
    - (Angiostrongylus sp. [Dog])
    - Hypercortisolism (Cushing's Disease) [Dog]
    - DIC
    - Cardiomyopathy
    - Protein-losing nephropathy
    - Acute pancreatitis
    - Septicaemia/Endotoxaemia
    - Immune haemolytic anaemia
    - Bone trauma/surgery
    - Hyperviscosity syndrome

Neurological Causes

Vasovagal Hypertension

- Excitement
- Cough
- Sneezing
- Labour contractions
- Seizures
- Faecal/Urinary Evacuation
- Carotid sinus reflex stimulation (collar)

Further Causes

- Traumatic brain injury
- CNS haemorrhage
- Brain tumours
- Cerebral circulatory disturbances
- Narcolepsy

Further Causes

Metabolic Causes

- Hypoglycaemia
- Metabolic Acidosis

- Hypo-/Hypercalcaemia
- Hypo-/Hypernatraemia
- Hypo/Hyperkalaemia
- Hypocortisolism (Addison's Disease) [Dog]

Hyperviscosity Syndrome

- Plasmocytoma (multiple myeloma) [esp Dog]
- Lymphatic leukaemia [Cat]
- FIP Coronavirus [Cat]
- Lupus erythematosus
- Dehydration
- Rheumatoid Arthritis

- (Leishmania sp. [esp Dog])
- (Ehrlichia sp. [esp Dog])
- Polycythaemia vera

Drugs

- ACE Inhibitors
- Hydralazine
- Calcium channel blocker
- Nitroglycerin
- Acepromazine
- Anticonvulsants
- Antiarrhythmics
- Diuretics

Diagnostic Approach

Syncope

1. Case History

2. General Examination

3. Neurological Examination

4. ECG
- Carotid sinus pressure

5. X-Ray Study
- Thorax
- Abdomen

6. Ultrasound
- Heart (Doppler Echocardiography)

7. Blood Tests
- Hct, Ery, Leuc, Hb
- TP, Alb, Glob
- GPT, AP, Urea, Crea, BG
- Na, K, Ca, Mg
- Diff BC
- Blood Gas Analysis (BGA)

- α HBDH
- Troponin
- ANP

MICROBIAL SEROLOGY
- FeLV-/FIV Antigen [Cat]
- Dirofilaria Antigen [Dog]

FUNCTION TESTS
- T_4, fT_4 [Cat]
- T_3 Suppression test [Cat]

FURTHER SEROLOGY
- Serum Digitalis level (Therapeutic control)

8. Urinalysis
- Urinary output/volume
- Urine dip stick
- Specific gravity

9. Further Tests
- Examination of the ocular fundus

- Blood Pressure measure (indirect/direct)
- Non-selective angiocardiography
- Analysis of body cavity fluid

Cyanosis

Blue discolouration of the skin and mucous membranes as a result of insufficient oxygen saturation

Common Causes	
Dog	**Cat**
Central Cyanosis	
+++ Mitral valve insufficiency	+++ Hypertrophic cardiomyopathy
++ Dilated cardiomyopathy	++ Restrictive cardiomyopathy
++ Congenital heart disease	++ Feline asthma
++ Tracheal collapse	++ Pulmonary disease
++ Pulmonary disease	++ Congenital heart disease
Peripheral Cyanosis	
+ Exposure to the cold	++ Exposure to the cold

Central Cyanosis

Laryngeal Disease

- Foreign body
- Glottal oedema
- Abscess
- Tonsillitis/Tonsillar carcinoma
- Overlong soft palate [esp Dog]
- Laryngeal tumours
- Laryngeal paralysis/collapse
- Granulomatous laryngitis

Tracheobronchial Disease

- Tracheal collapse [Dog]
- Tracheobronchitis
- Allergic bronchitis
- Foreign body
- Tracheal hypoplasia [Dog]

Pulmonary Disease

- Pneumonia
  - Viral
  - Bacterial
  - Mycotic
  - Rickettsial
  - Parasitic
  - Allergic
  - Aspiration pneumonia
  - Foreign body
- Lung tumours

- Pulmonary oedema
- Pulmonary contusion/ haemorrhage
- Thromboembolism of the pulmonary artery
- Pulmonary fibrosis
- Atelectasis/Emphysema
- Lung lobe torsion [Dog]

Thoracic Disease

- Pleural effusion
- Pneumothorax
- Mediastinal tumours
- Pleuritis/Mediastinitis
- Diaphragmatic hernia
- Rib fracture
- Diaphragmatic paralysis

Congenital Heart Disease

- Patent ductus arteriosus (PDA)
- (Sub)Aortic stenosis
- Stenosis of the pulmonary artery
- Atrial septal defect (ASD)
- Ventricular septal defect (VSD)
- Valvular dysplasia
- Endocardial fibroelastosis
- Tetralogy of Fallot
- Persistent right aortic arch

Heart Valve Disease

- Mitral valve insufficiency
- Valvular pulmonary stenosis
- Tricuspid valve insufficiency
- Valvular aortic stenosis

Acquired Heart Disease

- Primary Cardiomyopathy

- Dilated cardiomyopathy
- Hypertrophic cardiomyopathy [esp Cat]
- Restrictive cardiomyopathy
- Secondary cardiomyopathy
  - Carnitine/Taurine deficiency
  - Metabolic disease
- Heart tumours
- Myocarditis/Endocarditis
- Atrial rupture/Papillary muscle rupture
- Myocardial infarction

Pericardial Disease

- Pericarditis
- Pericardial tumours
- Pericardial rupture

Further Causes

- Shock
- Anaesthetic incident (Hypoxia)
- Drowning
- Anaemia/ Methaemoglobinaemia

Peripheral Cyanosis

- Exposure to the cold
- Thrombophlebitis
- Venous compression (Tumours)
- Venous thrombosis

Caudal Body Part

- Patent ductus arteriosus with R-L Shunt

Diagnostic Approach

Cyanosis

1. Case History

2. General Examination

3. ECG

4. X-Ray Study
- Thorax
- Abdomen

5. Ultrasound
- Heart (Doppler Echocardiography)

6. Blood Tests
- Hct, Ery, Leuc, Hb
- Na, K, Ca
- TP, Alb, Glob
- GPT, AP, Urea, Crea, BG
- Blood Gas Analysis (BGA)
- Diff BB
- α HBDH
- Troponin

- ANP

MICROBIAL SEROLOGY
- FeLV-/FIV Antigen [Cat]
- Dirofilaria Antigen [Dog]

FURTHER SEROLOGY
- Serum Methaemoglobin

7. Urinalysis
- Urinary output/volume
- Urine dip stick
- Specific gravity
- Urine sediment

8. Further Tests
- Non-selective angiocardiography
- Bronchoscopy ± Tracheobronchial lavage
- cytology
- bacterial culture
- fungal culture
- Analysis of body cavity fluid

3 Respiratory Principal Symptoms

Further Relevant Principal Symptoms

Respiratory Sounds

Inspiratory breathing sounds that are audible without the use of
a stethoscope
Stridor: Whistling type, often inspiratory stenotic sound of the upper
airways
Stertor: Snoring

Common Causes			
Dog		Cat	
+++	Brachycephalic Syndrome	+++	Rhinitis/Sinusitis
++	Rhinitis/Sinusitis	++	Nasopharyngeal foreign bodies

Common Causes			
Dog		Cat	
++	Tracheal collapse		
++	Infectious Tracheobronchitis	++	Brachycephalic Syndrome
+	Tonsillitis/Tonsillar carcinoma	++	Feline asthma
+	Laryngeal paralysis	+	Nasopharyngeal Polyps

Endonasal Causes

Rhinitis/Sinusitis

- Viral Rhinitis
  - Feline Herpes virus [Cat]
  - Feline Calici virus [Cat]
  - Canine Herpes virus [Dog]
  - Canine Adenovirus I, II [Dog]
  - Parainfluenza virus [Dog]
  - Canine Distemper virus [Dog]
- Bacterial Rhinitis
  - Pasteurella sp.
  - Bordetella sp.
  - Staphylococcus sp.
  - Pseudomonas sp.
  - Chlamydia sp. [Cat]
  - E. coli
  - Mycoplasma sp.
- Mycotic Rhinitis
  - Cryptococcus sp. [esp Cat]
  - Aspergillus sp.
  - Rhinosporidium sp. [Dog]
- Endonasal foreign body
  - Blade of grass [Cat]
  - Grain seeds/ears
- Parasitic Rhinitis
  - Capillaria sp.
  - (Linguatula sp.)
  - (Pneumonyssus sp.)
  - (Cuterebra sp.)
- Immunoreactive Rhinitis
  - Atopy/Inhalation allergy
  - IgA deficiency
  - FeLV/FIV [Cat]
- Oronasal fistula
  - Dental abscess
  - Cleft palate (congenital, traumatic)

Endonasal Tumours

- Adenocarcinoma
- Lymphosarcoma
- Squamous cell carcinoma
- Osteosarcoma
- Chondrosarcoma
- Fibrosarcoma
- Melanoma
- Myxosarcoma
- Nasopharyngeal Polyps [Cat]

Brachycephalic Syndrome

- Narrowing of the nares
- Anomalies of the nasal concha
- Short pharyngeal cavity
- Mucosal hyperplasia
- Overlong soft palate
- Laryngeal collapse
- Tracheal hypoplasia

Laryngeal Causes

Laryngitis

- Granulomatous Laryngitis

* Foreign body

Laryngeal Tumours

* Squamous Cell Carcinoma
* Lymphosarcoma
* Adenocarcinoma
* Rhabdomyosarcoma
* Leiomyosarcoma
* Mast cell tumour
* Haemangiosarcoma
* Osteosarcoma

Laryngeal Paralysis

* Iatrogenic: Thyroidectomy
* Paralysis of the recurrent laryngeal nerve [Dog]
* Thyroid carcinoma
* Polyneuropathy
  - Hypothyroidism
  - Hypocortisolism (Addison's Disease)
  - Myasthenia gravis
* Congenital Deformity

Laryngospasm/Glottal Oedema

* Insect sting allergy
* Drug allergy
* Endotracheal Intubation
* Smoke inhalation/Irritants
* Foreign bodies
* Mast cell tumour
* Aspiration of gastric acid

Further Causes

* Tonsillitis/Tonsillar carcinoma
* Peritonsillar abscess
* Overlong soft palate

Tracheal Causes

Intraluminal Stenosis

* Foreign body
* Tracheal collapse
* Accumulation of secretion (obstructive bronchitis)
  - Mucus
  - Pus
  - Blood
* Tracheal hypoplasia
* Stricture
* Bronchiectasia
* Tracheal tumours
  - Squamous cell carcinoma
  - Lymphosarcoma

Extraluminal Stenosis

* Left atrial cardiac enlargement
* Mediastinitis
* Lymphadenopathy
* Megaoesophagus
* Oesophageal foreign body
* Tracheal tumours
  - Thyroid carcinoma
  - Thymoma

Tracheobronchitis

* Viral Tracheobronchitis
  - Canine distemper virus [Dog]
  - Cat flu [Cat]
  - Feline Herpes virus [Cat]
  - Feline Calici virus [Cat]
  - Kennel Cough [Dog]
  - Canine Herpes virus [Dog]
  - Canine Adenovirus I, II [Dog]
  - Parainfluenza virus [Dog]

- Canine Reovirus I, II, III [Dog]
- Bacterial Tracheobronchitis
  - Bordetella sp.
  - Pasteurella sp.
  - Pseudomonas sp.
  - Streptococcus sp.
  - Staphylococcus sp.
  - Chlamydia sp. [Cat]
  - E. coli
  - Mycoplasma sp. [esp Cat]
  - Klebsiella sp.
- Parasitic Tracheobronchitis
  - Filaroides sp. [esp Dog]
  - Capillaria sp.
  - Pneumocystis sp.
- Cryptosporidium sp. [Cat]
- (Pneumonyssus sp.)
- Aelurostrongylus sp. [Cat]
- Angiostrongylus sp. [Dog]
- (Crenosoma sp. [Dog])
- Immunoreactive Tracheobronchitis
  - Feline asthma [Cat]
  - Eosinophilic bronchitis
- Further Causes
  - Smoke Inhalation
  - Foreign bodies
  - Endotracheal intubation
  - Dyskinesia of the ciliated epithelium
  - Aspiration of gastric acid

Diagnostic Approach

Respiratory Sounds

1. **Case History**

2. **General Examination**

3. **Oropharyngeal Examination**

4. **X-Ray Study**
   - Thorax
   - Throat
   - Skull

5. **Endoscopy**
   - Rhinoscopy (ortho-/retrograde)
     ± endonasal swab sample
     ± retrograde flush sample
     - Bacterial culture
     - Fungal culture
     - Cytology
   - Laryngo-/Bronchoscopy

   ± Tracheobronchial lavage
     - Bacterial-/Fungal Culture
     - Cytology

6. **Blood Tests**
   - Hct, Ery, Leuc, Hb
   - Diff BC

   MICROBIAL SEROLOGY
   - FeLV-/FIV Antigen [Cat]
   - Aspergillus Antibodies [Dog]
   - Cryptococcus Antibodies [Cat]

7. **Further Tests**
   - Ultrasound of the throat
   - Parasitological faecal examination
     - Flotation
     - Baermann-Wetzel method

Dyspnoea

Respiratory distress	
Common Causes	
Dog	**Cat**
+++ Pneumothorax	+++ Pneumothorax
++ Pulmonary oedema	++ Pulmonary oedema
++ Pulmonary haemorrhage	++ Pulmonary haemorrhage
++ Pneumonia	++ Pleural effusion
++ Pleural effusion	++ Feline Asthma
++ Pulmonary tumours	+ Pulmonary tumours
+ Diaphragmatic elevation	

Endonasal Causes

Rhinitis/Sinusitis

- Viral Rhinitis
  - Feline Herpes virus [Cat]
  - Feline Calici virus [Cat]
  - Canine Herpes virus [Dog]
  - Canine Adenovirus I, II [Dog]
  - Parainfluenza virus [Dog]
  - Canine Distemper virus [Dog]
- Bacterial Rhinitis
  - Pasteurella sp.
  - Bordetella sp.
  - Staphylococcus sp.
  - Pseudomonas sp.
  - Chlamydia sp. [Cat]
  - E. coli
  - Mycoplasma sp.
- Mycotic Rhinitis
  - Cryptococcus sp. [esp]
  - Aspergillus sp.
  - Rhinosporidium sp. [Dog]
- Endonasal foreign body
  - Blade of grass [Cat]
  - Grain seeds/ears
- Parasitic Rhinitis
  - Capillaria sp.
  - (Linguatula sp.)
  - (Pneumonyssus sp.)
  - (Cuterebra sp. [Dog])
- Immunoreactive Rhinitis
  - Atopy/Inhalation allergy
  - IgA Deficiency
  - FeLV/FIV [Cat]
- Oronasal fistula
  - Dental abscess
  - Cleft palate (congenital, traumatic)

Endonasal Tumours

- Adenocarcinoma
- Lymphosarcoma
- Squamous cell carcinoma
- Osteosarcoma
- Chondrosarcoma

- Fibrosarcoma
- Melanoma
- Myxosarcoma
- Nasopharyngeal Polyps [Cat]

Brachycephalic Syndrome

- Narrowing of the nares
- Anomalies of the nasal concha
- Short pharyngeal cavity
- Mucosal hyperplasia
- Overlong soft palate
- Laryngeal collapse
- Tracheal hypoplasia

Laryngeal Causes

Laryngitis

- Granulomatous Laryngitis
- Foreign body

Laryngeal Tumours

- Squamous Cell Carcinoma
- Lymphosarcoma
- Adenocarcinoma
- Rhabdomyosarcoma
- Leiomyosarcoma
- Mast cell tumour
- Haemangiosarcoma
- Osteosarcoma

Laryngeal Paralysis

- Iatrogenic: Thyroidectomy
- Paralysis of the recurrent laryngeal nerve [Dog]
- Thyroid carcinoma
- Polyneuropathy
  - Hypothyroidism
  - Hypocortisolism (Addison's Disease)
  - Myasthenia gravis
- Congenital Deformity

Laryngospasm/Glottal Oedema

- Insect sting allergy
- Drug allergy
- Endotracheal Intubation
- Smoke inhalation/Irritants
- Foreign bodies
- Mast cell tumour
- Aspiration of gastric acid

Further Causes

- Tonsillitis/Tonsillar carcinoma
- Peritonsillar abscess
- Overlong soft palate

Tracheal Causes

Intraluminal Stenosis

- Foreign body
- Tracheal collapse
- Accumulation of secretion (obstructive bronchopneumonia)
  - Mucus/pus/blood
- Tracheal hypoplasia
- Stricture
- Bronchiectasia
- Tracheal tumours
  - Squamous cell carcinoma
  - Lymphosarcoma

Extraluminal Stenosis

- Left atrial cardiac enlargement
- Mediastinitis
- Lymphadenopathy
- Megaoesophagus
- Oesophageal foreign body

- Tracheal tumours
  - Thyroid carcinoma
  - Thymoma

Tracheobronchitis

- Viral Tracheobronchitis
  - Canine distemper virus [Dog]
  - Cat flu [Cat]
  - Feline Herpes virus [Cat]
  - Feline Calici virus [Cat]
  - Kennel Cough [Dog]
  - Canine Herpes virus [Dog]
  - Canine Adenovirus I, II [Dog]
  - Parainfluenza virus [Dog]
  - Canine Reovirus I, II, III [Dog]
- Bacterial Tracheobronchitis
  - Bordetella sp.
  - Pasteurella sp.
  - Pseudomonas sp.
  - Streptococcus sp.
  - Staphylococcus sp.
  - Chlamydia sp. [Cat]
  - E. coli
  - Mycoplasma sp. [esp Cat]
  - Klebsiella sp.
- Parasitic Tracheobronchitis
  - Filaroides sp. [esp Dog]
  - Capillaria sp.
  - Pneumocystis sp.
  - Cryptosporidium sp. [Cat]
  - (Pneumonyssus sp.)
  - Aelurostrongylus sp. [Cat]
  - Angiostrongylus sp. [Dog]
  - (Crenosoma sp. [Dog])
- Immunoreactive Tracheobronchitis
  - Feline asthma [Cat]

- Eosinophilic bronchitis
- Further Causes
  - Smoke Inhalation
  - Foreign bodies
  - Endotracheal intubation
  - Dyskinesia of the ciliated epithelium
  - Aspiration of gastric acid

Pulmonary Causes

Pneumonia

- Viral Pneumonia
  - Canine Distemper virus [Dog]
  - CAV-1 (Hepatitis c. c.) [Dog]
  - Cat flu [Cat]
  - Kennel Cough [Dog]
  - FIP Coronavirus [Cat]
  - FeLV/FIV [Cat]
- Bacterial Pneumonia
  - Bordetella sp.
  - E. coli
  - Klebsiella sp.
  - Pseudomonas sp.
  - Pasteurella sp.
  - Staphylococcus sp.
  - Streptococcus sp.
  - Mycoplasma sp.
  - Mycobacterium spp.
- Rickettsial Pneumonia
  - (Ehrlichia sp. [Dog])
  - (Rickettsia sp. [Dog])
- Parasitic Pneumonia
  - Toxoplasma sp.
  - Pneumocystis sp.
  - Capillaria sp.
  - Filaroides sp. [esp Dog]
  - (Crenosoma sp. [Dog])
  - Aelurostrongylus sp. [Cat]

- Angiostrongylus sp. [Dog]
- (Dirofilaria sp. [esp Dog])
- (Paragonimus sp. [esp Dog])
- Larva migrans
- Mycotic Pneumonia
  - Cryptococcus sp. [esp Cat]
  - (Histoplasma sp.)
  - (Blastomyces sp.)
  - (Coccidioides sp.)
  - Facultative pathogenic fungi
- Immunoreactive Pneumonia
  - Atopy/Inhalation allergy
  - Bacterial/Fungal/Parasite allergy
  - Drug allergy
  - Lupus erythematosus
- Toxic Pneumonia
  - Smoke inhalation/Irritants
  - Uraemia
  - Aspiration pneumonia
- Other Causes
  - IgA Deficiency
  - Dyskinesia of the ciliated epithelium
  - Foreign body

Pulmonary Oedema

↑ Hydrostatic Pressure
- Left Sided Heart Failure
  - Dilated Cardiomyopathy
  - Hypertrophic Cardiomyopathy
  - Restrictive Cardiomyopathy
  - Mitral Valve insufficiency
  - (Sub)Aortic stenosis
  - Ventricular septal defect
  - Patent ductus arteriosus
- Anaphylaxis

- Hyperthyroidism [Cat]
- Hypertension [esp Cat]
- Cardiac arrhythmias
- Papillary muscle rupture
- Overinfusion

↓ Hydrostatic Pressure
- Hypoalbuminaemia + overinfusion

↑ Permeability
- Pneumonia
- Aspiration pneumonia
- Smoke inhalation/Irritant gases
- Uraemia
- Endotoxins
- DIC
- Pulmonary contusion
- Seizures
- Acute Pancreatitis
- Head trauma
- Anaphylaxis
- Snake venom
- O_2 Intoxication
- Drowning
- Electrical shock

Pulmonary Tumours

- Tumour metastasis
  - Thyroid carcinoma
  - Mammary carcinoma
  - Haemangiosarcoma
  - Squamous cell carcinoma
  - Transitional cell carcinoma
  - Melanoma
  - Lymphosarcoma
  - Malignant Histiocytosis [Bernese Mountain Dog]
  - Adenocarcinoma
- Primary tumours
  - Adenocarcinoma
  - Squamous cell carcinoma

Pulmonary Thromboembolism

- Parasites in the pulmonary artery
  - Aelurostrongylus sp. [Cat]
  - Dirofilaria sp. [esp Dog]
  - Angiostrongylus sp. [Dog]
- Larva migrans
- Cardiomyopathy
- Septicaemia/Endocarditis
- Anaesthesia/Lateral recumbency
- Surgery
- DIC
- Hyperviscosity syndrome
- Glomerulonephritis
- Renal amyloidosis
- Hypercortisolism (Cushing's Disease)
- Hypothyroidism
- Pancreatitis
- Immune haemolytic Anaemia

Other Causes

- Pulmonary haemorrhage
  - Pulmonary contusion
  - Lung lobe torsion
  - Foreign body
  - Coagulopathy
  - Pneumonia
  - Pulmonary abscess
  - Pulmonary tumours
- Atelectasis
- Emphysema
- Pulmonary fibrosis

Pleural/Mediastinal Causes

Pleural Effusion

Transudate
- Congestive Heart Failure (Right sided heart failure)

- Hypoalbuminaemia

Modified Transudate
- Congestive Heart Failure
- Tumours
- Diaphragmatic hernia
- Pancreatitis
- Autoimmune Diseases
- Hepatic cirrhosis

Exudate
- FIP Coronavirus [Cat]
- Tumours
- Pyothorax
  - Chlamydia sp.
  - Actinomyces sp.
  - Nocardia sp.
  - Pasteurella sp.
  - Bacteroides sp.
  - Fusobacterium sp.
  - Pneumonia
  - Foreign body perforation
  - Oesophageal perforation
  - Tumour necrosis
  - Thoracocentesis
- Diaphragmatic hernia
- Lung lobe torsion

Blood
- Lung lobe torsion
- Trauma
- Coagulopathy
- Tumours

Chyle
- Congestive Heart Failure [esp Cat]
- Tumours
- Trauma (rupture of the thoracic duct)
- Lymphangiectasia [Dog]
- Diaphragmatic hernia
- Lung lobe torsion
- Dirofilaria sp. [esp Dog]

Pneumothorax

- Traumatic Causes
  - Thoracic penetration
  - Thoracocentesis
  - Pressure ventilation
  - Oesophageal penetration
  - Tracheal penetration
  - Perforating rib fracture
  - Pulmonary contusion/
    Pleural tear
- Spontaneous Causes
  - Pneumonia
  - Bullous emphysema
  - Larva migrans
  - Mycotic Granuloma
  - Pulmonary tumour
  - Pulmonary abscess
  - Pulmonary cysts
  - Foreign body

Mediastinal Tumours

- Lymphadenopathy
- Lymphosarcoma [esp Cat]
- Heart base tumour
  (Chemodectoma) [Dog]
- Thyroid carcinoma
- Thymoma
- Mediastinal cysts
- Mesothelioma

Diaphragmatic elevation

- Diaphragmatic rupture
- Diaphragmatic hernia
- Gastric dilation/ volvulus
  [Dog]
- Hepatomegaly
- Paralysis of the phrenic nerve
- Intraabdominal tumour
- Profound abdominal effusion

Other Causes

- Anaemia/
  Methaemoglobinaemia
- Central nervous dysfunction of
  the respiratory centre
  - Heat stroke
  - Head injury
  - Brain tumours
  - Ischaemia
  - Encephalitis
- Drug related/toxic respiratory
  depression
  - Morphine/Morphine
    derivatives
  - Barbiturates
  - Curare
  - Acetylsalicylic acid
  - Beta blockers
  - Metaldehyde poisoning
  - Nicotine poisoning
  - Alpha Naphtylthiourea
    (ANTU) poisoning
  - Organophosphate poisoning
  - Phosphorus poisoning
- Metabolic Acidosis
  (with compensatory
  hyperventilation)
  **Normochloraemic
  Acidosis**
  - Diabetic ketoacidosis
  - Uraemic acidosis
  - Lactacidosis
  - Acetylsalicylic acid
  - Ethylene glycol poisoning
  Hyperchloraemic Acidosis
  - Diarrhoea
  - Renal tubular acidosis
  - Potassium sparing
    Diuretics (Spironolactone,
    Triamterene, Amiloride)

- Carboanhydrase inhibitor (Acetazolamide)
- Hypocortisolism (Addison's Disease) [Dog]
- Ammonium chloride
- Calcium chloride
- Parenteral nutrition (Arginine, Lysine, Histidine)
- Anaphylaxis
- Pain
- Hysteria
- Obesity (Pickwickian Syndrome)

Diagnostic Approach

Dyspnoea

1. **Case History**

2. **General Examination**

3. **Pharyngeal Examination**

4. **X-Ray Study**
- Thorax
- Throat
- Abdomen

5. **Ultrasound**
- Heart (Doppler Echocardiography)
- Thorax
- Abdomen

6. **Thoracocentesis (in case of effusion)**
- Fluid Analysis
  - Colour
  - Specific gravity
  - TP
  - Rivalta Test [Cat]
  - Alb/Glob Ratio
  - LDH
  - Bilirubin
  - Crea
  - Amylase, Lipase
  - Ether clearance test
  - Cholesterol, Triglyceride

- Leucocyte number
- Differential cell profile
- Tumour cytology
- Bacterial culture
- Fungal culture

7. **Blood Tests**
- Hct, Ery, Leuc, Hb
- TP, Albumin, Globulin
- Na, K, Ca
- GPT, AP, Urea, Crea, BG
- MCH, MCV, MCHC
- Diff BC
- Amylase, Lipase [Dog]
- Blood Gas Analysis (BGA)

MICROBIAL SEROLOGY
- FeLV-/FIV Antigen [Cat]
- Dirofilaria Antigen [Dog]

FUNCTION TESTS
- T_4, fT_4

COAGULATION
- Prothrombin time (PT/Quick)
- (Activated) partial Thromboplastin time (PTT/aPTT)
- Thrombocyte number

8. **Urinalysis**
- Urine dip stick

- Specific gravity
- Urine sediment

9. Faecal Examination
- Flotation
- Baermann–Wetzel Method

10.Endoscopy
- Bronchoscopy

± Tracheobronchial lavage
- Bacterial culture
- Fungal culture
- Cytology

11.Further Tests
- Canine Distemper virus Antigen (conjunctival smear) [Dog]

Cough

Tussis

Common Causes	
Dog	Cat
+++ Infectious Causes	+++ Allergic Causes
++ Allergic Causes	++ Tumours
++ Cardiac Causes	++ Infectious Causes
++ Tumours	
++ Tracheal collapse	
++ Foreign body	

Productive Cough

Mucous/Pus

- Bacterial Bronchopneumonia
  - Bordetella sp.
  - E. coli
  - Klebsiella sp.
  - Pseudomonas sp.
  - Pasteurella sp.
  - Staphylococcus sp.
  - Streptococcus sp.
  - Mycoplasma sp. [esp Cat]
  - Mycobacterium sp.
- Foreign body
  - Nasopharynx [esp Cat]
  - Larynx
  - Trachea
  - Bronchus
- Aspiration pneumonia
  - Vomitus
  - Regurgitation/ Megaoesophagus
  - Reflux oesophageitis
  - Laryngeal paralysis
  - Anaesthesia
  - Drug/Contrast medium application
  - Force feeding
- Tonsillitis/Tonsillar carcinoma
- Allergic Bronchopneumonia
  - Eosinophilic Pneumonia
  - Feline Asthma [Cat]

- – Atopy/Inhalation allergy
- – Bacterial/Fungal/ Parasitic allergy
- – Drug allergy
- – Lupus erythematosus
- Nasopharyngeal polyps [Cat]
- Rickettsial bronchopneumonia
  - – (Ehrlichia sp. [Dog])
  - – (Rickettsia sp. [Dog])
- Parasitic Bronchopneumonia
  - – Toxoplasma sp.
  - – Pneumocystis sp.
  - – Capillaria sp.
  - – Filaroides sp. [esp Dog]
  - – (Crenosoma sp. [Dog])
  - – Aelurostrongylus sp. [Cat]
  - – Angiostrongylus sp. [Dog]
  - – Dirofilaria sp. [esp Dog]
  - – (Paragonimus sp. [esp Dog])
  - – Larva migrans
- Mycotic Bronchopneumonia
  - – Cryptococcus sp. [esp Cat]
  - – Facultative pathogenic fungi
  - – (Histoplasma sp.)
  - – (Blastomyces sp.)
  - – (Coccidioides sp.)
- Toxic bronchopneumonia
  - – Smoke inhalation/Irritant gases
  - – Uraemia
- Pulmonary tumours
  - **Primary Tumours**
  - – Adenocarcinoma
  - – Squamous cell carcinoma
  - **Tumour Metastasis**
  - – Thyroid carcinoma
  - – Mammary carcinoma
  - – Haemangiosarcoma
  - – Osteosarcoma
  - – Squamous cell carcinoma

- – Transitional cell carcinoma
- – Melanoma
- – Lymphosarcoma [esp Cat]
- – Malignant Histiocytosis [Bernese Mountain Dog]
- – Adenocarcinoma
- Dyskinesia of the ciliated epithelium
- Bronchiectasia
- Pulmonary oedema
  - – Left sided heart failure
  - – Hyperthyroidism [Cat]
  - – Arterial hypertension [esp Cat]
  - – Cardiac arrhythmias
  - – Pneumonia

Blood

- Foreign body
  - – Nasopharynx [esp Cat]
  - – Larynx
  - – Trachea
  - – Bronchus
- Trauma
  - – Larynx/Trachea
  - – Pulmonary contusion
  - – Lung lobe torsion
  - – Endotracheal intubation
  - – Bronchoscopy
  - – Aspiration biopsy of the lung
- Pulmonary thromboembolism
  - – Dirofilaria sp. [esp Dog]
  - – Angiostrongylus sp. [Dog]
  - – Aelurostrongylus sp. [Cat]
  - – Larva migrans
  - – Cardiomyopathy
  - – Septicaemia/Endocarditis
  - – Surgery
  - – DIC
  - – Hyperviscosity syndrome
  - – Glomerulonephritis

- Renal amyloidosis
- Hypercortisolism (Cushing's Disease) [Dog]
- Hypothyroidism [Dog]
- Pancreatitis
- Immune haemolytic anaemia
• Coagulopathy
  - Dicoumarol/Warfarin poisoning
  - DIC
  - Acetylsalicylic acid
  - Heparin
• Bronchopneumonia/ Pulmonary abscess
• Pulmonary Tumours
  - Primary Tumours
  - Adenocarcinoma
  - Squamous cell carcinoma
  - Tumour metastasis
  - Thyroid carcinoma
  - Mammary carcinoma
  - Haemangiosarcoma
  - Osteosarcoma
  - Squamous cell carcinoma
  - Transitional cell carcinoma
  - Melanoma
  - Lymphosarcoma [esp Cat]
  - Malignant Histiocytosis [Bernese Mountain Dog]
  - Adenocarcinoma
• Pulmonary Oedema

Dry, Tickly Cough

• Viral Tracheobronchitis
  - Canine distemper virus [Dog]

- Cat Flu [Cat]
- Feline Herpes virus [Cat]
- Feline Calici virus [Cat]
- Kennel Cough [Dog]
- Canine Herpes virus [Dog]
- Canine Adenovirus I, II [Dog]
- Parainfluenza virus [Dog]
- Canine Reovirus I, II, III [Dog]
• Tracheal collapse [Dog]
• Brachycephalic syndrome
• Allergic Tracheobronchitis
  - Feline Asthma [Cat]
  - Eosinophilic Bronchitis
  - Atopy/Inhalation allergy
• Bronchial Compression
  - Left atrial cardiac enlargement
  - Mediastinal lymph-adenopathy
  - Heart base tumour (Chemodectoma) [Dog]
  - Thyroid carcinoma
  - Thymoma
• Tracheal hypoplasia
• Overlong soft palate [esp Dog]
• Laryngeal paralysis
• Bacterial Tracheobronchitis
• Parasitic Tracheobronchitis

Diagnostic Approach

Cough

1. Case History

2. General Examination

3. Pharyngeal Examination

4. X-Ray Study
- Thorax
- Throat
- Abdomen

5. Ultrasound
- Heart (Doppler Echocardiography)
- Thorax
- Abdomen

6. Thoracocentesis (in case of effusion)
- Fluid Analysis
  - Colour
  - Specific gravity
  - TP
  - Rivalta Test [Cat]
  - Alb/Glob Ration
  - LDH
  - Bilirubin
  - Crea
  - Amylase, Lipase
  - Ether clearance test
  - Cholesterol, Triglycerides
  - Leucocyte number
  - Differential cell profile
  - Tumour cytology
  - Bacterial culture
  - Fungal culture

7. Blood Tests
- Hct, Ery, Leuc, Hb
- TP, Albumin, Globulin
- Na, K, Ca

- GPT, AP, Urea, Crea, BG
- MCH, MCV, MCHC
- Diff BC
- Amylase, Lipase [Dog]
- Blood Gas Analysis (BGA)
- α HBDH
- Troponin
- ANP

MICROBIAL SEROLOGY
- FeLV-/FIV Antigen [Cat]
- Dirofilaria Antigen [Dog]

FUNCTION TESTS
- T_4, fT_4

COAGULATION
- Prothrombin time (PT/Quick)
- (Activated) partial Thromboplastin time (PTT/aPTT)
- Thrombocyte number

8. Urinalysis
- Urine dip stick
- Specific gravity
- Urine sediment

9. Faecal Examination
- Flotation
- Baermann-Wetzel Method

10. Endoscopy
- Bronchoscopy
  ± Tracheobronchial lavage
  - Bacterial culture
  - Fungal culture
  - Cytology

11. Further Tests
- Canine Distemper virus Antigen (Conjunctival smear) [Dog]

Lung Sounds

Audible sounds of the lung via auscultation
Inspiratory Sounds: Extrathoracic respiratory tract obstruction/stenosis
Expiratory Sounds: Intrathoracic respiratory tract obstruction/stenosis

Bronchial Respiratory Sound

Loud

- Tracheobronchitis
- Allergic bronchitis/feline asthma
- Respiratory tract obstruction
- Pulmonary fibrosis
- Pulmonary tumours

Quiet

- Normal finding

Vesicular Respiratory Sound

Loud

- Hyperventilation
  - Excitement
  - Pain
  - Metabolic acidosis
  - Anaemia
  - Dyspnoea
- Atelectasis
  (paradoxical conduction)

Quiet

- Normal finding
- Emphysema
- Pulmonary tumours
- Mediastinal tumours
- Pneumonia/Pulmonary abscess

Absent

- Pneumothorax
- Thoracic effusion
- Obesity
- Diaphragmatic hernia
- Lung lobe torsion [Dog]
- Atelectasis
- Severe Pneumonia

Rattling Sound

Dry Rattling Sound (Whistling, Wheezing, Humming)

- Respiratory Tract Obstruction
  - Tracheal collapse [Dog]
  - Tracheal hypoplasia
  - Laryngeal paralysis
  - Glottal oedema
  - Foreign body
  - Tumours
- Chronic obstructive Bronchitis
- Allergic Bronchitis/ Feline Asthma
- Chronic Pneumonia

Wet Rattling Sound (Rough/Fine Bubbles)

- Pulmonary oedema
- Pneumonia

Diagnostic Approach

Lung Sounds

1. **Case History**

2. **General Examination**

3. **Pharyngeal Examination**

4. **X-Ray Study**
- Thorax
- Throat
- Abdomen

5. **Ultrasound**
- Heart (Doppler Echocardiography)
- Thorax
- Abdomen

6. **Thoracocentesis (in case of effusion)**
- Fluid analysis
  - Colour
  - Specific gravity
  - TP
  - Rivalta Test [Cat]
  - Alb/Glob Ratio
  - LDH
  - Bilirubin
  - Crea
  - Amylase, Lipase
  - Ether clearance test
  - Cholesterol, Triglycerides
  - Leucocyte number
  - Differential cell count
  - Tumour cytology
  - Bacterial culture
  - Fungal culture

7. **Blood Tests**
- Hct, Ery, Leuc, Hb
- TP, Albumin, Globulin

- Na, K, Ca
- GPT, AP, Urea, Crea, BG
- MCH, MCV, MCHC
- Diff BC
- Amylase, Lipase [Dog]
- Blood Gas Analysis (BGA)

MICROBIAL SEROLOGY
- FeLV-/FIV Antigen [Cat]
- Dirofilaria Antigen [Dog]

FUNCTION TESTS
- T_4, fT_4

COAGULATION
- Prothrombin time (PT/Quick)
- (Activated) partial Thromboplastin time (PTT/aPTT)
- Thrombocyte number

8. **Urinalysis**
- Urine dip stick
- Specific gravity
- Urine sediment

9. **Faecal Examination**
- Flotation
- Baermann-Wetzel Method

10. **Endoscopy**
- Bronchoscopy
  - ± Tracheobronchial lavage
    - Bacterial culture
    - Fungal culture
    - Cytology

11. **Further Tests**
- Canine Distemper virus Antigen (Conjunctival smear) [Dog]

Nasal Discharge

Rhinorrhoea: Secretion from the nose, often in combination with sneezing and retching

Common Causes	
Dog	**Cat**
Unilateral Discharge	
+++ Dental abscess ++ Aspergillus rhinitis/sinusitis ++ Intranasal foreign body	+++ Nasopharyngeal foreign body ++ Endonasal tumours
Bilateral Discharge	
+++ Viral/bacterial rhinitis ++ Aspergillus rhinitis/sinusitis	+++ Viral/bacterial rhinitis ++ Cryptococcus rhinitis/sinusitis ++ Nasopharyngeal foreign body

Unilateral Discharge

Seromucous Discharge

- Trauma
- Nasopharyngeal foreign body [esp Cat]
- Endonasal tumour
  - Adenocarcinoma
  - Lymphosarcoma
  - Squamous cell carcinoma
  - Osteosarcoma
  - Fibrosarcoma
  - Melanoma
  - Myxosarcoma
  - Nasopharyngeal polyps [Cat]

Mucopurulent Discharge

- Nasopharyngeal foreign body [esp Cat]
- Oronasal fistula
  - Dental abscess
  - Cleft palate congenital/ traumatic
- Mycotic Rhinitis
  - Cryptococcus sp. [esp Cat]
  - Aspergillus sp. [Dog]
  - Sporothrix sp. [Cat]
  - Rhinosporidium sp. [Dog]
- Parasitic Rhinitis
  - Capillaria sp.
  - (Linguatula sp.)
  - (Pneumonyssus sp.)
  - (Cuterebra sp.)
  - Fly larvae
- Endonasal tumours
  - Adenocarcinoma
  - Lymphosarcoma
  - Squamous cell carcinoma
  - Canine transmissible venereal tumour [Dog]
  - Chondrosarcoma
  - Osteosarcoma

- Fibrosarcoma
- Melanoma
- Nasopharyngeal Polyps [Cat]

Haemorrhagic Discharge (Epistaxis)

- Trauma
- Nasopharyngeal foreign body [esp Cat]
- Oronasal fistula
  - Dental abscess
  - Cleft palate (congenital/traumatic)
- Mycotic Rhinitis
  - Cryptococcus sp. [esp Cat]
  - Aspergillus sp. [Dog]
  - Sporothrix sp. [Cat]
  - Rhinosporidium sp. [Dog]
- Parasitic Rhinitis
  - Capillaria sp.
  - (Linguatula sp.)
  - (Cuterebra sp.)
  - Fly larvae
- Endonasal tumours
  - Adenocarcinoma
  - Lymphosarcoma
  - Squamous cell carcinoma
  - Canine transmissible venereal tumour [Dog]
  - Chondrosarcoma
  - Osteosarcoma
  - Fibrosarcoma
  - Melanoma
  - Myxosarcoma
  - Nasopharyngeal polyps [Cat]

Bilateral Discharge

Seromucous Discharge

- Brachycephalic syndrome

- Narrowing of the nares
- Anomalies of the nasal concha
- Short pharyngeal cavity
- Mucosal hyperplasia
- Overlong soft palate
- Laryngeal collapse
- Tracheal hypoplasia
- Viral Rhinitis (in absence of bacterial secondary infection)
  - Feline Herpes virus [Cat]
  - Feline Calici virus [Cat]
  - Canine Herpes virus [Dog]
  - Canine Adenovirus I, II [Dog]
  - Parainfluenza virus [Dog]
  - Canine distemper virus [Dog]
- Allergic Rhinitis
  - Atopy/Inhalation allergy
- Dyskinesia of the ciliated epithelium
- (Severe pulmonary oedema)

Mucopurulent Discharge

- Nasopharyngeal foreign body [esp Cat]
- Viral Rhinitis (with bacterial secondary infection)
  - Feline Herpes virus [Cat]
  - Feline Calici virus [Cat]
  - Canine Herpes virus [Dog]
  - Canine Adenovirus I, II [Dog]
  - Parainfluenza virus [Dog]
  - Canine distemper virus [Dog]
- Bacterial Rhinitis
  - Pasteurella sp.
  - Bordetella sp.

- Staphylococcus sp.
- Pseudomonas sp.
- Chlamydia sp. [Cat]
- E. coli
- Mycoplasma sp. [esp Cat]
• Bacterial Bronchopneumonia
  - Bordetella sp.
  - E. coli
  - Klebsiella sp.
  - Pseudomonas sp.
  - Pasteurella sp.
  - Staphylococcus sp.
  - Streptococcus sp.
  - Mycoplasma sp. [esp Cat]
  - Mycobacterium sp.
• Oronasal fistula
  - Cleft palate (congenital/ traumatic)
• Mycotic Rhinitis
  - Cryptococcus sp. [esp Cat]
  - Aspergillus sp. [esp Dog]
  - Rhinosporidium sp. [Dog]
• Nasopharyngeal polyps [Cat]
• IgA Deficiency

Haemorrhagic Discharge (Epistaxis)

• Head/Thoracic trauma
• Chronic sneezing
  - Viral Rhinitis
  - Bacterial Rhinitis
  - Mycotic Rhinitis
  - Parasitic Rhinitis
• Foreign body
  - Nasopharynx [esp Cat]
  - Larynx
  - Trachea
  - Bronchi/Lung

- Oesophagus/stomach
• Coagulopathy
  - See Epistaxis
• Hyperviscosity syndrome
  - Multiple Myeloma
  - Lymphatic leukaemia [Cat]
  - FIP Coronavirus [Cat]
  - Lupus erythematosus
  - Polycythaemia vera
  - Dehydration
  - (Leishmania sp. [esp Dog])
  - (Ehrlichia sp. [Dog])
• Tumours
  - Nasopharynx
  - Larynx
  - Trachea
  - Bronchi/Lung
  - Oesophagus/Stomach
• Arterial Hypertension
  - Idiopathic
  - Renal failure
  - Hypercortisolisms (Cushing's Disease) [Dog]
  - Diabetes mellitus
  - Hyperthyroidism [Cat]
  - Central nervous disease
  - Hyperaldosteronism [Dog]
  - Phaeochromocytoma
• Vasculitis
  - FIP Coronavirus [Cat]
  - Canine Coronavirus [Dog]
  - Septicaemia/Endotoxaemia
  - Lupus erythematosus
  - Rheumatoid Disease
  - Polyarteritis nodosa
  - Uraemia

- Drug allergy
- Food allergy
- (Leishmania sp. [esp Dog])
- (Ehrlichia sp. [Dog])
- Dirofilaria sp. [esp Dog]
- Angiostrongylus sp. [Dog]

Diagnostic Approach

Nasal Discharge

1. **Case History**

2. **General Examination**

3. **Dental/ Pharyngeal Examination**

4. **Endoscpy**
- Rhinoscopy
  - ± Nasal flush (retrograde)
  - – Bacterial culture
  - – Fungal culture
  - – Cytology
  - ± Smear of the nasal mucous membrane
  - – Bacterial culture
  - – Fungal culture
  - – Cytology
  - ± Biopsy of the nasal mucous membrane
  - – Bacterial culture
  - – Fungal culture
  - – Cytology

5. **X-Ray Study**
- Skull/Tympanic bulla
- Throat
- Thorax

6. **Blood Tests**
- Hct, Ery, Leuc
- Diff BC
- TP, Alb, Glob
- GPT, AP, Urea, Crea, BG
- FIP Profile [Cat]
  - – TP
  - – Alb/Glob Ratio
  - – Bili
  - – GOT
  - – Serum electrophoresis

MICROBIAL SEROLOGY
- FeLV-/FIV Antigen [Cat]
- Aspergillus Antibodies [Dog]
- Cryptococcus Antibodies [Cat]

COAGULATION (IN CASE OF EPISTAXIS)
- Bleeding time
- Prothrombin time (PT/Quick)
- (Activated) partial Thromboplastin time (PTT/ aPTT)
- Fibrin degradation products (FDP)
- Thrombocyte number

7. **Further Tests**
- Canine Distemper antigen [Dog] (Conjunctival smear)

Epistaxis

Nose bleeds

Common Causes	
Dog	**Cat**
+++ Trauma	+++ Trauma
+++ Dicoumarol poisoning	++ Cat flu
++ Haemophilia A/B	++ FeLV/FIV- and FIP-associated
++ Von Willebrand Disease	+ Immune thrombocytopenia
++ DIC	+ Arterial Hypertension
++ Aspergillus-Rhinitis	+ Hyperviscosity syndrome
++ Infectious thrombocytopenia	+ Nasopharyngeal foreign bodies
++ Immune thrombocytopenia	+ Nasopharyngeal tumours
++ Intranasal tumours	
++ Intranasal foreign body	

Unilateral Epistaxis

Intranasal Causes

- Trauma
- Nasopharyngeal foreign body [esp Cat]
- Oronasal fistula
  - Dental abscess
  - Cleft palate (congenital/ traumatic)
- Mycotic Rhinitis
  - Cryptococcus sp. [esp Cat]
  - Aspergillus sp. [Dog]
  - Sporothrix sp. [Cat]
  - Rhinosporidium sp. [Dog]
- Parasitic Rhinitis
  - Capillaria sp.
  - (Linguatula sp.)
  - (Cuterebra sp.)
  - Fly larvae

- Intranasal tumours
  - Adenocarcinoma
  - Lymphosarcoma
  - Squamous cell carcinoma
  - Canine transmissible venereal tumour [Dog]
  - Chondrosarcoma
  - Osteosarcoma
  - Fibrosarcoma
  - Melanoma
  - Myxosarcoma
  - Nasopharyngeal polyps [Cat]

Bilateral Epistaxis

Intranasal Causes

- Same causes as in unilateral epistaxis

Coagulopathies

Thrombocytopenia

* Bone marrow disease
  - Infectious causes
  - Toxic causes
  - Immunoreactive causes
  - Bone marrow tumours
* DIC
  - Septicaemia/Endotoxaemia
  - Gastric dilation/volvulus [Dog]
  - Pyometra
  - Urinary tract infection
  - Haemorrhagic enteritis
  - Splenic torsion [esp Dog]
  - Acute Pancreatitis
  - Shock
  - Cardiac failure
  - Hepatic failure
  - Haemolysis
  - Snake venom
  - Heat stroke
  - Electric shock
  - Burns
  - FIP Coronavirus [Cat]
  - Tumour Disease
  - Dirofilaria sp. [esp Dog]
* Immune thrombocytopenia
  - Infection
  - Drugs
  - Lupus erythematosus
* Infectious thrombocytopenia
  - FeLV/FIV [Cat]
  - FIP Coronavirus [Cat]
  - Parvovirus
  - Canine Distemper virus [Dog]
  - CAV-1 (Hepatitis c. c.) [Dog]
  - Canine Herpes virus [Dog]
  - Leptospira sp. [Dog]
  - Salmonella sp.
  - Haemobartonella sp. [Cat]
  - Babesia sp. [esp Dog]
  - (Ehrlichia sp. [Dog])
  - (Histoplasma sp.)
* Splenomegaly
* Chronic haemorrhage
* Thrombosis

Thrombocytopathy

* Aquired thrombocytopenia
  - Drugs
  - Uraemia
  - Hepatic failure
  - Acute Pancreatitis
  - Bone tumours
  - Hyperviscosity syndrome
* Congenital thrombocytopathy
  - Von Willebrand Disease [esp Dog]
  - Chediak-Higashi Syndrome [Cat]
  - Thrombasthenia (Glanzmann) [Dog]
  - Platelet aggregation defect
  - Cyclic Neutropenia [Grey Collie]

Plasmatic Coagulopathy

* Congenital coagulopathy
  - Factor VIII Deficiency (Haemophilia A)
  - Factor IX Deficiency (Haemophilia B)
  - Von Willebrand Disease [esp Dog]
  - Factor VII Deficiency [Dog]
  - Factor X Deficiency [Dog]
  - Factor XI Deficiency [Dog]
  - Factor XII Deficiency (Hagemann) [Cat]

- Vitamin K dependent
  Coagulopathy [Cat]
- Vitamin K Deficiency/
  Antagonism
  - Hepatic failure
  - Malabsorption syndrome
  - Obstructive jaundice
  - Imbalanced intestinal flora
    (Antibiotics)
  - Dicoumarol poisoning
    (Rodenticides)
  - Indandione poisoning
    (Thrombosis prophylaxis)
- DIC

Arterial Hypertension

- Idiopathic
- Renal failure
- Hyperthyroidism [Cat]
- Hypercortisolism (Cushing's
  Disease) [Dog]
- Diabetes mellitus
- Central nervous Disease
- Hyperaldosteronism [Dog]
- Phaeochromocytoma

Hyperviscosity Syndrome

- Multiple Myeloma
- Lymphatic Leukaemia [Cat]
- FIP Coronavirus [Cat]
- Dehydration
- (Leishmania sp. [esp Dog])
- (Ehrlichia sp. [Dog])
- Lupus erythematosus
- Polycythaemia vera

Vasculitis

- FIP Coronavirus [Cat]
- Canine Coronavirus [Dog]
- Septicaemia/Endotoxaemia
- Lupus erythematosus
- Rheumatoid Disease
- Polyarteritis nodosa
- Uraemia
- Drug/Food allergy
- (Leishmania sp. [esp Dog])
- (Ehrlichia sp. [Dog])
- Dirofilaria sp. [esp Dog]
- Angiostrongylus sp. [Dog]

Diagnostic Approach

Epistaxis

1. **Case History**

2. **General Examination**

3. **Pharyngeal Examination**

4. **Blood Tests**
- Hct, Ery, Leuc, Hb
- TP, Alb, Glob
- GPT, AP, Urea, Crea, BG
- FIP Profile [Cat]

- TP
- Alb/Glob Ratio
- Bili
- GOT
- Serum electrophoresis
- Diff BC
- MCV, MCV, MCHC
- Na, K, Ca

Microbial Serology
- FeLV-/FIV Antigen [Cat]
- Aspergillus Antibodies
- Cryptococcus-Antibodies [Cat]
- Leishmania Antibodies [Dog]
- Ehrlichia Antibodies [Dog]

Coagulation
- Bleeding time
- Prothrombin time (PT/Quick)
- (Activated) partial Thromboplastin time (PTT/ aPTT)
- Thrombocyte number
- Fibrin degradation product (FDP)
- Autoantibodies against thrombocytes
- Von Willebrand Factor
- Determine factors II-XII

Immunoserology
- ANA Test

Function Tests
- T_4 [Cat]
- T_3 Suppression test [Cat]

5. Urinalysis
- Urine dip stick
- Specific gravity
- Urine sediment
- Bence-Jones Proteins

6. X-Ray Study
- Skull/Tympanic bulla
- Thorax
- Abdomen

7. Endoscopy
- Rhinoscopy
  - ± Nasal flush (retrograde)
    - Bacterial culture
    - Fungal culture
    - Cytology
  - ± Smear of the nasal mucous membrane
    - Bacterial culture
    - Fungal culture
    - Cytology
  - ± Biopsy of the nasal mucous membrane
    - Bacterial culture
    - Fungal culture
    - Cytology

8. Further Tests
- Bone marrow biopsy
  - Cytology
- Blood pressure measure (indirect/ direct)
- Ultrasound
  - Abdomen
  - Heart

Reverse Sneezing

Sudden inspiratory sneezing attacks with dyspnoea (1–2 min) of unknown origin. The attack can be disrupted by massaging the larynx or briefly holding the nostrils closed

Common Causes

Dog		Cat	
+	Nasopharyngeal spasm	+++	Nasopharyngeal foreign body
+	Overlong soft palate		
+	Pharyngeal foreign body	+	Cat flu Rhinitis/ Sinusitis
+	Tracheal collapse		
+	Laryngeal collapse	+	Nasopharyngeal polyps
+	Tonsillitis/Tonsillar carcinoma		

Diagnostic Approach

Reverse Sneezing

1. **Case History**

2. **General Examination**

3. **Pharyngeal Examination**

4. **Endoscopy**
Rhinoscopy
  - (orthograde/retrograde)
  - Laryngo-/Bronchoscopy

4 Gastrointestinal Principal Symptoms

Further Relevant Principal Symptoms

Anal Pruritus

Frequent licking and scooting of the anus

Common Causes	
Dog	**Cat**
+++ Blocked anal sacs	+++ Blocked anal sacs
+++ Anal gland abscess	+++ Anal gland abscess
++ Proctitis	++ Proctitis
+ Perianal fistulas	++ Urinary Tract Infections
+ Perianal tumours	
+ Urinary Tract Infections	

Perianal Disease

- Blocked anal sacs
- Anal gland abscess
- Perianal fistulas [Dog]
- Perineal hernia [Dog]
- Perianal wounds
- Perianal tumours
  - Rectal carcinoma
  - Rectal polyp
  - Anal sac adenoma/ carcinoma
  - Anal gland adenoma/ carcinoma
  - Hepatoid adenoma/ carcinoma [Dog]

Proctitis

- Intestinal parasites
  - Tapeworms
  - Trichuris sp. [Dog]
  - Ancylostoma sp.
  - Uncinaria sp.
  - Balantidium sp. [Dog]
  - (Entamoeba sp. [Dog])
- Bacterial proctitis
- Tumours

Other Causes

- Urinary Tract Disease [Bitch/ Cat]
- Vaginal disease
- Rectal prolapse

Diagnostic Approach

Anal Pruritus

1. **Case History**

2. **General Examination**

3. **Rectal Examination**
   ± Rectal smear/cytology

4. Faecal Examination
- Plain Examination
- Flotation
- Sticky tape impression preparation (anus)

5. Urinalysis
(Bitches Only and Cats)
- Urine dip stick

- Specific Gravity
- Urine sediment

6. X-Ray Study
- Abdomen/pelvis
- Contrast enema

7. Endoscopy
- Colonoscopy ± Biopsy

Diarrhoea

The passing of loose or liquid bowel movements

Common Causes		
Dog		Cat
+++ Food poisoning/intolerance	+++	Parasitic enteritis
	++	Viral enteritis
++ Viral enteritis	++	Immunoreactive enteritis
++ Parasitic enteritis	++	Hyperthyroidism
++ Immunoreactive enteritis	++	Intestinal tumours
++ Intestinal tumours	+	Partial bowel obstruction
+ Motility disturbances	+	Organ failure
+ Partial bowel obstruction		
+ Organ failure		

Acute Diarrhoea

Small Intestinal Diarrhoea

- Viral Enteritis
  - Parvovirus
  - Coronavirus
  - Rotavirus
  - FeLV/FIV [Cat]
  - Canine Distemper virus [Dog]
- Foreign body
- Food poisoning/ Enterotoxins [esp Dog]
  - Staphylococcus Enterotoxin
  - E. coli Enterotoxin
  - Clostridium Enterotoxin
- Partial bowel obstruction
  - Foreign body
  - Intestinal parasites
  - Intestinal tumours
  - Invagination
  - Incarceration (hernia)
- Parasitic Enteritis
  - Giardia sp.
  - Toxocara/Toxascaris sp.
  - Ancylostoma sp.

- Uncinaria sp.
- Strongyloides sp.
- Isospora sp.
- Cryptosporidium sp.
- Toxoplasma sp.
• Toxic Causes
  - NSAID/Glucocorticoids
  - Cytostatics
  - Antibiotics
  - Antiparasitics
  - Digitalis glycosides
  - Household agents
  - Toxic plants
  - Heavy metal poisoning
  - Organophosphate poisoning
  - Ethylene glycol poisoning
• Bacterial Enteritis
  - Salmonella sp.
  - Bacillus sp.
  - Campylobacter sp.
  - Yersinia sp.
  - Shigella sp.
  - E. coli
  - Clostridium sp.
• Food intolerance
• Other Causes
  - Acute pancreatitis [esp Dog]
  - Acute renal failure
  - Acute hepatic failure
  - Diabetic ketoacidosis

Chronic Diarrhoea

Small Intestinal Diarrhoea

• Food Intolerance
  - Gluten [Irish Setter]
  - Lactose
  - High caloric/low fibre diets
  - Food allergy

• Partial bowel obstruction
  - Foreign body
  - Intestinal parasites
  - Intestinal tumours
  - Invagination
  - Incarceration (Hernia)
• Viral Enteritis
  - FeLV/FIV [Cat]
  - FIP Coronavirus [Cat]
• Parasitic Enteritis
  - Giardia sp.
  - Cryptosporidium sp.
  - Toxoplasma sp.
  - Isospora sp.
  - Toxocara/Toxascaris sp.
  - Ancylostoma sp.
  - Uncinaria sp.
  - Strongyloides sp.
• Immunoreactive Enteritis
  - Lymphoplasmacellular enteritis
  - Eosinophilic enteritis
  - Granulomatous enteritis
• Intestinal tumours
  - Adenocarcinoma
  - Lymphosarcoma [esp Cat]
  - Fibrosarcoma
  - Leiomyoma/ Leiomyosarcoma
  - Gastrinoma (Zollinger-Ellison syndrome)
  - Mast cell tumour [Dog]
• Extraenteral Causes
  - Exocrine pancreatic insufficiency
  - Hyperthyroidism [Cat]
  - Chronic renal failure
  - Chronic hepatic failure
  - Congestive heart failure
  - Diabetes mellitus

- – Mast cell tumour [Dog]
- Bacterial Enteritis
  - – Dysbacteriosis/bacterial overgrowth
  - – Salmonella sp.
  - – Campylobacter sp.
  - – Yersinia sp.
  - – Clostridium sp.
- Mycotic Enteritis
  - – Aspergillus sp.
  - – Candida sp.
  - – (Histoplasma sp.)
- Ulcerative enteritis (Duodenal ulcers)
- Lymphangiectasia [Dog]

Large Intestinal Diarrhoea

- Food intolerance
  - – Low fibre
  - – Food allergy
- Partial colonic obstruction
  - – Foreign body
  - – Intestinal tumours
  - – Invagination
  - – Rectal diverticulum
  - – Prostatic enlargement [Dog]
- Parasitic colitis
  - – Trichuris sp. [Dog]
  - – Ancylostoma sp.

- – Uncinaria sp.
- – Balantidium sp. [Dog]
- – (Entamoeba sp. [Dog])
- Immunoreactive colitis
  - – Lymphoplasmacellular colitis
  - – Eosinophilic colitis
  - – Granulomatous colitis
  - – Ulcerative colitis
- Colonic tumours
  - – Adenocarcinoma
  - – Lymphosarcoma [esp Cat]
  - – Leiomyoma/ Leiomyosarcoma
  - – Polyp
- Viral colitis
  - – FeLV/FIV [Cat]
  - – FIP Coronavirus (Colonic granulomata) [Cat]
- Bacterial Enteritis
  - – Dysbacteriosis/bacterial overgrowth
  - – Salmonella sp.
  - – Campylobacter sp.
  - – Clostridium sp.
- Mycotic colitis
  - – (Histoplasma sp.)
- Other causes
  - – Irritable colon (psychogenic)
  - – Coprostasis (paradoxic diarrhoea)

Diagnostic Approach

Acute Diarrhoea

1. **Case History**

2. **General Examination**

3. **Blood Tests**
- Hct, Leuc, TP

- BG
- Na, K, Ca

4. **Faecal Examination**
- Plain Examination

- Flotation
- Giardia sp. detection
- Bacterial culture

5. X-Ray Study
- Abdomen
- Intestinal contrast medium study

Diagnostic Approach

Chronic Diarrhoea

1. Case History

2. General Examination

3. Blood Tests
- Hct, Ery, Leuc
- Na, K, Ca
- TP, Alb, Glob
- GPT, AP, Urea, Crea, BG
- TLI Test
- Diff BC
- Cholesterol
- Serum Cobalamin (Vit. B$_{12}$)
- Serum Folic acid
- FIP Profile [Cat]
  - TP
  - Alb/Glob Ratio
  - Bili
  - GOT
  - Serum electrophoresis

MICROBIAL SEROLOGY
- FeLV-/FIV Antigen [Cat]

FUNCTION TESTS
- T$_4$, fT$_4$
- T$_3$ Suppression Test [Cat]
- Xylose Test [Dog]

4. Urinalysis
- Urine dip stick
- Specific gravity
- Urine sediment

5. Faecal Examination
- Plain Examination
- Flotation
- Giardia sp. detection
- Bacterial culture
- Fat content (Sudan Staining)
- Chymotrypsin
- Elastase

6. X-Ray Study
- Abdomen
- Intestinal contrast medium study
- Contrast medium enema

7. Ultrasound
- Abdomen ± biopsy

8. Endoscopy
- Gastro-/Duodenoscopy ± biopsy
- Colonoscopy ± biopsy

9. Further Tests
- Rectal Examination ± Colonic Smear/cytology

Clinical Distinguishing Features of Small/Large Intestinal Diarrhoea

Criteria	Small Intestine	Large Intestine
Increased faecal volume	+	–
Flatulence	(+)	–
Borborygmi	(+)	–
Steatorrhoea	(+)	–
Polydipsia	(+)	–
Weight loss	(+)	–
Tenesmus	–	+
Increased Elimination Frequency	–	+
Mucous	–	+
"Scooting"	–	(+)
Faecal consistency	thin/watery	mushy
Blood quality	dark/melaena	light, fresh
Affected general well being	+	–/+
Vomitus	(+)	–/+

Dysphagia

Chewing and swallowing disturbance with a normally maintained appetite

Common Causes	
Dog	**Cat**
+++ Dental Disease	+++ Dental Disease
++ Stomatitis	++ Stomatitis
++ Disease of the jaw	++ Disease of the jaw
++ Tonsillitis/Tonsillar carcinoma	++ Tonsillitis/Tonsillar carcinoma
++ Motility Disorders	++ Motility Disorders

Chewing Disorder

Dental Disease

- Dental fracture
- Dental abscess
- Dental calculus/decay
- Feline Odontoclastic Resorptive Lesions (FORL) [Cat]
- Periodontitis
- Persistent deciduous teeth
- Dental malposition
- Dental root remnants (broken teeth)

Oropharyngeal Tumours

- Papilloma
- Fibroma/Fibrosarcoma
- Squamous cell carcinoma
- Melanoma
- Epulis/Gingival hyperplasia [esp Dog]
- Tonsillar carcinoma
- Salivary gland carcinoma
- Nasopharyngeal polyps [Cat]

Salivary Gland Disease

Gl. parotis
Gl. zygomatica
Gl. mandibularis
Gl. sublingualis
- Sialoadenitis
- Sialocele/Mucocele/Ranula
- Salivary gland adenoma/carcinoma
- Sialolithiasis

Oronasal Fistula

- Dental abscess

- Foreign body
- Cleft palate (congenital/traumatic)
- Congenital defects of the soft palate

Stomatitis/Gingivitis/Glossitis

- Viral Causes
  - FeLV/FIV [Cat]
  - Feline Calici virus [Cat]
  - Feline Herpes virus [Cat]
  - FIP Coronavirus [Cat]
- Bacterial Causes
  - Streptococcus sp.
  - Staphylococcus sp.
  - Neisseria sp.
  - E. coli
  - Pasteurella sp.
  - Acinetobacter sp.
  - Leptospira sp. [Dog]
  - Actinomyces sp.
  - Nocardia sp.
  - Mycobacterium sp. [Dog]
  - Fusobacterium sp.
  - Spirochetes
- Immunoreactive Causes
  - Eosinophilic granuloma
  - Plasma cell gingivitis/stomatitis
  - Lupus erythematosus
  - Pemphigus vulgaris
- Metabolic Causes
  - Uraemia
  - Hypothyroidism [Dog]
  - Diabetes mellitus
- Toxic Causes
  - Lead poisoning
  - Household agents
  - Poisonous plants
  - Cytostatics

- Chemical burn
- Other Causes
  - Foreign body/abscess
- Mycotic Causes
  - Candida sp.

Lymphadenopathy

Ln. parotideus
Ln. mandibulares
Ln. retropharyngeus lateralis
Ln. retropharyngeus medialis

- Bacterial infections (local/generalised)
- Tumour disease
- Viral infections
- Rickettsial infections
- Systemic mycotic infection

Orthodontic Disease

- Lower jaw luxation
- Upper/Lower jaw fracture
- Bone tumour
- Craniomandibular osteopathy
- Osteomyelitis
- Fracture of the hyoid bone
- Temporomandibular joint disease

Masticatory Muscle Disease (Temporomandibular Myositis)

- Congenital Causes
  - Muscular dystrophy [Dog]
  - Dermatomyositis [Dog]
  - Glycogen storage disease
- Inflammatory Causes
  - Toxoplasma sp.
  - Neospora sp. [Dog]
  - Lyme Borrelia sp. [Dog]
  - Leptospira sp. [Dog]

- Immunoreactive Causes
  - Eosinophilic Myositis [Dog]
- Metabolic Causes
  - Vitamin E Deficiency
  - Hypokalaemia [esp Cat]
  - Hypercortisolism (Cushing's Disease) [Dog]
  - Glucocorticoid long term therapy
  - Hypothyroidism [Dog]

Neurological Disease

- Encephalitis/Meningoencephalitis
- Brain tumours
- Cervical spine disease
- Paralysis
  - Trigeminal nerve (V) (Masticatory muscle)
  - Facial nerve (VII) (orofacial musculature)
  - Hypoglossal nerve (XII) (Glossal musculature)
  - Glossopharyngeal nerve (XI) (Pharynx/Larynx musculature/oesophagus)
  - Vagal nerve (X) (Pharynx/Laryngeal musculature/oesophagus, palate)
- Polyneuropathy

Congenital Causes

  - Axonopathy
  - Demyelinisation disease
  - Lysosomal storage disease

Inflammatory Causes

  - Polyradiculoneuritis
  - Polyneuritis

- FeLV/FIV [Cat]
- Toxoplasma sp.
- Neospora sp. [Dog]

Immunoreactive Causes

- Lupus erythematosus
- Myasthenia gravis

Metabolic Causes

- Hypothyroidism [Dog]
- Diabetes mellitus
- Paraneoplastic syndrome (Insulinoma)

Toxic Causes

- Organophosphate poisoning (chronic)
- Lead poisoning
- Cytostatics
- Lindane
- Botulism
- Tick paralysis

Other Causes

- Nerve compression syndrome
- Feline Dysautonomia [esp Cat]
- Loss of smell/taste
- Psychogenic Causes
  - Stress
  - Depression/Grief
- Traumatic Causes
  - Bitten off tongue
  - Torn frenulum
  - Burns
  - Cleft palate

- Foreign body
- Pain

Difficulty Swallowing

Pharyngeal Disease

- Pharyngitis (same causes as Stomatitis)
- Tonsillitis
- Tonsillar carcinoma
- Foreign body
- Peritonsillar abscess

Oesophageal Disease

- Oesophagitis
  - Spirocerca Granulomata [Dog]
  - Reflux oesophageitis [Dog]
  - Chronic vomitus
- Oesophageal stenosis
  - Foreign body
  - Oesophageal tumours
  - Oesophageal stricture
  - Hiatus hernia
  - (Spirocerca Granulomata [Dog])
- Motility disturbances/ Megaoesophagus
  - Cricopharyngeal achalasia
  - Oesophageal diverticulum
  - Persistent right aortic arch
  - Oesophageal foreign body
  - Oesophageal tumours
  - Oesophageal stricture
  - Hiatus hernia
  - Myasthenia gravis

- Polyneuritis
- Polymyositis
- Lupus erythematosus
- Feline dysautonomia [esp Cat]
- Botulism
- Tetanus [esp Dog]
- Canine Distemper Virus [Dog]
- Lead poisoning
- Thallium poisoning
- Organophosphate poisoning
- Acrylamide poisoning
- Hypocortisolism (Addison's Disease) [Dog]
- Hypothyroidism [Dog]
- Thymoma
- Bilateral vagal nerve paralysis
- Paralysis of the glossopharyngeal nerve
- (Trypanosoma cruzi [Dog])
- (Spirocerca Granulomata [Dog])

Diagnostic Approach

Dysphagia

1. **Case History**

2. **General Examination**

3. **Oropharyngeal and Jaw Examination**

4. **Neurological Examination**
- Cranial Nerves

5. **X-Ray Study**
- Skull
  - Tympanic bulla
  - Upper/lower jaw
  - Teeth
- Throat
- Thorax
- Contrast Swallowing study/ Fluoroscopy

6. **Blood Tests**
- Hct, Ery, Leuc, Hb
- TP, Alb, Glob
- GPT, AP, Urea, Crea, BG

- Diff BC
- Na, K, Ca, P
- Chol, CK

MICROBIAL SEROLOGY
- FeLV-/FIV Antigen [Cat]

IMMUNOSEROLOGY
- ANA Test
- Autoantibodies against acetylcholine receptors (Myasthenia gravis detection)

FUNCTION TESTS
- Adrenal gland function tests [Dog]
  - Dexamethasone Suppression test
  - ACTH Stimulation test
  - Cortisol/Creatinine Ratio
- T_4, fT_4

7. **Urinalysis**
- Urine dip stick

- Specific gravity
- Urine sediment

8. Endoscopy
- Oesophago-/Gastroscopy

9. Further Tests
- Electromyography (EMG)
- Muscle biopsy
- Spinal tap/analysis

Vomitus

Retrograde evacuation of the stomach

Common Causes			
Dog		**Cat**	
+++	Food intolerance	+++	Food intolerance
++	Ingestion of grass (cause or effect?)	++	Ingestion of grass (cause or effect
++	Gastritis	++	Gastritis
++	Gastric/Intestinal ulcer	++	Gastric/Intestinal ulcer
++	Gastrointestinal obstruction	++	Gastrointestinal obstruction
++	Motility disturbances	++	Motility disturbances
+	Organ failure	+	Organ failure

Acute Vomitus

Acute Gastritis

- Foreign body
- Food intolerance/ Enterotoxins
- Viral Gastroenteritis
  - Parvovirus
  - Coronavirus
  - Rotavirus
  - FeLV/FIV [Cat]
  - Canine Distemper Virus [Dog]
- Parasitic gastroenteritis
  - Olulanus sp. [Cat]
  - Physaloptera sp.
  - Giardia sp.
  - Toxocara/Toxascaris sp.
  - Ancylostoma sp.
  - Stenocephala sp.
  - Strongyloides sp.
  - Isospora sp.
  - (Spirocerca sp. [Dog])
- Toxic Gastroenteritis
  - Beta$_2$ Agonists
  - Apomorphine [Dog]
  - Xylazine
  - Syrup of ipecac [Cat]
  - Ephedrine
  - Local anaesthetics
  - Tricyclic antidepressants

- Loperamide
- Bromocriptine
- Cytostatics
- Tetracyclines
- Chloramphenicol
- Antiparasitics
- Digitalis Glycosides
- Household agents
- Toxic plants
- Heavy metal poisoning
- Organophosphate poisoning
- Ethylene glycol poisoning
- Acetylsalicylic acid
- Paracetamol
- Ibuprofen
- Indomethacin
- Bacterial gastroenteritis
  - Dysbacteriosis/bacterial overgrowth
  - Salmonella sp.
  - Campylobacter sp.
  - Yersinia sp.
  - Shigella sp.
  - E. coli
  - Clostridium sp.
  - Helicobacter sp.
  - Gastrospirilium sp.
- Food intolerance/allergy
- Other causes
  - Uraemia
  - CNS Trauma

Gastrointestinal Obstruction

- Gastric dilation/volvulus [Dog]
- Mechanical Ileus
  - Foreign body
  - Intestinal parasites
  - Intestinal tumours
  - Invagination
  - Incarceration (Hernia)

- Volvulus
- Pyloric stenosis
- Constipation

Other Causes

- Acute pancreatitis
- Acute renal failure
- CNS Disease

Chronic Vomitus

Chronic Gastroenteritis

- Food intolerance/allergy
- Parasitic gastroenteritis
- Immunoreactive gastroenteritis (Inflammatory Bowel Disease)
  - Lymphoplasmacellular gastroenteritis
  - Eosinophilic gastroenteritis
  - Granulomatous gastroenteritis
- Gastric/Duodenal ulcer
- Foreign body
- Food intolerance/Enterotoxins
- Viral gastroenteritis
- Bacterial gastroenteritis
- Lymphangiectasia [Dog]
- Paraneoplastic syndrome
  - Mast cell tumour [Dog]
  - Gastrinoma
- Mycotic gastroenteritis
  - (Histoplasma sp.)
  - (Aspergillus sp.)
  - (Candida sp.)

Gastrointestinal Motility Disturbance

- Pyloric stenosis [Dog]
- Gastroenteritis
- Gastric/Duodenal ulcer

- Gastric/Intestinal tumour
- Gastropexy [Dog]
- Postoperative intestinal atony
- Peritonitis
- Uraemia
- Hypokalaemia [esp Cat]
- Hypothyroidism [Dog]
- Diabetic ketoacidosis
- Pancreatitis
- Hepatic encephalopathy
- Feline dysautonomia [esp Cat]

Gastric/Intestinal Tumours

- Adenocarcinoma
- Lymphosarcoma [esp Cat]
- Polyps
- Leiomyoma/Leiomyosarcoma
- Fibrosarcoma

Other Causes

- Pancreatitis

- Congestive cardiac failure
- Chronic renal failure
- Chronic hepatic failure
- Hyperthyroidism [Cat]
- Diabetes mellitus
- Hypokalaemia [esp Cat]
- Hypercalcaemia
- Hypocortisolism (Addison's Disease) [Dog]
- Metabolic Acidosis
- Partial intestinal obstruction
  - Foreign body
  - Intestinal tumours
  - Invagination
  - Incarceration (Hernia)
- Vestibular Disturbances
- Central nervous Disease
  - Encephalomeningitis
  - Cerebral oedema
  - Brain tumours
- Constipation

Diagnostic Approach

Vomitus

1. **Case History**

2. **General Examination**

3. **X-Ray Study**
- Abdomen
- Thorax
- Intestinal contrast study

4. **Blood Tests**
- Hct, Ery, Leuc
- TP, Alb, Glob
- GPT, AP, Urea, Crea, BG
- Na, K, Ca

- Amylase, Lipase [Dog]
- Diff BC
- Cholesterol
- Serum bile acids
- Serum Gastrin
- Ammonium
- FIP Profile [Cat]
  - TP
  - Alb/Glob Ratio
  - Bili
  - GOT
  - Serum electrophoresis

MICROBIAL SEROLOGY
- FeLV-/FIV Antigen [Cat]

FUNCTION TESTS
- T_4, fT_4
- T_3 Suppression Test [Cat]
- Adrenal gland function test [Dog]
  - Dexamethasone Suppression test
  - ACTH Stimulation test
  - Cortisol/Creatinine Ratio

5. Urinalysis
- Urinary output/volume
- Urine dip stick
- Specific gravity
- Urine sediment

6. Faecal Examination
- Plain examination
- Flotation
- Bacterial culture
- Fungal culture

7. Ultrasound
- Abdomen ± liver biopsy
- Heart (Doppler Echocardiography)

8. Endoscopy
- Oesophago-/Gastro-/Duodenoscopy ± Biopsy

9. Further Tests
- Laparotomy
- Spinal tap/analysis

Clinical Distinguishing Features of Vomitus/ Regurgitation

Criteria	Vomitus	Regurgitation
Time period after food intake	delayed	Immediate or delayed
Attempts to swallow	once	several
Bile	+	
pH-level	< 5.0	neutral
Mucous		+
Weight loss		+
Dyspnea/Cough		+
Metabolic Alkalosis/Acidosis	+	
Hypokalaemia/Hypochloraemia	+	

Haematemesis

Vomitus of blood

Common Causes		
Dog		Cat
+++ Foreign body		+++ Foreign body
++ Gastric/intestinal ulcer		++ Gastric/intestinal ulcer
++ Gastric/intestinal tumour		++ Gastric/intestinal tumour

Gastrointestinal Causes

Acute Causes

- Foreign body
- Traumatic blood vessel/organ rupture
- Oesophageal varices

Chronic Causes

- Foreign body
- Chronic vomitus
- Gastric/intestinal ulcer
  - Helicobacter sp.
  - Gastrospirilium sp.
  - NSAID
  - Glucocorticoids
  - Uraemia
  - Stress
  - Mast cell tumour [esp Dog]
  - Gastrinoma (Zollinger-Ellison Syndrome)
  - Gastroenteritis
- Gastric/Intestinal tumour
  - Adenocarcinoma
  - Lymphosarcoma [esp Cat]

Other Causes

- Swallowed blood
  - Epistaxis
  - Haemorrhage into the respiratory tract
  - Haemorrhage into the oral cavity
- Coagulopathy

Diagnostic Approach

Haematemesis

1. **Case History**

2. **General Examination**

3. **Pharyngeal Examination**

4. **Blood Tests**
- Hct, Ery, Leuc, Hb
- TP, Alb, Glob
- GPT, AP, Urea, Crea

- Amylase, Lipase [Dog]

COAGULATION
- Bleeding time
- Prothrombin time (PT/Quick)
- (Activated) partial Thromboplastin time (PTT/ aPTT)
- Fibrin degradation products (FDP)
- Thrombocyte number

MICROBIAL SEROLOGY
- FeLV-/FIV Antigen [Cat]

- Helicobacter Antibodies

5. X-Ray Study
- Abdomen
- Thorax
- Throat

6. Endoscopy
- Gastro-/Duodenoscopy ± Biopsy
- Bronchoscopy
- Rhinoscopy ± Biopsy

Copremesis

Vomitus of faecal matter

Common Causes	
Dog	**Cat**
+++ Foreign body ileus	+++ Foreign body ileus
++ Invagination	++ Invagination
++ Intestinal parasites	++ Intestinal parasites
++ Intestinal tumours	++ Intestinal tumours

Gastrointestinal Obstruction

Mechanical Ileus

- Foreign body
- Intestinal parasites

- Intestinal tumours
- Invagination
- Incarceration (Hernia)
- Volvulus
- Constipation

Diagnostic Approach

Copremesis

1. Case History

2 General Examination

3. X-Ray Study
- Abdomen
- Intestinal contrast medium study

4. **Blood Tests**	• TP
• Hct, Ery, Leuc, Hb	• Na, K, Ca

Emaciation

> Weight loss reaching cachexia/marasmus

Common Causes	
Dog	Cat
+++ Dysphagia	+++ Dysphagia
++ Diabetes mellitus	++ Hyperthyroidism
++ Malabsorption syndrome	++ Diabetes mellitus
++ Maldigestion syndrome	++ Malabsorption syndrome
++ Tumour cachexia	++ Maldigestion syndrome
++ Chronic renal failure	++ Tumour cachexia
	++ Chronic renal failure

Impaired Food Intake

General Causes

- Quantitative/qualitative malnutrition
- Dysphagia
- Anorexia
- Chronic vomitus
- Chronic regurgitation
- Chronic diarrhoea
- Motility disturbances
- Muscle weakness

Impaired Food Utilisation

Malabsorption Syndrome

- Viral Enteritis
  - Parvovirus
  - Rota-/Coronavirus
  - FeLV/FIV [Cat]
  - Canine Distemper virus [Dog]

- Bacterial Enteritis
  - Salmonella sp.
  - Campylobacter sp.
  - Yersinia sp.
  - Shigella sp.
  - E. coli
  - Clostridium sp.
  - Helicobacter sp.
  - Dysbacteriosis
- Parasitic Enteritis
  - **Protozoa**
    - Giardia sp.
    - Toxoplasma sp.
    - Cystoisospora sp.
    - Cryptosporidium sp.
    - (Entamoeba sp. [Dog])
  - **Roundworms**
    - Toxocara spp.
    - Toxascaris sp.
    - Ancylostoma sp.
    - Uncinaria sp.
    - Trichuris sp. [Dog]

- Strongyloides sp.
- (Spirocerca sp. [Dog])
- **Tapeworms**
  - Dipylidium sp.
  - Joyeuxiella sp.
  - Diphyllobothrium sp. [Dog]
  - Spirometra sp. [Dog]
  - Echinococcus sp.
  - Taenia spp.
  - Mesocestoides sp.
- Food Intolerance
  - Lactose
  - Gluten [Dog]
  - Food allergy
- Immunoreactive Enteritis (Inflammatory bowel disease)
  - Lymphoplasmacellular Enteritis
  - Eosinophilic Enteritis
  - Granulomatous Enteritis
- Intestinal tumours
  - Lymphosarcoma
  - Adenocarcinoma
  - Fibrosarcoma
  - Leiomyoma/ Leiomyosarcoma
  - Undifferentiated sarcoma
  - Gastrinoma (Zollinger-Ellison Syndrome)
- Gastric/Intestinal ulcer
- Mycotic Enteritis
  - (Candida sp.)
  - (Histoplasma sp.)
  - (Aspergillus sp.)
- Toxic Enteritis
  - Enterotoxins
  - Drugs
  - Poisoning
- Lymphangiectasia [Dog]

Maldigestion Syndrome

- Exocrine pancreatic insufficiency
- Bile acid deficiency

Endocrine Causes

- Diabetes mellitus
- Hypocortisolism (Addison's Disease) [Dog]

Organ Failure

- Cardiac failure
- Hepatic failure
  - Portosystemic Shunt
  - Cirrhosis
- Renal failure

Calorie Loss

Protein Loss

- Protein-losing enteropathy
- Protein-losing nephropathy
- Exsudative body cavity effusions
- Chronic haemorrhage
- Burns

Energy Loss

- Hyperthyroidism [Cat]
- Fever
- Pregnancy
- Lactation
- Systemic infection
- Tumour cachexia
- Exposure to the cold

Diagnostic Approach

Emaciation

1. **Case History**

2. **General Examination**

3. **Oral/ Pharyngeal Examination**

4. **Blood Tests**
   - Hct, Ery, Leuc, Hb
   - TP, Alb, Glob
   - GPT, AP, Urea, Crea, BG
   - Amylase, Lipase
   - TLI Test
   - Bile acids
   - Ammonium
   - Diff BC
   - Na, K, Ca, P
   - Vit. B_{12}
   - FIP Profile [Cat]
     - TP
     - Alb/Glob Ratio
     - Bili
     - GOT
     - Serum electrophoresis

MICROBIAL SEROLOGY
   - FeLV-/FIV Antigen [Cat]

FUNCTION TESTS
   - T_4, fT_4
   - T_3 Suppression test [Cat]
   - Adrenal gland function test [Dog]
     - Dexamethasone Suppression test
     - ACTH Stimulation test
     - Cortisol/Creatinine Ratio

5. **Urinalysis**
   - Urine dip stick
   - Specific gravity
   - Urine sediment

6. **Faecal Examination**
   - Plain examination
   - Flotation
   - Chymotrypsin
   - Elastase

7. **X-Ray Study**
   - Abdomen
   - Thorax
   - Skull (in cases of dysphagia)

8. **Ultrasound**
   - Heart (Doppler Echocardiography)
   - Abdomen (± Liver biopsy)

9. **Endoscopy**
   - Gastro-/Duodenoscopy ± Biopsy

10. **Further Tests**
    - Analysis of body cavity fluid
    - Spinal tap/analysis

Hypersalivation

Excessive production of spittle

Common Causes			
Dog		**Cat**	
+++	Dental Disease	+++	Dental Disease
++	Stomatitis/Pharyngitis	++	Stomatitis/Pharyngitis
++	Malocclusion syndrome	++	Malocclusion syndrome
++	Organophosphate poisoning	++	Organophosphate poisoning
+	(Rabies)	+	(Rabies)

Oropharyngeal Causes

Malocclusion Syndrome

- Lip anomalies
- Dental malposition
- Jaw anomaly (Prognatism/ Brachygnathism)

Dental Disease

- Dental fracture
- Dental abscess
- Tartar/decay
- Feline odontoclastic resorptive lesion (FORL)[Cat]
- Periodontitis
- Persistent deciduous teeth
- Dental malposition
- Dental root remnants (broken teeth)

Oral/Pharyngeal Tumours

- Papilloma
- Fibroma/Fibrosarcoma
- Squamous cell carcinoma
- Melanoma
- Epulis/Gingival hyperplasia [esp Dog]
- Tonsillar carcinoma
- Salivary gland carcinoma
- Nasopharyngeal polyps [Cat]

Salivary Gland Disease

Gl. parotis
Gl. zygomatica
Gl. mandibularis
Gl. sublingualis

- Sialoadenitis
- Sialocele/Mucocele/Ranula
- Salivary gland adenoma/ carcinoma
- Sialolithiasis

Oronasal Fistula

- Dental abscess
- Foreign body
- Cleft palate (congenital/ trauma)

Stomatitis/Gingivitis/Glossitis/Tonsillitis

- Viral Causes
  - FeLV/FIV [Cat]
  - Feline Calici virus [Cat]
  - Feline Herpes virus [Cat]
  - (FIP Coronavirus [Cat])
- Bacterial Causes
  - Streptococcus sp.
  - Staphylococcus sp.
  - Neisseria sp.
  - E. coli
  - Pasteurella sp.
  - Acinetobacter sp.
  - Leptospira sp. [Dog]
  - Actinomyces sp.
  - Nocardia sp.
  - Mycobacterium sp. [Dog]
  - Fusobacterium sp.
  - Spirochetes
- Immunoreactive Causes
  - Eosinophilic Granuloma
  - Plasma cell gingivitis/stomatitis
  - Lupus erythematosus
  - Pemphigus vulgaris
- Metabolic Causes
  - Uraemia
  - Hypothyroidism [Dog]
  - Diabetes mellitus
- Toxic Causes
  - Lead poisoning
  - Household agents
  - Toxic plants
  - Cytostatics
  - Chemical burn
- Other Causes
  - Foreign body/abscess
- Mycotic Causes
  - Candida sp.

Other Causes
Poisoning

- Organophosphates
- Carbamates
- Pyrethrin/Pyrethroid
- Ivermectin
- Household agents
- Toxic plants/animals

Psychoneural Reflex Response

- Excitement
- Pain
- Pawlow Reflex
- Taste aversion (bitter)
- Hyperthermia
- Kinetosis/Motion sickness
- Nausea

Orthodontic Disease

- Mandibular luxation
- Maxillary/Mandibular fracture
- Bone tumours
- Craniomandibular osteopathy
- Osteomyelitis
- Hyoid bone fracture
- Temporomandibular disease

Masticatory Muscle Disease/Temporomandibular Myositis

- Congenital Causes
  - Muscular dystrophy [Dog]
  - Dermatomyositis [Dog]
  - Glycogen storage disease
- Inflammatory Causes
  - Toxoplasma sp.
  - Neospora sp. [Dog]
  - Lyme Borreliosis sp. [Dog]
  - Leptospira sp. [Dog]

- Immunoreactive Causes
  - Eosinophilic Myositis [Dog]
- Metabolic Causes
  - Vitamin E Deficiency
  - Hypokalaemia [esp Cat]
  - Hypercortisolism (Cushing's Disease) [Dog]
  - Glucocorticoid long term therapy
  - Hypothyroidism [Dog]

Neurological Disease

- Encephalitis/ Meningoencephalitis
- Brain Tumours
- Cervical spine disease
- Paralysis
  - Trigeminal nerve (V) (Masticatory muscle)
  - Facial nerve (VII) (orofacial musculature)
  - Hypoglossal nerve (XII) (Glossal musculature)
  - Glossopharyngeal nerve (XI) (Pharyngeal/Laryngeal musculature/oesophagus)
  - Vagal nerve (X) (Pharyngeal/Laryngeal musculature/oesophagus, hard palate)
- Polyneuropathy
  Congenital Causes
  - Axonopathy
  - Demyelinisation disease
  - Lysosomal storage disease
  Inflammatory Causes
  - Polyradiculoneuritis
  - Polyneuritis
  - FeLV/FIV [Cat]
  - Toxoplasma sp.
  - Neospora sp. [Dog]
  Immunoreactive Causes
  - Lupus erythematosus
  - Myasthenia gravis
  Metabolic Causes
  - Hypothyroidism [Dog]
  - Diabetes mellitus
  - Paraneoplastic syndrome (Insulinoma)
  Toxic Causes
  - Organophosphate poisoning (chronic)
  - Lead Poisoning
  - Cytostatics
  - Lindane
  - Botulism
  - Tick paralysis
  Other Causes
  - Nerve compression syndrome
  - Feline dysautonomia [esp Cat]
- Loss of smell/taste

Other Causes

- Seizures
- Traumatic Causes
  - Bitten off tongue
  - Torn Frenulum
  - Burns
  - Cleft palate
  - Foreign body
- Oesophageal foreign body

Diagnostic Approach

Hypersalivation

1. Case History

2. General Examination

3. Oral/Pharyngeal/ Jaw Examination

4. Neurological Examination
- Cranial nerves
  - Facial symmetry (VII)
  - Facial sensation(V)
  - Menace reflex (II, VII)
  - Blink reflex (V, VII)
  - Corneal reflex/ Eye movement (V, VI, VII/III, IV, VI)
  - Pupillary reflex (III, Sympathetic nerve)
  - Swallowing reflex/glossal motor function (X, XI, XII/ XII)

5. X-Ray Study
- Skull
  - Tympanic bulla
  - Maxilla/Mandible
  - Teeth
- Throat
- Thorax
- Contrast swallowing study/ Fluoroscopy

6. Blood Tests
- Hct, Ery, Leuc, Hb
- TP, Alb, Glob
- GPT, AP, Urea, Crea, BG
- Diff BC
- Na, K, Ca, P
- Chol, CK

MICROBIAL SEROLOGY
- FeLV-/FIV Antigen [Cat]

IMMUNOSEROLOGY
- ANA Test
- Autoantibodies against acetylcholine receptors (Myasthenia gravis detection)

FUNCTION TESTS
- Adrenal gland function test [Dog]
  - Dexamethasone Suppression test
  - ACTH Stimulation test
  - Cortisol/Creatinine Ratio
- T_4, fT_4

7. Urinalysis
- Urine dip stick
- Specific gravity
- Urine sediment

8. Endoscopy
- Oesophagoscopy/Gastroscopy

9. Further Tests
- Muscle biopsy
- Spinal tap/analysis

Coprophagia

Ingestion of faeces

Common Causes	
Dog	Cat
+++ Idiopathic	Rare
++ Maldigestion syndrome	
+ Endocrinopathies	
+ Intestinal parasites	

Psychogenic Causes

- Playing habit
- Behavioural disorder
- Boredom

Organic Causes

Malabsorption syndrome

- Intestinal parasites
  Protozoa
  - Giardia sp.
  - Toxoplasma sp.
  - Cystoisospora sp.
  - Cryptosporidium sp.
  - (Entamoeba sp. [Dog])
  Roundworms
  - Toxocara spp.
  - Toxascaris sp.
  - Ancylostoma sp.
  - Uncinaria sp.
  - Trichuris sp. [Dog]
  - Strongyloides sp.
  - (Spirocerca sp. [Dog])
  Tapeworms
  - Dipylidium sp.
  - Joyeuxiella sp.
  - Diphyllobothrium sp. [Dog]
  - Spirometra sp. [Dog]
  - Echinococcus sp.
  - Taenia spp.
  - Mesocestoides sp.

Maldigestion syndrome

- Exocrine pancreatic insufficiency
- Bile acid deficiency

Endocrine Causes

- Hypercortisolism (Cushing's Disease) [Dog]
- Diabetes mellitus
- Hyperthyroidism [Cat]

Other Causes

- Malnutrition?
- Glucocorticoid long-term therapy

Diagnostic Approach

Coprophagia

1. Case History

2. General Examination

3. Blood Tests
- Hct, Ery, Leuc, Hb
- TP, Alb, Glob
- GPT, AP, Urea, Crea, BG
- TLI Test
- Amylase, Lipase [Dog]
- Bile acids
- Diff BC
- Na, K, Ca, P

FUNCTION TESTS
- Adrenal gland function test [Dog]
  - Dexamethasone Suppression test
  - ACTH Stimulation test
  - Cortisol/Creatinine Ratio
- T_4, fT_4

4. Faecal Examination
- Plain examination
- Flotation
- Chymotrypsin
- Elastase

Faeces, bloody

Melena/tarry stools: dark, digested blood contained in faeces (upper gastrointestinal haemorrhage)
Haematochezia: bright, undigested blood contained in faeces (lower gastrointestinal haemorrhage)
Haemorrhagic diarrhoea: bright and dark blood contained in faeces (upper and lower gastrointestinal haemorrhage)

Common Causes	
Dog	**Cat**
Melena	
+++ Gastric/Duodenal ulcer	+++ Gastric/Duodenal ulcer
++ Gastric/Intestinal tumour	++ Gastric/Intestinal tumour
Haematochezia	
+++ Colitis/Proctitis	+++ Colitis/Proctitis
++ Tumours of the large intestine	++ Tumours of the large intestine
++ Perianal disease	++ Perianal disease

Haemorrhagic Diarrhoea
+++ Viral gastroenteritis

Melaena

Gastric Haemorrhage

- Foreign body
- Gastric ulcer
  - Helicobacter sp.
  - Gastrospirilium sp.
  - NSAID/Glucocorticoids
  - Uraemia
  - Stress
  - Shock
  - Pancreatitis
  - Mast cell tumour [Dog]
  - Gastrinoma (Zollinger-Ellison Syndrome)
  - Acute Gastritis
  - Hypocortisolism (Addison's Disease) [Dog]
- Gastric tumours
  - Adenocarcinoma
  - Lymphosarcoma [esp Cat]
  - Fibrosarcoma
  - Leiomyoma/Leiomyosarcoma

Haemorrhage of the Small Intestine

- Foreign body
- Duodenal tumours
  - Adenocarcinoma
  - Lymphosarcoma [esp Cat]
  - Fibrosarcoma
  - Leiomyoma/Leiomyosarcoma
- Invagination

- Duodenal ulcer
  - Helicobacter sp.
  - Gastrospirilium sp.
  - NSAID/Glucocorticoids
  - Uraemia
  - Stress
  - Shock
  - Pancreatitis
  - Mast cell tumour [Dog]
  - Gastrinoma (Zollinger-Ellison Syndrome)
  - Acute gastroenteritis

Other Causes

- Raw meat diet
- Swallowed blood
  - epistaxis
  - respiratory haemorrhage
  - haemorrhage in the oral cavity
- Coagulopathy
- Shock

Haematochezia

Colonic Haemorrhage

- Foreign body
- Trauma
- Invagination
  - Ileocolon
  - Caecocolon
- Parasitic colitis
  - Trichuris sp. [Dog]
  - Ancylostoma sp.
  - Lymphoplasmacellular colitis

- – Eosinophilic colitis
- – Granulomatous colitis
- – Ulcerative colitis [Dog]
- Colonic tumours
  - – Adenocarcinoma
  - – Lymphosarcoma [esp Cat]
  - – Leiomyoma/
    Leiomyosarcoma
  - – Polyp
- Food intolerance
  - – Lack of crude fibre

Anorectal Haemorrhage

- Foreign body
- Perianal wounds
- Anal gland abscess
- Perianal fistula [Dog]
- Perianal tumours [esp Dog]
- Rectal tumours

- – Rectal adenocarcinoma
- – Polyp

Haemorrhagic Diarrhoea

Haemorrhagic Gastroenteritis

- Viral Gastroenteritis [Dog]
  - – Parvovirus
  - – Coronavirus
- Food intoxication/
  Enterotoxins
- Immunoreactive Causes
- Bacterial gastroenteritis
  - – Clostridium sp. [esp Dog]
  - – E. coli
  - – Salmonella sp.
- Other Causes
  - – DIC
  - – Intestinal obstruction
  - – Septicaemia

Diagnostic Apparoach

Faeces, bloody

1. Case History

2. General Examination

3. Pharyngeal Examination

4. Rectal Examination
± Colonic smear/cytology

5. Blood Tests
- Hct, Ery, Leuc, Hb
- TP, Alb, Glob
- GPT, AP, Urea, Crea
- Amylase, Lipase

COAGULOPATHY
- Bleeding time

- Prothrombin time (PT/Quick)
- (Activated) partial
  Thromboplastin time (PTT/
  aPTT)
- Fibrin degradation products
  (FDP)
- Thrombocyte number

MICROBIAL SEROLOGY
- FeLV-/FIV Antigen [Cat]
- Helicobacter Antibodies

6. Faecal Examination
- Plain examination
- Flotation

- Parvovirus Antigen [Dog]
- Bacterial culture

7. Urinalysis
- Urine dip stick
- Specific gravity
- Urine sediment

8. X-Ray Study
- Abdomen

9. Ultrasound
- Abdomen ± biopsy

10. Endoscopy
- Gastro-/Duodenoscopy
  ± biopsy
- Coloscopy ± biopsy

11. Further Tests
- Laparotomy

Rectal Tenesmus

Frequent and painful evacuation of faecal matter in small amounts

Common Causes			
Dog		**Cat**	
+++	Colitis	+++	Colitis
++	Constipation	++	Constipation
++	Anal gland abscess	++	Anal gland abscess
++	Prostatic hyperplasia	++	Colorectal tumours
+	Perineal hernia		
+	Colorectal tumours		

Obstructive Causes

Intraluminal Intestinal Obstruction

- Perineal hernia [Dog]
- Colorectal tumours
  - Adenocarcinoma
  - Lymphosarcoma [esp Cat]
  - Leiomyoma/ Leiomyosarcoma
  - Polyp
- Invagination
  - Ileocolon
  - Caecocolon
- Rectal diverticulum

- Anal stricture
- Atresia ani
- Faecal clumping around the anus
- Rectal prolapse

Extraluminal Intestinal Obstruction

- Prostatic enlargement [Dog]
  - Prostatic hyperplasia
  - Prostatitis/Prostatic abscess
  - Prostatic cysts
  - Paraprostatic cyst
  - Prostatic carcinoma

- Pelvic fractures
- Pathological pregnancy

Other Causes
Colitis/Proctitis

- Food Intolerance
  - Lack of crude fibre
  - Food allergy
- Bacterial colitis
  - Dysbacteriosis/bacterial overgrowth
  - Salmonella sp.
  - Campylobacter sp.
  - Clostridium sp.
- Parasitic colitis
  - Trichuris sp. [Dog]
  - Ancylostoma sp.
  - Uncinaria sp.
  - Balantidium sp. [Dog]
  - Cystoisospora sp.
  - (Entamoeba sp. [Dog])
- Immunoreactive colitis (Inflammatory bowel disease)
  - Lymphoplasmacellular colitis
  - Eosinophilic colitis
  - Granulomatous colitis
  - Ulcerative colitis
- Psychogenic colitis
  - Irritable colon
- Partial colonic obstruction

- Foreign body
- Intestinal tumour
- Invagination
- Rectal diverticulum
- Viral colitis
  - FeLV/FIV [Cat]
  - FIP Coronavirus [Cat]
- Mycotic colitis
  - (Histoplasma sp.)

Perianal Disease

- Anal sac abscess
- Perianal fistula [Dog]
- Perineal hernia [Dog]
- Perianal wounds
- Perianal tumours
  - Rectal carcinoma
  - Rectal polyp
  - Anal gland adenoma/carcinoma
  - Anal sac adenoma/carcinoma
  - Hepatoid gland adenoma/carcinoma [Dog]

Further Causes

- Constipation (esp feeding of bones)
- Urinary Tract Disease

Diagnostic Approach
Rectal Tenesmus

1. **Case History**
2. **General Examination**
3. **Rectal Examination**
   ± Colonic smear/cytology
   ± Sticky tape impression

4. X-Ray Study
- Abdomen
- Pelvis
- Contrast enema
- Intestinal contrast medium passage

5. Blood Tests
- Hct, Ery, Leuc

MICROBIAL SEROLOGY
- FeLV-/FIV Antigen [Cat]

6. Urinalysis
- Urine dip stick
- Specific gravity
- Urine sediment

7. Faecal Examination
- Plain examination
- Flotation
- Bacterial culture

8. Ultrasound
- Abdomen

9. Endoscopy
- Coloscopy ± biopsy

Faecal Incontinence

Involuntary defaecation as a result of primary or secondary sphincter incompetence

Common Causes	
Dog	Cat
+++ Intervertebral disc prolapse	+++ Pelvic fractures
++ Cauda equina syndrome	++ Spinal trauma
++ Pelvic fractures	++ Perianal Disease
++ Perianal Disease	

Neurological Causes

Lumbosacral Spinal Cord Lesion (L4–S3)

- Traumatic Causes
  - Disc prolapse
  - Vertebral fracture/luxation
  - Haemorrhage/Haematoma
  - Fibrocartilaginous embolism
  - Thromboembolism
- Congenital causes
  - Deformed spinal column (ie hemivertebra/wedge shaped vertebra)
  - Meningocele
- Infectious Causes
  - Discospondylitis/ Osteomyelitis
  - Abscess
  - Myelitis

- Immunoreactive Causes
  - Granulomatous Meningoencephalomyelitis
- Degenerative Causes
  - Spondylosis deformans
  - Disc prolapse
  - Lumbosacral stenosis (Cauda equina syndrome) [Dog]
  - (Dura mater ossification)
- Tumours/Tumour metastasis
  - Osteosarcoma
  - Chondrosarcoma
  - Multiple Myeloma [esp Dog]
- Other Causes
  - Hypervitaminosis A [Cat]

Peripheral Nerve Lesion

- Pudendal nerve lesion
  - Perianal surgery
  - Tumours
  - Pelvic fractures

Polyneuropathy

- Infectious Causes
  - FeLV-/FIV [Cat]
  - Toxoplasma sp.
  - Neospora sp. [Dog]
- Immunoreactive Causes
  - Lupus erythematosus
- Metabolic Causes
  - Diabetes mellitus
  - Hypercortisolism (Cushing's Disease) [esp Dog]
  - Hypothyroidism [Dog]

- Toxic Causes
  - Organophosphate poisoning (chronic)
  - Lead poisoning
  - Cytostatics
  - Lindane
  - Botulism toxin
  - Tick toxin (Tick paralysis)
- Congenital Causes
  - Axonopathy
  - Demyelinisation diseases
  - Lysosomal storage disease
  - Spinal muscular atrophy
- Other causes
  - Nerve root compression syndrome
  - (Feline dysautonomia [Cat])
  - Polyneuritis/ Polyradiculoneuritis [Dog]

Other Causes

- Perianal Disease
  - Anal sac abscess
  - Perianal fistula [Dog]
  - Perianal tumours
  - Perineal hernia [Dog]
  - Perianal wounds
- Acute Diarrhoea
- Psychogenic Causes
  - Fear/Excitement
  - Senility
  - Irritable colon
- Constipation
- Urinary Tract Disease

Diagnostic Approach

Faecal Incontinence

1. Case History

2. General Examination (incl. rectal)

3. Neurological Examination
- Awareness/behaviour
- Body/Limb posture
- Locomotion
- Muscle tone/strength
- Spinal reflexes
  - Bicipital reflex (C6–C8)
  - Tricipital reflex (C7–T1)
  - Patellar reflex (L4–L6)
  - Withdrawal reflex (C6–T1 and L6–S1)
  - Cutaneous trunci reflex (C7–T1)
  - Anal sphincter reflex (S1–S3)
  - Urinary bladder – can it be expressed?

4. X-Ray Study
- Abdomen
- Pelvis
- Lumbar Spine
  ± Myelography

5. Blood Tests
- Hct, Ery, Leuc

- Na, K, Ca
- CK
- Urea, Crea
- Diff BC

MICROBIAL SEROLOGY
- FeLV-/FIV Antigen [Cat]

6. Urinalysis
- Urinary output/volume
- Urine dip stick
- Specific gravity
- Urine sediment
  - Bacteria
  - Erythrocytes, leucocytes
  - Epithelial cells
  - Casts
  - Crystals
  - Tumour cytology
- Bacterial culture (Cystocentesis)

7. Faecal Examination
- Plain examination
- Flotation
- Bacterial culture

8. Further Tests
- Colonoscopy ± biopsy
- Spinal tap/analysis

Meteorism/Flatulence

Gastric/Intestinal flatulence: Increased intestinal gas content with/without flatulence (wind), with/without borborygmi (rolling/gurgling intestinal sounds)

Common Causes	
Dog	Cat
+++ Bloating food	+++ Milk in absence of lactase
++ Malabsorption syndrome	++ Malabsorption syndrome
++ Maldigestion syndrome	++ Maldigestion syndrome
++ Motility disturbance	++ Motility disturbance

Aerophagia

- Rushed food intake
  - Food jealousy
- Hypersalivation

↑ Intestinal Gas formation

Bloating Food

- Soya beans
- Cabbage
- Spoilt food
- Milk in lactase
  deficiency

Malabsorption Syndrome

- Viral enteritis
  - Parvovirus
  - Rota-/Coronavirus
  - FeLV/FIV [Cat]
  - Canine distemper virus
    [Dog]
- Bacterial enteritis
  - Salmonella sp.
  - Campylobacter sp.
  - Yersinia sp.
  - Shigella sp.
  - E. coli
  - Clostridium sp.
  - Helicobacter sp.
  - Dysbacteriosis
- Parasitic enteritis

Protozoa

- Giardia sp.
- Toxoplasma sp.
- Cystoisospora sp.
- Cryptosporidium sp.
- (Entamoeba sp. [Dog])

Roundworms

- Toxocara spp.
- Toxascaris sp.
- Ancylostoma sp.
- Uncinaria sp.
- Trichuris sp. [Dog]
- Strongyloides sp.
- (Spirocerca sp. [Dog])

Tapeworms

- Dipylidium sp.
- Joyeuxiella sp.
- Diphyllobothrium sp. [Dog]
- Spirometra sp. [Dog]
- Echinococcus sp.
- Taenia spp.
- Mesocestoides sp.
- Immunoreactive enteritis
  (Inflammatory bowel disease)
  - Lymphoplasmacellular
    enteritis
  - Eosinophilic enteritis
  - Granulomatous enteritis

- Mycotic enteritis
  - (Candida sp.)
  - (Histoplasma sp.)
  - (Aspergillus sp.)

Maldigestion Syndrome

- Exocrine pancreatic insufficiency
- Bile acid deficiency

Motility Disturbances

Mechanical Ileus (Intestinal Obstruction) Intraluminal intestinal obstruction

- Foreign body
- Invagination
- Intestinal parasites
  - Roundworms
  - Tapeworms
- Intestinal tumours
  - Adenocarcinoma
  - Lymphosarcoma
  - Leiomyoma/ Leiomyosarcoma
  - Fibrosarcoma
  - Polyp

Extraluminal intestinal obstruction

- Abdominal tumours
- Incarceration (hernia)
- Volvulus
- Pelvic fractures
- Pathological pregnancy
- Lymphadenopathy
- Adhesions

Paralytic Ileus (Intestinal atony)

- Mechanical Ileus (advanced stage)
- Abdominal trauma
- Peritonitis
- Spinal cord disease
- Shock
- Acute pancreatitis
- Uraemia
- Hypokalaemia
- Diabetic ketoacidosis
- Intestinal tumours
- Gastroenteritis
- Idiopathic megacolon
- Organ failure
  - Congestive heart failure
  - Liver failure
  - Kidney failure
- Hepatoencephalopathy
- Feline dysautonomia [Cat]
- Polyneuropathy
- Mesenterial infarction
- Hypothyroidism [Dog]
- Postoperative intestinal paralysis
- Drugs
  - Atropine
  - Butylscopolamine
  - Laxative misuse
- Heavy metal poisoning
  - Lead
  - Thallium

Diagnostic Approach

Meteorism

1. Case History

2. General Examination

3. X-Ray Study
- Abdomen
- Intestinal contrast medium passage
- Contrast enema

4. Blood Tests
- Hct, Ery, Leuc
- Na, K, Ca
- TP, Alb, Glob
- GPT, AP, Urea, Crea, BG
- Amylase, Lipase [Dog]
- TLI Test
- Cholesterol
- Serum Cobalamin (Vit. B12)
- Serum Folic acid
- Serum bile acids
- Serum Gastrin
- Diff BC
- FIP Profile [Cat]
  - TP
  - Alb/Glob Ratio
  - Bili
  - GOT
  - Serum electrophoresis

MICROBIAL SEROLOGY
- FeLV-/FIV Antigen [Cat]

FUNCTION TESTS
- T_4, fT_4
- TSH-/TRH Stimulation Test [Dog]
- PABA-Xylose Test [Dog]

5. Urinalysis
- Urine dip stick
- Specific gravity
- Urine sediment

6. Faecal Examination
- Plain examination
- Flotation
- Bacterial culture
- Fat content (Sudan staining)
- Chymotrypsin

7. Ultrasound
- Abdomen ± biopsy

8. Endoscopy
- Gastro-/Duodenoscopy ± biopsy
- Colonoscopy ± biopsy

9. Further Tests
- Colonic smear/cytology

Halitosis

Unpleasant odour noticeable on the breath, foetor ex oris

Common Causes	
Dog	Cat
+++ Dental Disease	+++ Dental Disease
++ Food retention	++ Food retention
++ Uraemia	++ Uraemia
++ Diabetic ketoacidosis	++ Diabetic ketoacidosis
++ Tumour in the oral cavity	++ Tumour in the oral cavity

Oropharyngeal Causes

Stomatitis/Gingivitis/Glossitis/Tonsillitis

- Viral Causes
  - FeLV/FIV [Cat]
  - Feline Calici virus [Cat]
  - Feline Herpes virus [Cat]
- Bacterial Causes
  - Streptococcus sp.
  - Staphylococcus sp.
  - Neisseria sp.
  - E. coli
  - Pasteurella sp.
  - Acinetobacter sp.
  - Leptospira sp. [Dog]
  - Actinomyces sp.
  - Nocardia sp.
  - Mycobacterium sp. [Dog]
  - Fusobacterium sp.
  - Spirochetes
- Immunoreactive causes
  - Eosinophilic granuloma
  - Plasmacell gingivitis/stomatitis
  - Lupus erythematosus
  - Pemphigus vulgaris
- Metabolic Causes
  - Uraemia
  - Hypothyroidism [Dog]
  - Diabetes mellitus
- Toxic Causes
  - Lead Poisoning
  - Household agents
  - Poisonous plants
  - Cytostatics
  - Chemical burns
- Other causes
  - Foreign body/abscess
- Mycotic Causes
  - Candida sp.

Dental Disease

- Dental fracture
- Dental abscess
- Dental calculus/decay
- Feline odontoclastic resorptive lesions (FORL) [Cat]
- Periodontitis
- Persistent deciduous teeth
- Dental malposition/food retention
- Root remnants (broken teeth)

Oropharyngeal tumours

- Papilloma
- Fibroma/Fibrosarcoma
- Squamous cell carcinoma
- Melanoma

- Epulis/Gingival hyperplasia [esp Dog]
- Tonsillar carcinoma
- Lymphoma/Lymphosarcoma
- Mast cell tumour
- Salivary gland carcinoma
- Nasopharyngeal polyps [Cat]

Salivary Gland Disease

Gl. parotis
Gl. zygomatica
Gl. mandibularis
Gl. sublingualis

- Sialoadenitis
- Sialocele/Mucocele/Ranula
- Salivary gland adenoma/carcinoma
- Sialolithiasis

Oronasal fistula

- Dental abscess
- Foreign body

- Cleft palate (congenital/traumatic)

Other Causes

- Lip anomalies [esp Dog]

Other Causes

Gastrointestinal Causes

- Coprophagia
- Megaoesophagus
- Gastric tumours
- Gastritis

Metabolic Causes

- Uraemia
- Diabetic ketoacidosis

Respiratory Causes

- Rhinitis/Sinusitis
- Bronchopneumonia

Diagnostic Approach

Halitosis

1. **Case History**

2. **General Examination**

3. **Examination of the Oral Cavity and Pharynx**

4. **Blood Tests**
   - Hct, Ery, Leuc
   - Urea, Crea, BG

5. **X-Ray Study**
   - Skull (+ Tympanic bulla)
   - Throat
   - Thorax

6. **Endoscopy**
   - Rhinoscopy ± Biopsy
   - Gastroscopy ± Biopsy
   - Bronchoscopy ± Tracheobronchial lavage

Constipation

> **Coprostasis:** Accumulation of faecal matter in the colon

Common Causes	
Dog	**Cat**
+++ Feeding of bones	+++ Pelvic fractures (healed)
++ Pelvic fractures (healed)	++ Colorectal tumours
++ Colorectal tumours	++ Idiopathic megacolon
++ Perineal hernia	++ Hypokalaemia
++ Lumbosacral spinal cord lesion	++ Feline dysautonomia

Painful defaecation

Bone Diseases

- Spinal disease
- Hip joint disease
- Disease of the hind limbs
- Pelvic fractures

Perianal Disease

- Anal sac abscess
- Perianal fistula [Dog]
- Perineal hernia [Dog]
- Perianal wounds
- Perianal tumours
  - Rectal carcinoma
  - Rectal polyp
  - Anal sac adenoma/ carcinoma
  - Anal gland adenoma/ carcinoma
  - Hepatoid adenoma/ carcinoma [Dog]

Obstructive Causes

Intraluminal Intestinal Obstruction

- Perineal hernia [Dog]
- Colorectal tumours
  - Adenocarcinoma
  - Lymphosarcoma [esp Cat]
  - Leiomyoma/ Leiomyosarcoma
  - Polyp
- Rectal diverticulum
- Anal stricture
- Atresia ani
- Faecal clumping around the anus
- Rectal prolapse

Extraluminal Intestinal Obstruction

- Pelvic fractures (healed)
- Prostatic enlargement [Dog]
  - Prostatic hyperplasia

- Prostatitis/prostatic abscess
- Prostatic cysts
- Paraprostatic cyst
- Prostatic carcinoma
• Pelvic tumours
• Lymphadenopathy
  - Lnn. sublumbales
• Pathological pregnancy
• Condition after Tripleosteotomy (pelvic narrowing)

Neurological Causes

Lumbosacral Spinal Cord Lesion (L4–S3)

• Traumatic Causes
  - Disc prolapse
  - Vertebral fracture/luxation
  - Haemorrhage/Haematoma
  - Fibrocartilaginous embolism
  - Thromboembolism
• Congenital Causes
  - Lumbosacral stenosis (Cauda equina syndrome) [Dog]
  - Deformed spinal column (ie hemivertebra/wedge shaped vertebra)
  - Meningocele
• Infectious Causes
  - Discospondylitis/ Osteomyelitis
  - Abscess
  - Myelitis
• Immunoreactive Causes
  - Granulomatous meningoencephalomyelitis
• Degenerative Causes
  - Spondylosis deformans

- Disc prolapse
- Lumbosacral stenosis (Cauda equina syndrome) [Dog]
- (Dura mater ossification)
• Tumours
  - Osteosarcoma
  - Chondrosarcoma
  - Multiple myeloma [esp Dog]
  - Lymphosarcoma
  - Meningeoma
  - Tumour metastasis
• Other Causes
  - Hypervitaminosis A [Cat]

Peripheral Nerve Lesion

• Pelvic nerve

Polyneuropathy

• Infectious Polyneuropathy/ Polyneuritis
  - FeLV/FIV [Cat]
  - Neospora sp. [Dog]
  - Toxoplasma sp.
• Immunoreactive Polyneuropathy
  - Lupus erythematosus
  - Myasthenia gravis
• Endocrine polyneuropathy
  - Hypercortisolism (Cushing's Disease) [Dog]
  - Hypothyroidism [Dog]
  - Diabetes mellitus
  - Hypoglycaemia (Insulinoma)
• Toxic polyneuropathy
• Feline dysautonomia [Cat]

Other Causes

Constipating Foods

* Bones
* Dry food in combination with insufficient water intake
* Cocoa
* Bananas
* Nutmeg

Drugs

* Butylscopolamine
* Atropine
* Loperamide
* Diuretics
* Sucralfate
* Antihistamines
* Iron preparations
* Calcium channel blockers
* Barium sulfate
* Antacids (Aluminium hydroxide)
* Diphenoxylate

Poisoning

* Rodenticides (Cholecalciferol)
* Heavy metals
  – Lead
  – Copper
  – Thallium

Metabolic Causes

* Dehydration
* Hypothyroidism [Dog]
* Hypokalaemia
* Hypercalcaemia

Other Causes

* Lack of exercise
* Environmental disturbance affecting defaecation
  – Unhygienic cat litter
* Congenital megacolon (Hirschsprung Disease)

Diagnostic Approach

Constipation

1. **Case History**

2. **General Examination**

3. **Neurological Examination**
* Spinal Reflexes
  – Bicipital reflex (C6–C8)
  – Triceps reflex (C7–T1)
  – Patellar reflex (L4–L6)
  – Withdrawal reflex (C6–T1 and L6–S1)
  – Cutaneous trunci reflex (C7–T1)
  – Anal sphincter reflex (S1–S3)
  – Urinary bladder – can it be expressed?

4. **X-Ray Study**
* Abdomen
* Pelvis
* Intestinal contrast medium passage (after colonic evacuation)

- Contrast enema (after colonic elimination)

5. Blood Tests
- Hct, Ery, Leuc
- Na, K, Ca
- TP
- GPT, AP, Urea, Crea
- Diff BC
- Cholesterol [Dog]

6. Urinalysis
- Urine dip stick
- Specific gravity
- Urine sediment

7. Ultrasound
- Abdomen

8. Endoscopy
- Colonoscopy ± biopsy

9. Further Examination
- Laparotomy

Polyphagia

Pathological increase of appetite

Common Causes	
Dog	Cat
+++ Over supply	+++ Hyperthyroidism
++ Food jealousy	++ Diabetes mellitus
++ Glucocorticoid therapy	++ Glucocorticoid therapy
++ Hypercortisolism (Cushing's Disease)	++ Malabsorption syndrome
++ Diabetes mellitus	++ Maldigestion syndrome
++ Malabsorption syndrome	
++ Maldigestion syndrome	

With Weight Gain

Physiological Causes
- Lack of exercise
- Over supply

Endocrine Causes
- Hypothalamic dysfunction
- Hypercortisolism (Cushing's Disease)
- Hyperinsulinism/Insulinoma
- Hypogonadism/castration

Drugs
- Glucocorticoid long term therapy
- Anabolic steroids
- Anticonvulsants
- β Blockers [Dog]

With Weight Loss

Physiological Causes

- Lactation
- Exposure to the cold
- Exercise
- Caloric Malnutrition

Endocrine Causes

- Hyperthyroidism
- Diabetes mellitus

Malabsorption Syndrome

- Viral Enteritis
  - Parvovirus
  - Rota-/Coronavirus
  - FeLV/FIV [Cat]
  - Canine Distemper Virus [Dog]
- Bacterial Enteritis
  - Salmonella sp.
  - Campylobacter sp.
  - Yersinia sp.
  - Shigella sp.
  - E. coli
  - Clostridium sp.
  - Helicobacter sp.
  - Dysbacteriosis (Antibiosis)
- Parasitic Enteritis

Protozoa
  - Giardia sp.
  - Toxoplasma sp.
  - Cystoisospora sp.
  - Cryptosporidium sp.
  - (Entamoeba sp. [Dog])

Roundworms
  - Toxocara spp.
  - Toxascaris sp.
  - Ancylostoma sp.
  - Uncinaria sp.
  - Trichuris sp. [Dog]
  - Strongyloides sp.
  - (Spirocerca sp. [Dog])

Tapeworms
  - Dipylidium sp.
  - Joyeuxiella sp.
  - Diphyllobothrium sp. [Dog]
  - Spirometra sp. [Dog]
  - Echinococcus sp.
  - Taenia spp.
  - Mesocestoides sp.
- Food Intolerance
  - Lactose
  - Gluten [Dog]
  - Food allergy
- Immunoreactive Enteritis (Inflammatory bowel disease)
  - Lymphoplasmacellular enteritis
  - Eosinophilic enteritis
  - Granulomatous enteritis
- Intestinal tumours
  - Lymphosarcoma [esp Cat]
  - Adenocarcinoma
  - Fibrosarcoma
  - Leiomyoma/ Leiomyosarcoma
  - Undifferentiated sarcoma
  - Gastrinoma (Zollinger-Ellison Syndrome)
- Duodenal ulcer
- Toxic Enteritis
  - Enterotoxins
  - Drugs
  - Poisoning
- Lymphangiectasia [Dog]
- Mycotic Enteritis
  - Candida sp.
  - Aspergillus sp.
  - (Histoplasma sp.)

Maldigestion Syndrome

- Exocrine pancreatic insufficiency
- Bile acid deficiency

Other Causes

- Hypoalbuminaemia
  - Protein-losing enteropathy
  - Protein-losing nephropathy

- Portosystemic shunt
- Liver cirrhosis
- Cachexia
- Burns
- Exsudative body cavity effusions
- Chronic haemorrhage
- Hypothalamic tumour
- Feline lymphocytic cholangitis [Cat]

Diagnostic Approach

Polyphagia

1. **Case History**

2. **General Examination**

3. **Oral Cavity/ Pharyngeal Examination**

4. **Blood Tests**
- Hct, Ery, Leuc, Hb
- TP, Alb, Glob
- GPT, AP, Urea, Crea, BG
- Amylase, Lipase
- TLI Test
- Bile acids
- Ammonium
- Diff BC
- Na, K, Ca, P
- FIP Profile [Cat]
  - TP
  - Alb-/Glob Ratio
  - Bili
  - GOT
  - Serum electrophoresis
- Vit. B$_{12}$

MICROBIAL SEROLOGY
- FeLV-/FIV Antigen [Cat]

FUNCTION TESTS
- T$_4$, fT$_4$
- T$_3$ Suppression Test [Cat]
- Adrenal gland function test [Dog]
  - Dexamethasone Suppression test
  - ACTH Stimulation test
  - Cortisol/Creatinine Ratio

5. **Urinalysis**
- Urine dip stick
- Specific gravity
- Urine sediment

6. **Faecal Examination**
- Plain examination
- Flotation
- Chymotrypsin
- Elastase

7. **X-Ray Study**
- Skull

- Abdomen
- Thorax

8. Ultrasound

- Abdomen ± Liver biopsy
- Heart (Doppler Echocardiography)

9. Endoscopy

- Gastro-/Duodenoscopy ± Biopsy

10. Further Tests

- Analysis of body cavity fluid
- Spinal tap/analysis

Regurgitation

Retrograde oesophageal evacuation/retching of undigested food

Common Causes	
Dog	Cat
+++ Idiopathic megaoesophagus	+++ Idiopathic megaoesophagus
++ Myasthenia gravis	++ Myasthenia gravis
++ Persistent right aortic arch	+ Feline dysautonomia
++ Oesophageal foreign body	
++ Hypothyroidism	
++ Hypocortisolism (Addison's Disease)	

Oesophageal Diseases

Megaoesophagus (Motility Disorders)

- Congenital malformation
- Idiopathic megaoesophagus
- Myasthenia gravis
- Feline dysautonomia [Cat]
- Chronic oesophageitis
- Chronic oesophageal stenosis
- Hypothyroidism [Dog]
- Hypocortisolism (Addison's Disease) [Dog]
- Lupus erythematosus
- Botulism
- Tetanus

- Canine distemper virus [Dog]
- Brain stem disease
- Bilateral vagal lesion
- Dermatomyositis [Dog]
- Glycogen storage disease
- Thymoma
- Lead poisoning
- Thallium poisoning
- Organophosphate poisoning (chronic)
- (Trypanosoma cruzi [Dog])

Oesophageal Stenosis

- Oesophageal foreign body
- Hiatus hernia
- Gastric dilation/volvulus [Dog]

- Persistent right aortic arch
- Oesophageal tumours
- Mediastinal tumours
- Oesophageal stricture
- Oesophageal diverticulum
- (Spirocerca granulomata [Dog])

Oesophageitis

- Reflux oesophageitis [esp Dog]
- Chronic vomitus
- Foreign body oesophageitis
- (Spirocerca–oesophageitis [Dog])

Diagnostic Approach

Regurgitation

1. **Case History**

2. **General Examination**

3. **Vomitus Analysis**
- Food – digestive stage
- pH
- Bile

4. **Pharyngeal Examination**

5. **X-Ray Study**
- Throat
- Thorax
- Contrast oesophagogram/ Fluoroscopy

6. **Blood Tests**
- Hct, Ery, Leuc, Hb
- Na, K, Ca, P
- TP, Alb, Glob
- GPT, AP, Urea, Crea, BG
- Diff BC
- Chol, CK

MICROBIAL SEROLOGY
- FeLV-/FIV-Antigen [Cat]

IMMUNOSEROLOGY
- Autoantibodies against Acetylcholine receptors (Myasthenia gravis detection)
- ANA Test

FUNCTION TESTS
- Adrenal gland function tests [Dog]
  - Dexamethasone Suppression test
  - ACTH Stimulation test
  - Cortisol/Creatinine Ratio
- T_4, fT_4
- TSH-/TRH Stimulation test [Dog]

FURTHER TESTS
- Prostigmin®-/Tensilon® Test (Myasthenia gravis detection)

7. **Endoscopy**
- Oesophago-/Gastroscopy ± Biopsy

8. **Further Tests**
- Canine distemper virus antigen [Dog] (Conjunctival smear)
- Muscle biopsy

5 Urological Principal Symptoms

Urine, Bloody

Haematuria: Excretion of blood in the urine
Haemoglobinuria: Excretion of haemoglobin in the urine
Myoglobinuria: Excretion of myoglobin in the urine

Common Causes	
Dog	Cat
+++ Cystitis/Urethritis	+++ Cystitis/Urethritis
++ Prostatic disease	++ FUS/FLUTD
++ Hypersexuality (male)	++ Urolithiasis
++ Urolithiasis	++ Urinary tract tumours
++ Urinary tract tumours	++ Trauma
++ Trauma	++ Coagulopathy
++ Coagulopathies	

Renal Haemorrhage

- Trauma
- Pyelonephritis
  - E. coli
  - Staphylococcus sp.
  - Streptococcus sp.
  - Proteus sp.
  - Klebsiella sp.
  - Enterobacter sp.
  - Pseudomonas sp.
  - (Dioctophyma sp.)

- Nephrolithiasis
  - Struvite
  - Ca Carbonate
  - Ca Phosphate
  - Oxalate
  - Cystine
  - Urate
- Renal tumours
  - Lymphosarcoma
  - Renal carcinoma
  - Nephroblastoma
  - Cystadenocarcinoma
- Renal cysts

Ureteral/Bladder/ Urethral Haemorrhage

- Trauma
- Cystitis/Urethritis
  - E. coli
  - Staphylococcus sp.
  - Streptococcus sp.
  - Proteus sp.
  - Klebsiella sp.
  - Enterobacter sp.
  - Pseudomonas sp.
  - Candida sp.
  - Capillaria sp.
  - Cytostatics
- Urolithiasis
  - Struvite
  - Ca Carbonate
  - Ca Phosphate
  - Oxalate
  - Cystine
  - Urate
- Urinary tract tumour
  - Transitional cell carcinoma
  - Leiomyoma
  - Fibroma/Fibrosarcoma
  - Rhabdomyosarcoma

- Squamous cell carcinoma
- Canine transmissible venereal tumour
- Polyp
- Papilloma
- FUS/FLUTD [Cat]

Haemorrhage of the Genital Tract

Prostatic Haemorrhage

- Trauma
- Prostatic hyperplasia
- Prostatitis/Prostatic abscess
- Prostatic cysts
- Prostatic carcinoma

Uterine Haemorrhage

- Trauma
- Proestrus
- Postpartal placental abruption

Vaginal /Penile haemorrhage

- Trauma
- Hypersexuality (haemorrhage of the erectile tissue) [Dog]
- Canine transmissible venereal tumour

Coagulopathies

Thrombocytopenia

- Bone marrow damage
  - Infectious Causes
  - Toxic Causes
  - Immunoreactive Causes
  - Bone marrow tumours
- DIC
  - Septicaemia/Endotoxaemia

- Gastric dilation/volvulus [Dog]
- Pyometra
- Urinary tract infection
- Haemorrhagic enteritis
- Splenic torsion [esp Dog]
- Acute pancreatitis
- Shock
- Heart failure
- Liver failure
- Haemolysis
- Snake venom
- Heat stroke
- Electrical shock
- Burns
- FIP Coronavirus [Cat]
- Tumour disease
- (Dirofilaria sp. [esp Dog])
• Immune thrombocytopenia
- Infection
- Drugs
- Lupus erythematosus
• Infectious Thrombocytopenia
- FeLV/FIV [Cat]
- FIP Coronavirus [Cat]
- Parvovirus
- Canine distemper virus [Dog]
- CAV-1 (Hepatitis c. c.) [Dog]
- Canine Herpes virus [Dog]
- Leptospira sp. [Dog]
- Salmonella sp.
- Haemobartonella sp. [Cat]
- Babesia sp. [esp Dog]
- (Ehrlichia sp. [Dog])
- (Histoplasma sp.)
• Splenomegaly
• Chronic haemorrhage
• Thrombosis

Thrombocytopathy

• Acquired Thrombocytopenia
- Drugs
- Uraemia
- Liver failure
- Acute pancreatitis
- Bone tumours
- Hyperviscosity syndrome
• Congenital thrombocytopathy
- Von Willebrand Disease [esp Dog]
- Chediak-Higashi Syndrome [Cat]
- Thrombasthenia (Glanzmann) [Dog]
- Platelet aggregation defect
- Cyclic neutropenia [Grey Collie]

Plasmatic Coagulopathy

• Congenital Coagulopathy
- Factor VIII deficiency (Haemophilia A)
- Factor IX deficiency (Haemophilia B)
- Von Willebrand Disease [esp Dog]
- Factor VII deficiency [Dog]
- Factor X Deficiency [Dog]
- Factor XI deficiency [Dog]
- Factor XII deficiency (Hagemannn) [Cat]
- Vitamin K dependent coagulopathy [Cat]
• Vitamin K deficiency/ antagonism

- Liver failure
- Malabsorption syndrome
- Obstructive icterus
- Damage of the intestinal flora (Antibiotics)
- Dicoumarol poisoning (Rodenticides)
- DIC

Haemoglobinuria
Haemolysis

- Viral haemolysis
  - FeLV/FIV [Cat]
- Bacterial haemolysis
  - Leptospira sp. [Dog]
- Parasitic haemolysis
  - Babesia sp. [Dog]
  - Haemobartonella sp. [Cat]
  - (Ehrlichia sp. [Dog])
  - (Hepatozoon sp. [Dog])
  - (Dirofilaria sp. [esp Dog])
  - (Cytauxzoon sp. [Cat])
- Immunoreactive Haemolysis
  - Neonatal isoerythrolysis [Cat]
  - Blood transfusion incompatibility
  - Autoimmune haemolysis
  - Dug allergy
- Toxic Causes
  - Phenacetin
  - Propylene glycol
  - Antiarrhythmics
  - Anticonvulsants
  - Cimetidine
  - Levamisole
  - Metronidazole
  - Griseofulvin

- Phenothiazide
- Methylene blue
- Vitamin K
- Benzocaine
- Methionine
- Dimethyl sulfoxide
- Zinc
- Cytostatics
- Paracetamol
- Onions/Garlic/Broccoli
- Snake venom
- Water enema [Cat]
- Heavy metal poisoning
- Toxic plants (esp Dieffenbachia sp.)
- Metabolic Causes
  - Hypophosphataemia
  - Pyruvate kinase deficiency [Dog]
  - Phosphofructokinase deficiency
  - Copper storage disease [Dog]
  - Feline porphyria [Cat]
- Other causes
  - Heat stroke
  - Electrical accident
  - Extreme performance
  - DIC
  - Vasculitis
  - Haemangiosarcoma

Myoglobinuria
Rhabdomyolysis

- Muscle trauma
- Lactacidosis (aching muscles)
- Seizures
- Myositis
  - Toxoplasma sp.
  - Neospora sp. [Dog]

- Eosinophilic myositis [esp Dog]
- Dermatomyositis [Dog]
- (Ehrlichia sp. [Dog])

Diagnostic Approach

Urine, bloody

1. **Case History**

2. **General Examination**

3. **Blood Tests**
- Hct, Ery, Leuc
- TP
- Na, K, Ca
- Urea, Crea
- Diff BC

MICROBIAL SEROLOGY
- FeLV-/FIV Antigen [Cat]

COAGULATION
- Thrombocyte number
- Prothrombin time (PT/Quick)
- (Activated) partial Thromboplastin time (PTT/aPTT)
- Fibrin degradation product (FDP)
- Bleeding time

4. **Urinalysis**
- Urinary output/volume
- Urine dipstick
- Specific gravity

- Urine sediment
  - Bacteria
  - Erys, Leuc
  - Epithelial cells
  - Casts
  - Crystals
  - Tumour cytology
  - Bacterial culture (Cystocentesis)

5. **X-Ray Study**
- Abdomen
- Pelvis
- Contrast urethrography
- Contrast-/double contrast urography
- Excretory urography

6. **Ultrasound**
- Abdomen ± Biopsy

7. **Further Tests**
- Vaginoscopy
- Laparotomy

Urinary Urgency

Dysuria, Stranguria, Tenesmus vesicae: Painful urination disorder
Pollakiuria: Frequent urination of small amounts

Common Causes	
Dog	**Cat**
+++ Cystitis/Urethritis	+++ Cystitis/Urethritis
++ Prostatic enlargement	++ FUS/FLUTD
++ Urolithiasis	++ Bladder tumours
++ Reflex dyssynergia	++ Pelvic fractures
++ Bladder tumours	
+ Pelvic fractures	

Obstructive Causes

Urolithiasis

pH alkaline
- Struvite
- Ca Carbonate
- Ca Phosphate
- Ammonium urate

pH acidic
- Oxalate
- Cystine
- Urate

Prostatic enlargement

- Prostatitis/Prostatic abscess
- Prostatic hyperplasia
- Prostatic cysts
- Paraprostatic cyst
- Prostatic carcinoma

Urinary Tract Tumours

- Transitional cell carcinoma
- Leiomyoma
- Fibroma/Fibrosarcoma
- Squamous cell carcinoma
- Canine transmissible venereal tumour [Dog]
- Polyp
- Papilloma
- Rhabdomyosarcoma

Other Causes

- Perineal hernia [Dog]
- Pelvic fractures
- FUS/FLUTD [Cat]
- Post-traumatic urethral stricture
- Vaginal/Uterine prolapse

Inflammatory Causes

Cystitis/Urethritis

- Bacterial cystitis
  - E. coli
  - Staphylococcus sp.
  - Streptococcus sp.
  - Proteus sp.
  - Klebsiella sp.
  - Enterobacter sp.
  - Pseudomonas sp.
  - Corynebacterium sp.
- FUS/FLUTD [Cat]

Other causes

  - Pyelonephritis
  - Vaginitis
  - Endometritis
  - Balanoposthitis
- Mycotic cystitis

- Candida sp.
- Parasitic cystitis
  - Capillaria sp.
- Toxic cystitis
  - Cytostatics

Other Causes

- Reflex dyssynergia [Dog]
  - (Synchronous sphincter spasm and detrusor spasm in the male dog)

- Traumatic Causes
  - Bladder trauma/rupture
- Perianal disease
- Faecal urgency/rectal tenesmus
- Vaginitis/Endometritis
- Balanoposthitis
- Congenital defect
  - Urachal fistula
  - Urethral fistula
  - Ectopic ureters

Diagnostic Approach

Urinary Urgency

1. **Case History**

2. **General Examination**

3. **Neurological Examination**
- Spinal Reflexes
  - Bicipital reflex (C6–C8)
  - Triceps reflex (C7–T1)
  - Patellar reflex (L4–L6)
  - Withdrawal reflex (C6–T1 and L6–S1)
  - Cutaneous trunci reflex (C7–T1)
  - Anal sphincter reflex (S1–S3)
  - Bladder – can it be expressed?

4. **Blood Tests**
- Hct, Ery, Leuc
- TP
- Na, K, Ca
- Urea, Crea
- Diff BC

MICROBIAL SEROLOGY
- FeLV/FIV Antigen [Cat]

5. **Urinalysis**
- Urinary output/volume
- Urine dip stick
- Specific gravity
- Urine sediment
  - Bacteria, yeast fungi
  - Erys, Leuc
  - Epithelial cells
  - Casts
  - Crystals
  - Tumour cytology
- Bacterial/fungal culture (cystocentesis)

6. **X-Ray Study**
- Abdomen
- Pelvis
- Contrast urethrography
- Contrast/Double contrast urography
- Excretory urography

7. Ultrasound	8. Further Tests
• Abdomen	• Laparotomy

Urinary Incontinence and Retention

Involuntary passing of urine (urine dribbling)
Paradoxic urinary incontinence with retention bladder
(overflow bladder)

Common Causes	
Dog	Cat
+++ Cystitis/Urethritis	+++ Cystitis/Urethritis
++ Oestrogen deficiency	++ FUS/FLUTD
(Ovariohysterectomy)	++ Spinal disease
++ Spinal disease	
++ Obstructive Causes	

Full Bladder

Neurological Causes

Sphincter spasm (UMN Lesion)
• Spinal lesion cranial of S1
  – Discopathy
  – Vertebral fracture/luxation
  – Haemorrhage/Haematoma
  – Fibrocartilaginous Embolism
  – Tumours
  – Atlantoaxial subluxation [Dog]
  – Cervical Instability/ Stenosis (Wobbler Syndrome) [Dog]
  – Degenerative myelopathy
  – Myelitis
• Cerebral Causes
  – Traumatic brain injury
  – Encephalomeningitis
  – Brain tumours/Tumour metastasis

  – Granulomatous meningoencephalitis (GME)

Detrusor atony (LMN Lesion)
• Sacral spinal lesion (S1–S3)
  – Fracture of the sacral bone
  – Lumbosacral stenosis (Cauda equina syndrome) [Dog]
• Lesion of the pelvic nerves
• Lesion of the pudendal nerve
• Dysautonomia (Key-Gaskell Syndrome) [Cat]
• Tail avulsion [Cat]

Reflex dyssynergia
• Synchronous sphincter spasm and detrusor spasm in the male dog

Obstructive Causes

• Urolithiasis
pH alkaline
  – Struvite

- Ca Carbonate
- Ca Phosphate

pH acidic
- Oxalate
- Cystine
- Urate
- FUS/FLUTD [Cat]
- Urinary tract tumours
  - Transitional cell carcinoma
  - Leiomyoma
  - Fibroma/Fibrosarcoma
  - Rhabdomyosarcoma
  - Squamous cell carcinoma
  - Canine transmissible venereal tumour [Dog]
  - Polyp
  - Papilloma
- Prostatic enlargement [Dog]
  - Prostatitis/Prostatic abscess
  - Prostatic hyperplasia
  - Prostatic cysts
  - Paraprostatic cyst
  - Prostatic carcinoma
- Other causes

- Post-traumatic urethral stricture
- Cystitis/Urethritis
- Pelvic fractures

Empty Bladder

- Sphincter atony
  - Oestrogen deficiency [esp Dog] (ovariohysterectomy)
  - Testosterone deficiency
  - Post-traumatic (Urinary catheter)
  - Post obstruction (bladder distension)
  - Pregnancy
- Detrusor spasm (irritable bladder)
  - Bacterial cystitis
  - Psychogenic
- Congenital causes
  - Ectopic ureters
  - Urachal fistula
  - Urethral fistula

Diagnostic Approach

Urinary Incontinence and Retention

1. **Case History**

2. **General Examination**

3. **Neurological Examination**
- Awareness/behaviour
- Body/limb posture and stance
- Locomotion
- Muscle tone/strength
- Spinal reflexes
  - Bicipital reflex (C6–C8)
  - Triceps reflex (C7–T1)
  - Patellar reflex (L4–L6)
  - Withdrawal reflex (C6–T1 and L6–S1)
  - Cutaneous trunci reflex (C7–T1)
  - Anal sphincter reflex (S1–S3)
  - Bladder – can it be expressed?

4. **Blood Tests**
- Hct, Ery, Leuc
- TP

- Na, K, Ca
- Urea, Crea
- Diff BC

MICROBIAL SEROLOGY
- FeLV-/FIV Antigen [Cat]

5. Urinalysis
- Urinary output/volume
- Urine dip stick
- Specific gravity
- Urine sediment
  - Bacteria
  - Erythrocytes, Leucocyte
  - Epithelial cells
  - Casts
  - Crystals

- – Tumour cytology
- Bacterial culture (Cystocentesis)

6. X-Ray Study
- Abdomen/Pelvis
- Spine ± Myelography
- Contrast urethrography
- Contrast/Double contrast urography
- Excretory urography

7. Ultrasound
- Abdomen

8. Further Tests
- Laparotomy
- Analysis of spinal tap fluid

Clinical Distinguishing Features of Urinary Incontinence/Retention with a Full Bladder

	Ability to empty the bladder manually	
	easy	difficult

Easy to catheterise	• Detrusor atony (LMN Lesion) (Overflow bladder)
	  – Sacral spinal lesion (S1–S3)
	  – Lesion of the pelvic nerve
	  – Lesion of the pudendal nerve
	  – Dysautonomia (Key-Gaskell Syndrome)
		• Reflex dyssynergia (Synchronous sphincter spasm and detrusor spasm in the male dog)

Difficult to catheterise		• Sphincter spasm (UMN Lesion)
		  – Spinal lesion cranial of S1
		  – Cerebral causes
		• Urinary tract obstruction

Urinary Tract Infections, Chronic Recurrent

Potential sources of error/causes with ongoing and repeated urinary tract infections

Therapeutic failure

- Choice of antibiotic
- Dosage error
- Too short treatment duration
- Bacterial resistancy

Reinfection/Superinfection

- Urinary tract obstruction
  - Urolithiasis
  - FUS/FLUTD [Cat]
  - Tumour of the urinary tract
  - Prostatic enlargement
  - Pelvic fractures
  - Post-traumatic urethral stricture
- Infection reservoir (source of infection)
  - Pyelonephritis
  - Vaginitis
  - Endometritis
  - Prostatitis [Dog]
  - Balanoposthitis
  - Abscess
  - Septicaemia
  - Urachal diverticulum
  - Urethrostomy
  - Rectovaginal fistula
  - Perianal disease
- Mycotic cystitis
  - Candida sp.
- Parasitic cystitis
  - Capillaria sp.
- Glucosuria
  - Diabetes mellitus
  - Chronic renal failure
- Frequent catheterisation
- Neurogenic urinary incontinence
- Immunosuppression
  - **Primary Immunosuppression**
  - **Secondary Immunosuppression**
  - FeLV/FIV [Cat]
  - Glucocorticoid long term therapy
  - Hypercortisolism (Cushing's Disease) [Dog]

Diagnostic Approach

Urinary Tract Infections, Chronic Recurrent

1. **Case History**

2. **General Examination**

3. **Blood Tests**
- Hct, Ery, Leuc
- Diff BC

- TP
- Na, K, Ca
- Urea, Crea

MICROBIAL SEROLOGY
- FeLV-/FIV Antigen [Cat]

4. Urinalysis
- Urinary output/volume
- Urine dip stick
- Specific gravity
- Urine sediment
  - Bacteria, Yeast fungi
  - Erys, Leuc
  - Epithelial cells
  - Casts
  - Crystals

  - Tumour cytology
- Bacterial/Fungal culture (Cystocentesis) (+ sensitivity)

5. X-Ray Study
- Abdomen
- Pelvis
- Contrast urethrography
- Contrast/double contrast urography
- Excretory urography

6. Ultrasound
- Abdomen

7. Further Tests
- Laparotomy

Oliguria/Anuria

Urinary output < 0.25ml/kg/h

Common Causes	
Dog	Cat
+++ Shock	+++ Shock
++ Urinary tract obstruction	++ Urinary tract obstruction
++ Acute renal failure	++ Acute renal failure
++ Chronic renal failure (final stage)	++ Chronic renal failure (final stage)

Prerenal Causes

- Hypovolaemia
  - Dehydration
  - Shock
  - Blood loss
- Congestive heart failure

Renal Causes

Acute Renal Failure

- Renal ischaemia
  - Trauma
  - Hypovolaemia
  - Hypotension
  - Anaesthesia

- Septicaemia
- Renal infarction
- Toxic nephritis
  Nephrotoxins
  - Haemoglobinuria/ Myoglobinuria
  - Amphotericin B
  - Aminoglycosides (esp Gentamicin)
  - Piperazine
  - Cephalosporines
  - Sulfonamides
  - Tetracyclines
  - NSAID
  - Cytostatics
  - Methoxyflurane
  - Mycotoxins
  - Ethylene glycol poisoning
  - Heavy metal poisoning
  - Toxic plants
  - Household agents
- Glomerulonephritis
  Immune Complex Disease
  - FeLV/FIV [Cat]
  - FIP Coronavirus [Cat]
  - CAV-1 (Hepatitis c. c.) [Dog]
  - Brucella sp. [Dog]
  - Lyme Borreliosis sp. [Dog]
  - Mycoplasma sp. [esp Cat]
  - Septicaemia/bacterial endocarditis
  - Chronic bacterial infection
  - (Leishmania sp. [esp Dog])
  - (Ehrlichia sp. [Dog])
  - (Dirofilaria sp. [esp Dog])
  - Pyometra
  - Prostatitis [Dog]
  - Pancreatitis
  - Tumour disease
  - Lupus erythematosus

- Rheumatoid arthritis
- Hypercortisolism (Cushing's Disease) [Dog]
- Glucocorticoid long term therapy
- Diabetes mellitus
- Pyelonephritis
  - E. coli
  - Staphylococcus sp.
  - Streptococcus sp.
  - Proteus sp.
  - Klebsiella sp.
  - Enterobacter sp.
  - Pseudomonas sp.
  - (Dioctophyma sp.)
- Interstitial nephritis
  - Leptospira sp. [Dog]
  - CAV-1 [Dog]
  - Klebsiella sp.
  - E. coli
  - Proteus sp.
  - Staphylococcus sp.
  - Streptococcus sp.

Chronic Renal Failure (End Stage)

- Interstitial nephritis
- Renal amyloidosis
- Glomerulonephritis
- Pyelonephritis
- Renal tumours
  - Lymphosarcoma [esp Cat]
  - Renal carcinoma
  - Nephroblastoma
  - Cystadenocarcinoma [Dog]
- Renal cirrhosis (fibrosis)
- Renal abscess/-haematoma
- Renal calcification
- Nephrolithiasis
  - Struvite
  - Ca Carbonate

- Ca Phosphate
- Oxalate
- Cystine
- Urate
- Renal cysts [Cat]

Postrenal Causes

Urinary Obstruction

- Urolithiasis
  pH alkaline
  - Struvite
  - Ca Carbonate
  - Ca Phosphate
  pH acidic
  - Oxalate
  - Cystine
  - Urate
- FUS/FLUTD [Cat]
- Urinary tumours
  - Transitional cell carcinoma
  - Leiomyoma
  - Fibroma/Fibrosarcoma
  - Rhabdomyosarcoma

- Squamous cell carcinoma
- Canine transmissible venereal tumour [Dog]
- Polyp
- Prostatic enlargement
  - Prostatitis/prostatic abscess
  - Prostatic hyperplasia
  - Prostatic cysts
  - Paraprostatic cyst
  - Prostatic carcinoma
- Other causes
  - Post-traumatic urethral stricture
  - Cystitis/urethritis
  - Pelvic fractures

Traumatic Causes

- Neurological micturition disturbance
- Bladder rupture/perforation
- Urethral perforation
- Ureteral avulsion

Diagnostic Approach

Oliguria/Anuria

1. Case History

2. General Examination

3. Neurological Examination
- Spinal reflexes
  - Bicipital reflex (C6–C8)
  - Triceps reflex (C7–T1)
  - Patellar reflex (L4–L6)
  - Withdrawal reflex (C6–T1 and L6–S1)
  - Cutaneous trunci reflex (C7–T1)
  - Anal sphincter reflex (S1–S3)
  - Bladder – can it be expressed?

4. Blood Tests
- Hct, Ery, Leuc
- TP, Alb, Glob
- Na, K, Ca
- Urea, Crea
- Diff BC

- FIP Profile [Cat]
  - TP
  - Alb/Glob Ratio
  - Bili
  - GOT
  - Serum electrophoresis
- Ethylene glycol detection
- FeLV-/FIV Antigen [Cat]
- Leptospira Antibodies [Dog]

5. Urinalysis
- Urinary output/volume
- Urine dip stick
- Specific gravity
- Urine sediment
  - Bacteria, Yeast fungi
  - Erys, Leuc
  - Epithelial cells
  - Casts
  - Crystals
  - Tumour cytology
- Bacterial/Fungal culture (Cystocentesis)

6. X-Ray Study
- Abdomen
- Pelvis
- Contrast urethrography
- Contrast/Double contrast urography
- Excretory urography

7. Ultrasound
- Abdomen ± renal biopsy

8. Further Tests
- Electrocardiogram (ECG)
- Laparotomy

Polydipsia/Polyuria

Polydipsia: increased water intake (Dog: > 90 ml/kg/day, Cat: > 45 ml/kg/day)
Polyuria: increased urination (Dog/Cat: > 45 ml/kg/day)

Common Causes	
Dog	Cat
+++ Pyometra	+++ Chronic renal failure
+++ Diabetes mellitus	
++ Diabetes insipidus	++ Diabetes mellitus
++ Glucocorticoid therapy	++ Hyperthyroidism
++ Hypercortisolism (Cushing's Disease)	
++ Chronic renal failure	
+ Liver disease	

Renal Causes

Chronic Renal Failure

- Glomerulonephritis
  - FeLV/FIV [Cat]
  - FIP Coronavirus [Cat]
  - CAV-1 (Hepatitis c. c.) [Dog]
  - Brucella sp. [Dog]
  - Lyme Borrelia sp. [Dog]
  - (Leishmania sp. [esp Dog])
  - (Ehrlichia sp. [Dog])
  - (Dirofilaria sp. [esp Dog])
  - Mycoplasma sp. [esp Cat]
  - Septicaemia/bacterial endocarditis
  - Chronic bacterial infection
  - Pyometra
  - Prostatitis [Dog]
  - Pancreatitis
  - Tumour disease
  - Lupus erythematosus
  - Rheumatoid arthritis
  - Hypercortisolism (Cushing's disease) [Dog]
  - Glucocorticoid long term therapy
  - Diabetes mellitus
- Pyelonephritis
  - E. coli
  - Staphylococcus sp.
  - Streptococcus sp.
  - Proteus sp.
  - Klebsiella sp.
  - Enterobacter sp.
  - Pseudomonas sp.
  - (Dioctophyma sp.)
- Interstitial nephritis
- Nephrotoxins
  - Haemoglobinuria/ Myoglobinuria
  - Amphotericin B
  - Aminoglycosides
  - Cephalosporines
  - Sulfonamides
  - Tetracyclines
  - NSAID
  - Cytostatics
  - Methoxyflurane
  - Mycotoxins
  - Ethylene glycol poisoning
  - Heavy metal poisoning
  - Toxic plants
  - Household agents
- Renal tumours
  - Lymphosarcoma [esp Cat]
  - Renal carcinoma
  - Nephroblastoma
  - Cystadenocarcinoma [Dog]
- Renal amyloidosis
- Nephrolithiasis
  - Struvite
  - Ca Carbonate
  - Ca Phosphate
  - Oxalate
  - Cystine
  - Urate
- Renal cysts

Other Causes

- Postobstructive diuresis
- Polyuric phase after acute renal failure

Extrarenal Causes

Drugs

- Glucocorticoids
- Anticonvulsants
  - Phenobarbital
  - Primidon

- Diuretics
- Continuous drip infusion
- Thyroid hormone supplementation
- Salty food
- Vitamin D

Metabolic Causes

- Hypercortisolism (Cushing's disease) [Dog]
- Diabetes mellitus
- Hyperthyroidism [Cat]
- Hypercalcaemia
- Hypokalaemia [esp Cat]
- Hyponatriaemia
- Hypoglycaemia (Insulinoma)

- Central/renal diabetes insipidus [esp Dog]
- Hypoaldosteronism [Dog]
- Hypocortisolism (Addison's disease) [Dog]
- Acromegaly (STH excess)
- Phaeochromocytoma

Other Causes

- Pyometra
- Fever
- Psychogenic Causes
- Acute hepatitis
- Liver cirrhosis/portocaval shunt
- Polycythaemia vera

Diagnostic Approach

Polydipsia/Polyuria

1. **Case History**

2. **General Examination**

3. **Blood Tests**
- Hct, Ery, Leuc
- Na, K, Ca, P
- TP, Alb, Glob
- GPT, AP, Urea, Crea
- BG
- Blood Sedimentation Rate (BSR)
- FIP Profile [Cat]
  - TP
  - Alb/Glob Ratio
  - Bili
  - GOT
  - Serum electrophoresis
- Diff BC

MICROBIAL SEROLOGY
- FeLV-/FIV Antigen [Cat]

FUNCTION TESTS
- Adrenal gland function test [Dog]
  - Dexamethasone Suppression test
  - ACTH Stimulation test
  - Cortisol/Creatinine Ratio
- T_4, fT_4
- T_3 Suppression test [Cat]
- Urine concentration test [Dog]
- Creatinine/Inulin Clearance Test
- ADH Test [Dog]
- Parathormone

4. **Urinalysis**
- Urinary output/volume
- Urine dip stick
- Specific gravity

- Urine sediment
  - Bacteria, Yeast fungi
  - Erys, Leuc
  - Epithelial cells
  - Casts
  - Crystals
  - Tumour cytology
- Bacterial/Fungal culture
  (Cystocentesis)

5. X-Ray Study
- Abdomen

- Pelvis
- Contrast urethrography
- Contrast/Double contrast urography
- Excretory urography

6. Ultrasound
- Abdomen ± renal biopsy

7. Further Tests
- Laparotomy

Renomegaly

Kidney enlargement: Renal diameter (Pole to pole) > 3–3.5 × lumbar vertebra L2 (vd radiographic plane)

Common Causes	
Dog	Cat
+++ Renal tumours	+++ Renal tumours
++ Hydronephrosis	++ Renal cysts
	++ FIP

Unilateral Renomegaly

- Trauma
  - Haematoma
- Renal tumours
  - Renal carcinoma [Dog]
  - Nephroblastoma
- Hydronephrosis
  - Urolithiasis
  - Ureteral stricture
  - Renal tumours
  - Pyelonephritis
- Compensatory renal hypertrophy
  - Cirrhotic kidney

  - Nephrectomy
  - Renal infarction
  - Renal dysplasia
- Renal abscess

Bilateral Renomegaly

- Renal tumours
  - Lymphosarcoma [Cat]
  - Cystadenocarcinoma [German Shepherd Dog]
- Nephritis
  - Leptospira sp. [Dog]
  - FIP Coronavirus [Cat]
- Hydronephrosis

- Urolithiasis
- Ureteral stricture
- Renal tumours
- Pyelonephritis

- Renal cysts
- Ethylene glycol poisoning
- Diabetes mellitus

Diagnostic Approach

Renomegaly

1. Case History
2. General Examination
3. Blood Tests
- Hct, Ery, Leuc
- TP, Alb, Glob
- Na, K, Ca
- Urea, Crea
- FIP Profile [Cat]
  - TP
  - Alb/Glob ratio
  - Bili
  - GOT
  - Serum electrophoresis
- Diff BC

MICROBIAL SEROLOGY
- FeLV-/FIV Antigen [Cat]
- Leptospira Antibodies [Dog]

4. Urinalysis
- Urinary output/volume
- Urine dip stick
- Specific gravity

- Urine sediment
  - Bacteria, Yeast fungi
  - Erys, Leuc
  - Epithelial cells
  - Casts
  - Crystals
  - Tumour cytology
- Bacterial/Fungal culture
  (Cystocentesis)

5. X-Ray Study
- Abdomen
- Pelvis
- Contrast urethrography
- Contrast/Double contrast
  urography
- Excretory urography

6. Ultrasound
- Abdomen ± renal biopsy

7. Further Tests
- Laparotomy

6 Principal Symptoms of the Reproductive Tract

Further Relevant Principal Symptoms

Miscarriage/Foetal Death

Premature termination of the pregnancy via delivery or foetal death

Common Causes	
Dog	**Cat**
+++ Systemic infections	+++ Systemic infections
++ Brucellosis	++ FeLV/FIV
++ Uterine disease	++ Uterine disease
++ Endocrinopathies	++ Endocrinopathies

Maternal Factors

Infectious Causes

- Viral causes
  - FeLV/FIV [Cat]
  - Canine/feline Herpes virus
  - Canine/feline Parvovirus
  - Canine distemper virus [Dog]
- Bacterial causes
  - Brucella sp. [Dog]
  - Mycoplasma sp.
  - E. coli
  - Salmonella sp.
  - Campylobacter sp.
  - Mycobacterium sp.
- Rickettsial causes
  - Coxiella sp. (Q Fever) [Dog]
- Parasitic causes
  - Toxoplasma sp.
- Endometritis/Pyometra
  - E. coli

Other Diseases

- Uterine diseases
  - Trauma

  - Glandular cystic endometrial hyperplasia
  - Uterine prolapse
  - Uterine torsion
  - Uterine rupture
  - Uterine adhesions
  - Congenital uterine malformation
  - Extrauterine pregnancy
  - Uterine tumours
- Endocrine Causes
  - Hypothyroidism [Dog]
  - Diabetes mellitus
  - Corpus luteum dysfunction
- Drugs
  - Chloramphenicol
  - Oestrogens
  - Glucocorticoids
  - Prostaglandins
  - Bromocriptine
  - Cytostatics
  - Ergotamine
  - Toxic plants

Foetal Factors

- Lethal genetic defects
- Lethal developmental disorders

Diagnostic Approach

Miscarriage/Foetal Death

1. Case History

2. General Examination

3. X-Ray Study
- Abdomen

4. Blood Tests
- Hct, Ery, Leuc
- Na, K, Ca
- TP, Alb, Glob
- GPT, AP, Urea, Crea, BG
- Diff BC

MICROBIAL SEROLOGY
- FeLV-/FIV Antigen [Cat]
- Brucella Antibodies [Dog]
- Toxoplasma Antibodies

FUNCTION TESTS
- T_4, fT_4

- TSH-/TRH Stimulation Test [Dog]
- Serum Progesteron

5. Urinalysis
- Urine dip stick
- Specific gravity
- Urine sediment

6. Endoscopy
- Vaginoscopy
  ± Vaginal smear
  − Cytology
  − Bacterial culture

7. Further Tests
- Histopathological examination of the placenta and dead foetuses

Fertility Disorders

Ovulation: Dog: ca. 48 h after LH Peak (2nd third of the oestrus)
Cat: 24–48 h after mating
Mating date: 2nd–4th day of the receptive period (Serum progesterone > 5 ng/ml)
Pregnancy diagnosis: Ultrasound from day 25, Palpation: from day 30, X-Rays: from day 50
Gestation period: Dog: 63 days; Cat: 60 days

Common Causes	
Dog	Cat
+++ Wrong mating date	+++ Infectious disease
++ Infectious disease	

Female Causes of Infertility

- Wrong mating date [Dog]
- Ovariectomy
- Ovariohysterectomy
- Rejection/aversion of partner
- Sexual immaturity
- Endometritis/pyometra
- Glandular cystic endometrial hyperplasia [Dog]
- Ovarian cysts
- Ovarian tumours
- Embryonic death/resorption
- Absent ovulation stimulus [Cat]
- Infectious causes
  - FeLV/FIV [Cat]
  - Canine/feline Herpes virus
  - Canine/feline Parvovirus
  - Canine distemper virus [Dog]
  - Brucella sp. [Dog]
  - Mycoplasma sp. [esp Cat]
  - E. coli
  - Salmonella sp.
  - Campylobacter sp.
  - Mycobacterium sp.
- Endocrine causes
  - Hypothyroidism [Dog]
  - Hypercortisolism (Cushing's Disease) [Dog]
- Uterine malformations
- Chromosomal defects
- Extrauterine pregnancy

Male Causes of Infertility

- Sexual immaturity
- Disruptive factors/pain
- Testicular hypoplasia/ degeneration
  - Orchitis
  - High age

- Endogenous/exogenous oestrogen
- Hypothyroidism [Dog]
- Hypercortisolism (Cushing's disease) [Dog]
- Klinefelter's syndrome (XXY)
- Ketoconazole
- Hypothalamic lesion
- Warmth/radiation
- Heavy metal poisoning
- Bilateral cryptorchism
- Orchitis/Epididymitis
  - Canine distemper virus [Dog]
  - FIP Coronavirus [Cat]
  - Brucella sp. [Dog]
  - Staphylococcus sp.
  - Streptococcus sp.
  - E. coli
  - Mycoplasma sp. [esp Cat]
  - (Ehrlichia sp. [Dog])
  - (Rickettsia sp. [Dog])
  - Autoimmune diseases
- Testicular tumours [esp Dog]
  - Sertoli cell tumour
  - Leydig cell tumour
  - Seminoma
- Prostatic disease [Dog]
- Balanoposthitis
- Penile/Preputial tumours
- Phimosis
- Systemic disease
- Drugs
  - Ketoconazole
  - Glucocorticoids
  - Anabolics
  - Antiparasitics
- Pathological retrograde ejaculation
- Spermatocele

Diagnostic Approach

Female Fertility Disturbances

1. Case History

2. General Examination

3. Endoscopy
- Vaginoscopy
  ± Vaginal smear
  - Cytology
  - Bacterial culture

4. Blood Tests
- Hct, Ery, Leuc
- Na, K, Ca
- TP, Alb, Glob
- GPT, AP, Urea, Crea, BG
- FIP Profile [Cat]
  - TP
  - Alb/Glob ratio
  - Bili
  - GOT
  - Serum electrophoresis
- Diff BC

MICROBIAL SEROLOGY
- FeLV-/FIV Antigen [Cat]

- Brucella Antibodies [Dog]
- Toxoplasma Antibodies
- Herpes virus Antibodies

FUNCTION TESTS
- Serum Progesterone
- T_4, fT_4
- TSH-/TRH Stimulation test [Dog]
- Adrenal gland function test [Dog]
  - Dexamethasone Suppression test
  - ACTH Stimulation test
  - Cortisol/Creatinine Ratio

5. Urinalysis
- Urine dip stick
- Specific gravity
- Urine sediment

6. Ultrasound
- Abdomen

Diagnostic Approach

Male Fertility Disturbances

1. Case History

2. General Examination

3. Penile/Preputial Examination
  ± Preputial smear
  - Cytology
  - Bacterial culture

4. Ejaculate Analysis
- Amount, colour, consistency
- Sperm density
- Sperm motility, Sperm vitality
- Sperm anomalies
- AP
- Leuco, Erys
- Bacterial culture
- Karyotyping

5. Blood Tests

- Hct, Ery, Leuc
- Na, K, Ca
- TP, Alb, Glob
- GPT, AP, Urea, Crea, BG
- FIP Profile [Cat]
  - TP
  - Alb/Glob ratio
  - Bili
  - GOT
  - Serum electrophoresis
- Diff BC

MICROBIAL SEROLOGY

- FeLV-/FIV Antigen [Cat]
- Brucella Antibodies [Dog]

FUNCTION TESTS

- Serum Testosterone

- T_4, fT_4
- TSH-/TRH stimulation test [Dog]
- Dexamethasone Screening test/ ACTH stimulation test [Dog]

6. Urinalysis

- Urine dip stick
- Specific gravity
- Urine sediment

7. Ultrasound

  $\pm$ Testicular biopsy
  - Cytology
  - Bacterial culture

Dystocia

Physiological Parturition:

1. Temperature drop of 1–1.5 °C shortly before parturition
2. Cervical opening stage
   - Opening contractions (6–12 h)
3. Foetal delivery
   - Active contractions (abdominal muscle pressure) (< 4 h)
   - Rupture of the foetal membrane
   - Delivery
4. After birth stage
   - Placental delivery variably one by one after each birth or all together (< 1 h)

Abnormal parturition (Dystocia):

1. Poor maternal general condition
2. Strong non-productive active contractions > 30 min
3. Time interval between rupture of the foetal membrane and delivery of the first foetus > 4 h
4. Time intervals in between deliveries > 2 h
5. Gestation > 70 d

Common Causes	
Dog	Cat
+++ Foetal factors	+++ Foetal factors
++ Obstructed birth canal	++ Obstructed birth canal
++ Uterine inertia	++ Uterine inertia

Maternal Factors

Uterine Inertia

- Exhaustion
- Hypoglycaemia
- Hypocalcaemia (Eclampsia)
- Dehydration
- Uterine rupture
- Diaphragmatic hernia
- Abdominal pain
- Systemic disease
- Nervousness
- Obesity
- Age (young/old)

Obstructed Birth Canal

- Narrow pelvis (brachycephalic dog breeds)
- Pelvic fractures (healed)
- Not fully dilated cervix
- Dry birth canal
- Uterine tumours
- Glandular cystic endometrial hyperplasia
- Uterine adhesions
- Uterine torsion
- Congenital uterine malformations

Foetal Factors

- Foetal oversize (uniparous delivery)
- Foetal position/pose anomalies
- Foetal death
- Foetal malformations

Diagnostic Approach

Dystocia

1. **Case History**

2. **General Examination**

3. **Endoscopy**
- Vaginoscopy (Cervical position)

4. **X-Ray Study**
- Pelvis
- Abdomen

5. **Ultrasound**

- Foetal vital signs
- Foetal position/pose anomalies

6. **Blood Tests**
- Hct
- TP, BG
- Na, K, Ca

7. **Further Tests**
- Digital Examination (obstructed birth canal)

Testicular Enlargement

Larger than normal size of testes uni or bilaterally

Common Causes	
Dog	Cat
+++ Testicular tumours	+++ Bite/scratch wounds
++ Scrotal dermatitis	++ Orchitis/Epididymitis
++ Orchitis/Epididymitis	

Testicular Disease

Orchitis/Epididymitis

- Viral orchitis
  - Canine distemper virus [Dog]
  - FIP Coronavirus [Cat]
- Bacterial orchitis
  - Brucella sp. [Dog]
  - Staphylococcus sp.
  - Streptococcus sp.
  - E. coli
  - Mycoplasma sp [esp Cat]
- Rickettsial orchitis
  - (Ehrlichia sp. [Dog])
  - (Rickettsia sp. [Dog])

- Autoimmune disease

Testicular Tumours

- Sertoli cell tumour [esp Dog]
- Leydig cell tumour [esp Dog]
- Seminoma [esp Dog]

Other Causes

- Haematoma
- Bite wounds
- Scrotal dermatitis [esp Dog]
- Scrotal hernia
- Testicular torsion [esp Dog]
- Spermatocele

Diagnostic Approach

Testicular Enlargement

1. **Case History**

2. **General Examination**

3. **Testicular palpation**

4. **Ultrasound**
   - Testicle/Epididymis

5. **Ejaculate Analysis**
   - Cytology
   - Bacterial culture

6. **Blood Tests**
   - Hct, Ery, Leuc
   - FIP Profile [Cat]

- TP
- Alb/Glob Ratio
- Bili
- GOT
- Serum electrophoresis

MICROBIAL SEROLOGY
- FeLV-/FIV Antigen [Cat]

- Brucella Antibodies [Dog]

7. Further Tests
- Testicular biopsy
  - Cytology
  - Bacterial culture

Mammary Discharge

Fluid secretion from the mammary gland in the female

Common Causes		
Dog		Cat
+++ Pregnancy		+++ Pregnancy
++ Pseudopregnancy		++ Mastitis
++ Mastitis		++ Ulcerating Mammary tumours
++ Ulcerating Mammary tumours		

Milk Secretion (Galactorrhoea)

- Pregnancy
- Pseudopregnancy
- Hypothyroidism [Dog]
- Pituitary gland tumour

Purulent Discharge

Mastitis

- Bacterial Mastitis
  - E. coli
  - Staphylococcus sp.
  - Streptococcus sp.

Ulcerating Mammary Tumour

- Adenocarcinoma

Haemorrhagic Discharge

Mastitis

- Bacterial Mastitis
  - E. coli
  - Staphylococcus sp.
  - Streptococcus sp.

Mammary Tumours

- Adenocarcinoma
- Squamous cell carcinoma
- Sarcoma
- Mixed tumour
- Myoepithelioma
- Haemangiosarcoma

Traumatic Causes

- Blunt/sharp trauma
- Foreign body
- Haematoma

Diagnostic Approach

Mammary Discharge

1. **Case History**

2. **General Examination**

3. **Palpation of the Mammary Gland**

4. **Fluid Analysis of the Mammary Discharge**
   - Cytology
   - Bacterial culture

5. **Ultrasound**
   - Uterus

   - – Pregnancy exclusion
   - Mammary Glands

6. **X-Ray Study**
   - Thorax (in presence of mammary tumours)

7. **Blood Tests**
   - Hct, Ery, Leuc
   - Diff BC

Mammary Enlargement

Increased size of the mammary gland in the female or male

Common Causes	
Dog	Cat
+++ Pregnancy	+++ Pregnancy
++ Pseudopregnancy	++ Malignant mammary tumours (ca. 90%)
++ Malignant mammary tumours (ca. 50%)	++ Mastitis
++ Precancerous mammary (ca. 25%)	++ Feline fibroadenomatosis
++ Benign mammary tumours (ca. 25%)	
+ Mastitis	

In the Female Animal

Mammopathy

- Milk
  - Pregnancy
  - Pseudopregnancy
- Bacterial Mastitis
  - E. coli
  - Staphylococcus sp.
  - Streptococcus sp.
- Mammary Tumours

Benign Mammary Tumours

  - Adenoma, complex Adenoma
  - Lipoma
  - Mixed tumour
  - Haemangioma
  - Cysts
  - Myoepithelioma
  - Fibroma
  - Osteoma
  - Chondroma

Malignant Mammary Tumours

  - Adenocarcinoma
  - Squamous cell carcinoma
  - Mixed tumour
  - Myoepithelial carcinoma
  - Complex carcinoma
  - Poorly differentiated carcinoma
  - Carcinosarcoma
  - Fibrosarcoma
  - Osteosarcoma
  - Chondrosarcoma
  - Liposarcoma
  - Lymphosarcoma
  - Lymphoma
  - Mast cell sarcoma
  - Mast cell tumour
- Other Causes
  - Foreign body
  - Abscess
  - Haematoma
  - Larva migrans granuloma

In the Male Animal

Gynaecomastia

- Testicular tumours (endogenous oestrogen) [esp Dog]
  - Sertoli cell tumour
  - Leydig cell tumour
  - Seminoma
- Orchitis
  - Canine distemper virus [Dog]
  - FIP Coronavirus [Cat]
  - Brucella sp. [Dog]
  - Staphylococcus sp.
  - Streptococcus sp.
  - E. coli
  - Mycoplasma sp. [esp Cat]
  - (Ehrlichia sp. [Dog])
  - Autoimmune disease
- Mammary tumours
- Drugs
  - Gestagens
  - Ketoconazole
  - Metronidazole
- Other Causes
  - Foreign body
  - Abscess
  - Haematoma

Diagnostic Approach

Mammary Enlargement

1. **Case History**

2. **General Examination**

3. **Palpation of the Mammary Gland**

4. **Fluid Analysis (of Mammary Discharge)**
- Cytology
- Bacterial culture

5. **Testicular Examination (Male)**
- Palpation

- Ultrasound

6. **X-Ray Study**
- Thorax (in presence of mammary tumours)

7. **Blood Tests**
- Hct, Ery, Leuc
- GPT, AP, Urea, Crea, BG

8. **Further Tests**
- Histopathological examination after mastectomy

Penile Prolapse

Paraphimosis: Penile strangulation caused during erection due to a too narrow preputial opening (phimosis)

Priapism: Painful and persistent erection in absence of a sexual stimulus

Paraphimosis

- Congenital phimosis
- Acquired phimosis
  - cicatricial stricture
- Preputial eversion
- Adhesions of hair on the glans penis
- Penile oedema
- Fracture of the penile bone
- Penile tumours
  - Canine transmissible venereal tumour
  - Squamous cell carcinoma
  - Haemangiosarcoma
  - Melanoma
  - Mast cell tumour
  - Papilloma

Priapismus

- Thrombosis of the erectile tissue

Diagnostic Approach

Penile Prolapse

1. Case History

2. General Examination

3. Penile Examination

4. X-Ray Study
- Penis

5. Ultrasound
- Erectile tissue

Postpartal Complications

Puerperal disorder

In the Mother

- Birth Injury
  - Perineal tear
  - Organ rupture (uterus, cervix, vagina, bladder, abdominal wall)
  - Bladder paralysis
  - Pelvic fractures
  - Luxation of the sacral bone
  - Uterine prolapse
  - Vaginal prolapse
  - Rectal prolapse
  - Pulmonary emphysema
  - Haemorrhage
- Placental subinvolution [Dog]
  - Eosinophilic collagenous accumulation
- Endometritis/Pyometra
- Endotoxicosis
  - Placental retention
  - Placental subinvolution
  - Endometritis/pyometra
- Bacterial Mastitis
  - E. coli
  - Staphylococcus sp.
  - Streptococcus sp.

- Eclampsia
  - Hypocalcaemic tetany
- Placental retention [Dog]
- Agalactia
- Disturbed nurturing behaviour
  - Exaggerated nurturing
  - Disinterest
  - Aggression/infanticide

In the Neonate

- Birth Injury
  - Contusions
  - Fractures
- Congenital deformations
- Low birth weight
- Undernourishment (Hypoglycaemia)
  - Agalactia
  - Mastitis
  - Maternal aggression
  - Congenital deformation (Cleft palate)
  - Weakness
  - Litter mates, competition
- Anaesthetic damage
  - Respiratory depression

- Neonatal septicaemia/
  Umbilical infection
  - E. coli
  - Streptococcus sp.
  - Staphylococcus sp.
- Viral infectious disease
  - Canine distemper virus [Dog]
  - CAV-1 (Hepatitis c. c.)
    [Dog]
  - Canine/feline Herpes virus
  - Canine/feline Parvovirus
  - Feline Calici virus [Cat]
  - FeLV/FIV [Cat]
  - Rota-/Coronavirus enteritis
- Bacterial infectious disease
  - Bordetella sp.
  - Pasteurella sp.
  - E. coli
  - Salmonella sp.
  - Campylobacter sp.
  - Brucella sp. [Dog]
- Parasitic infectious disease
  - Toxocara sp.
  - Toxascaris sp.
  - Ancylostoma sp.
  - Toxoplasma sp.
  - Isospora spp.
  - Cryptosporidium sp.
  - Giardia sp.
- Injuries caused by the mother
  - Bite injuries
  - Licking injuries
- Surfactant deficiency
  - Premature birth
- Neonatal isoerythrolysis [Cat]
  - Blood type A in neonate
    with blood type B in mother
- Primary immunosuppression

Diagnostic Approach

Postpartal Maternal Complications

1. **Case History**

2. **General Examination**

3. **Endoscopy**
- Vaginoscopy

4. **Milk Examination**
- Cytology
- Bacterial culture

5. **Blood Tests**
- Hct, Ery, Leuc
- Na, K, Ca
- TP, Alb, Glob
- GPT, AP, Urea, Crea, BG
- Blood Sedimentation (BSR)
- Diff BC

MICROBIAL SEROLOGY
- FeLV-/FIV Antigen [Cat]

6. **Urinalysis**
- Urine dip stick
- Specific gravity
- Urine sediment

7. **X-Ray Study**
- Abdomen

8. **Ultrasound**
- Abdomen

9. **Further Tests**
- Laparotomy
  (Ovariohysterectomy)

Diagnostic Approach

Postpartal Neonatal Complications

1. Case History

2. General Examination

3. Inspection of the orifices
- Congenital deformations

4. Blood Tests
- Hct, Ery, Leuc
- TP, BG
- Diff BC

MICROBIAL SEROLOGY
- FeLV-/FIV Antigen [Cat]

FURTHER EXAMINATIONS
- Blood culture
- Blood typing [Cat]

5. Urinalysis
- Urine dip stick
- Specific gravity
- Urine sediment

6. Faecal Examination
- Plain examination
- Flotation
- Bacterial culture
- Parvovirus Antigen

7. X-Ray Study
- Whole body

8. Ultrasound
- Heart
- Abdomen

9. Further Tests
- Maternal Examination
  - Milk examination
  - Faecal examination
- Comparison to litter mates
- Histopathological examination of dead neonates

Preputial Discharge

Common Causes	
Dog	Cat
+++ Seminal fluid	+++ Cystitis/Urethritis
++ Balanoposthitis	++ FUS/FLUTD
++ Cystitis/Urethritis	++ Urinary incontinence
++ Prostatitis	
++ Urinary incontinence	

Purulent Discharge

- Balanoposthitis [esp Dog]
  - Staphylococcus sp.
  - Streptococcus sp.
  - E. coli
  - Mycoplasma sp.
  - Moraxella sp.
  - Proteus sp.
  - Klebsiella sp.
  - Pseudomonas sp.
  - Corynebacterium sp.
  - Bacillus sp.
  - Acinetobacter sp.
- Cystitis/Urethritis
  - E. coli
  - Staphylococcus sp.
  - Streptococcus sp.
  - Proteus sp.
  - Klebsiella sp.
  - Enterobacter sp.
  - Pseudomonas sp.
  - Corynebacterium sp.
  - Candida spp.
  - Capillaria sp.
- Pyelonephritis
- Prostatitis/prostatic abscess [Dog]
- Penile/preputial tumours
  - Canine transmissible venereal tumour [Dog]
  - Squamous cell carcinoma
  - Haemangiosarcoma
  - Mast cell tumour
  - Melanoma
  - Papilloma
- Phimosis/paraphimosis

Haemorrhagic Discharge

Penile/Preputial Tumour

  - Canine transmissible venereal tumour [Dog]
  - Squamous cell carcinoma
  - Haemangiosarcoma
  - Mast cell tumour
  - Melanoma
  - Papilloma
- Urinary tract haemorrhage
  - Trauma
  - Pyelonephritis
  - Cystitis/Urethritis
  - Prostatic disease [Dog]
  - Nephrolithiasis/Urolithiasis
  - FUS/FLUTD [Cat]
  - Urinary tract tumours
  - Coagulopathies
- Trauma/foreign body
- Phimosis/Paraphimosis
- Balanoposthitis [esp Dog]

Urinary Incontinence

- Neurological Causes

Full Bladder

  - Sphincter spasm (UMN Lesion)
  - Detrusor atony (LMN Lesion)
  - Reflex dyssynergia [Dog]

Empty Bladder

  - Sphincter atony
  - Detrusor spasm (irritable bladder)

- Congenital Causes
- Obstructive Causes
  - Urolithiasis
  - Urinary tract tumours
- Prostatic enlargement [Dog]
- FUS/FLUTD [Cat]
- Post-traumatic urethral stricture

Diagnostic Approach

Preputial Discharge

1. Case History

2. General Examination

3. Penile Examination

4. Rectal Examination [Dog]

5. Analysis of Preputial Secretion/ Preputial Smear
- Cytology
- Bacterial culture

6. Blood Tests
- Hct, Ery, Leuc
- Urea, Crea
- Diff BC
- Na, K, Ca

MICROBIAL SEROLOGY
- FeLV-/FIV Antigen [Cat]

COAGULATION
- Bleeding time
- Prothrombin time (PT/Quick)
- (Activated) partial Thromboplastin time (PTT/ aPTT)

- Fibrin degradation product (FDP)
- Thrombocyte number

7. Urinalysis
- Urinary output/volume
- Urine dip stick
- Specific gravity
- Urine sediment
  - Bacteria
  - Erys, Leuc
  - Epithelial cells
  - Casts
  - Crystals
  - Tumour cytology
- Bacterial culture (Cystocentesis)

8. X-Ray Study
- Abdomen
- Pelvis
- Contrast urethrography
- Contrast/Double contrast urography
- Excretory urography

9. Ultrasound
- Abdomen ± Prostatic biopsy

Vaginal Discharge

Common Causes	
Dog	**Cat**
+++ Endometritis/Pyometra	+++ Endometritis/Pyometra
++ Urinary tract disease	++ Urinary tract disease
++ Peripartal complications	++ Vaginitis
++ Vaginitis	

Seromucous Discharge

- Physiological discharge
  - Late metoestrus
  - Late stage pregnancy
  - Postpartum
- Mucometra/hydrometra

Purulent Discharge

- Physiological discharge
  - Early metoestrus
- Endometritis/pyometra
  - E. coli
- Vaginitis
  - Juvenile vaginitis
  - Urinary incontinence
  - Urinary tract infections
  - Congenital deformations
  - Vaginal tumours
  - Herpes virus
  - E. coli
  - Pasteurella sp.
  - Streptococcus sp.
  - Chlamydia sp.
  - Brucella sp.
  - Pseudomonas sp.
  - Mycoplasma sp.
  - Abscess/haematoma
  - Foreign body

- Cystitis/Urethritis
  - E. coli
  - Staphylococcus sp.
  - Streptococcus sp.
  - Proteus sp.
  - Klebsiella sp.
  - Enterobacter sp.
  - Pseudomonas sp.
  - Corynebacterium sp.

Haemorrhagic Discharge

- Physiological discharge
  - Proestrus/oestrus
  - until ca. 6 weeks postpartum
- Birth injuries
- Uterine torsion
- Imminent miscarriage
- Foetal death
- Placental retention [Dog]
- Placental subinvolution [Dog]
- Vaginal tumours
  - Canine transmissible venereal tumour [Dog]
  - Leiomyoma
- Urinary tract haemorrhage
  - Trauma
  - Pyelonephritis
  - Cystitis/Urethritis
  - Nephrolithiasis/Urolithiasis

- FUS/FLUTD [Cat]
- Urinary tract tumours
- Coagulopathy

Urinary Incontinence

- Neurological Causes

Full bladder

- Sphincter spasm (UMN Lesion)
- Detrusor atony (LMN Lesion)

Empty bladder

- Sphincter atony
- Detrusor spasm (irritable bladder)
- Congenital causes
- Obstructive Causes
  - Urolithiasis
  - Urinary tract tumours
  - FUS/FLUTD [Cat]
  - Post-traumatic urethral stricture

Diagnostic Approach

Vaginal Discharge

1. **Case History**

2. **General Examination**

3. **Analysis of the vaginal secretion**

4. **Blood Tests**
- Hct, Ery, Leuc
- TP, BG
- Urea, Crea
- Blood Sedimentation (BST)
- Diff BC

MICROBIAL SEROLOGY
- FeLV-/FIV Antigen [Cat]

5. **Urinalysis**
- Urinary output/volume
- Urine dip stick
- Specific gravity
- Urine sediment

 - Bacteria
 - Erys, Leuc
 - Epithelial cells
 - Casts
 - Crystals
 - Tumour cytology
- Bacterial culture (Cystocentesis)

6. **Ultrasound**
- Abdomen

7. **X-Ray Study**
- Abdomen

8. **Endoscopy**
- Vaginoscopy
  ± Vaginal smear
  - Cytology
  - Bacterial culture

9. **Further Tests**
- Laparotomy/Ovario-hysterectomy

Vaginal Prolapse

Bulging or falling of the vagina and its nearby structures out
of its usual position

Common Causes		
Dog		**Cat**
+++	Genetic predisposition	+	Intra partum with uterine prolapse
++	Ovarian cysts	+	Ovarian cysts
++	Ovarian tumours		
+	Intra partum with uterine prolapse		

Causes

- Endogenous oestrogen
  - Proestrus/oestrus
  - Ovarian cysts
  - Ovarian tumours
  - End of pregnancy
- Exogenous oestrogen
  - Oestrogen therapy
  - Toxic plants
- Vaginal tumours
  - Canine transmissible venereal tumour [Dog]
  - Leiomyoma
  - Polyp
- Genetic family related breed predisposition [Dog]
- Intra partum with uterine prolapse

Diagnostic Approach

Vaginal Prolapse

1. **Case History**
2. **General Examination**
3. **Endoscopy**

- • Vaginoscopy
- ± Tumour biopsy
- − Cytology

Abnormal Cycle

Normal Cycle:	Dog	Cat
Proestrus:	7–9 days	1–2 days
Oestrus:	4–8 days	ca. 6 days (with coitus)
		14–21 days (without coitus)
Metoestrus:	4–6 weeks	
Anoestrus:	variable (3–5 months)	
Cycle length:	14–21 days	14–21 days
Interoestrus:	variable (ca. 7 months)	variable

Oestrus

Prolonged Oestrus

- Endogenous oestrogen
  - Ovarian cysts
  - Ovarian tumours
- Exogenous oestrogen
  - Synthetic oestrogens
  - Toxic plants

Absent Oestrus

- Error of observation
- Ovariectomy/ Ovariohysterectomy
- Silent heat
- Split oestrus [Dog]
- Immature/old age
- Ovarian dysfunction
- Hypothyroidism [Dog]
- Hypercortisolism (Cushing's Disease) [Dog]
- Systemic Disease
- Shortened photoperiod [Cat]
- Chromosomal defects
- Drugs

Interoestrus

Prolonged Interoestrus

- Pregnancy
- Pseudopregnancy [esp Dog]
- Malnutrition
- Glandular cystic endometrial hyperplasia [Dog]
- Old age
- Hypothyroidism [Dog]
- Hypercortisolism (Cushing's Disease) [Dog]
- Systemic Disease
- Shortened photoperiod [Cat]

Shortened Interoestrus

- Endogenous oestrogen
  - Ovarian cysts/tumours
- Exogenous oestrogen
  - Synthetic oestrogens
  - Toxic plants
- Split oestrus [Dog]
- Corpus luteum dysfunction (Luteolysis)

Diagnostic Approach

Abnormal Cycle

1. Case History

2. General Examination

3. Endoscopy
- Vaginoscopy
  ± Vaginal smear
  - Cytology
  - Bacterial culture

4. Blood Tests
- Hct, Ery, Leuc
- TP, Alb, Glob
- GPT, AP, Urea, Crea, BG
- Diff BC
- Na, K, Ca
- FIP Profile [Cat]
  - TP
  - Alb/Glob ratio
  - Bili
  - GOT
  - Serum electrophoresis

MICROBIAL SEROLOGY
- FeLV-/FIV Antigen [Cat]
- Brucella Antibodies [Dog]
- Toxoplasma Antibodies

FUNCTION TESTS
- Serum progesterone
- Serum oestradiol
- T_4, fT_4
- TSH-/TRH Stimulation test [Dog]
- Adrenal gland function test [Dog]
  - Dexamethasone Suppression test
  - ACTH Stimulation test
  - Cortisol/Creatinine Ratio

5. Urinalysis
- Urine dip stick
- Specific gravity
- Urine sediment

6. Ultrasound
- Abdomen

7 Neurological Principal Symptoms

Further Relevant Principal Symptoms

Ataxia

Coordination Disorder of Motion Sequences:
± Hypermetria + broad legged posture + intention tremor
   (cerebellar cause likely)
± Head tilt + nystagmus + circling movements (vestibular cause
   likely)
± Paresis (central or spinal cause likely)
± Hind limb weakness (metabolic causes, heart failure or
   neuromuscular causes likely)

Common Causes	
Dog	Cat
+++ Peripheral vestibular disorder	+++ Peripheral vestibular disorder
++ Metabolic causes	++ Metabolic causes
++ Spinal causes	++ Spinal causes
++ Cerebral causes	++ Cerebral causes
++ Neuromuscular causes	++ Neuromuscular causes

Peripheral Vestibular Disorder

Otitis media/interna

- Parasitic Otitis
  - Otodectes sp.
  - Notoedres sp. [Cat]
  - Demodex sp.
  - Sarcoptes sp.
- Bacterial Otitis
  - Staphylococcus sp.
  - Proteus sp.
  - Pseudomonas sp.
  - Lyme Borreliosis sp. [Dog]
- Mycotic Otitis
  - Malassezia sp.
  - Candida sp.
  - Aspergillus sp.
- Viral Otitis
  - Canine Distemper Virus [Dog]
  - FeLV/FIV [Cat]
  - FIP Coronavirus [Cat]
  - Herpes virus
- Immunoreactive otitis
  - Atopy/Inhalation allergy
  - Ear mite allergy
  - Bacterial allergy
  - Fungal allergy
  - Drug allergy (Neomycin ear ointments)

- Toxic causes
  - Aminoglycosides
  - Polymyxin B
  - Chloramphenicol
  - Diuretics
  - Cytostatics
  - Heavy metal poisoning
- Other causes
  - Foreign body
  - Trauma
  - Polyps [Cat]
  - Rhinitis

Middle Ear Tumours

- Middle ear polyps [Cat]
- Osteosarcoma
- Chondrosarcoma
- Fibrosarcoma
- Squamous cell carcinoma
- Vestibular Schwannoma
- Cholesteatoma
- Vestibulocochlearis neurinoma

Other Causes

- Vestibular circulatory disorder
- Geriatric vestibular syndrome
- Traumatic cause
  - Fracture of the petrous part in the temporal bone
  - Labyrinth contusion

- Polyneuropathy
  - esp hypothyroidism [Dog]

Central Vestibular Disorder
Congenital Causes

- Hydrocephalus
- Lissencephaly
- Lysosomal storage disease
- Degenerative encephalopathies
  - Dysmyelogenesis

Encephalitis/ Meningoencephalitis

- Viral encephalitis
  - (Rabies virus)
  - Pseudorabies Herpes virus
  - Canine distemper virus [Dog]
  - CAV-1 (Hepatitis c. c.) [Dog]
  - Canine/feline Herpesvirus
  - Canine/feline Parvovirus
  - FeLV/FIV [Cat]
  - FIP Coronavirus [Cat]
  - TBE Virus [Dog]
- Bacterial encephalitis
  - Lyme Borreliosis sp. [Dog]
  - Listeria sp. [Dog]
  - Aerobes + Anaerobes (Peripheral primary source of infection)
- Immunoreactive encephalitis
  - Granulomatous meningoencephalitis (GME)
  - Eosinophilic meningoencephalitis (EME)
- Parasitic encephalitis
  - Toxoplasma sp.
  - Neospora sp. [Dog]
  - (Encephalitozoon sp. [Dog])
  - Larva migrans
  - Toxocara sp.
  - Ancylostoma sp.
  - (Dirofilaria sp.)
- Rickettsial encephalitis
  - (Ehrlichia sp. [Dog])
  - (Rickettsia sp. [Dog])
- Mycotic encephalitis
  - Cryptococcus sp. [Cat]
  - Aspergillus sp. [Dog]
  - (Histoplasma sp.)
  - (Blastomyces sp.)
  - (Coccidioides sp.)
- Other causes
  - Feline spongiform encephalopathy [Cat]
  - Feline polioencephalomyelitis [Cat]
  - Foreign body/abscess

Brain tumour/Tumour metastasis

- Lymphosarcoma [esp Cat]
- Meningeoma [esp Cat]
- Neurinoma
- Glioma
- Medulloblastoma
- Plexus chorioideus papilloma
- Neuroblastoma

Other Causes

- Traumatic brain injury
- Cerebral circulatory disturbance
- Thiamine deficiency [Cat]

Cerebellar Causes

Cerebellar/Brain Stem Disease

- Cerebellar hypoplasia
  - Feline Parvovirus (in utero) [Cat]
  - Canine Herpes virus (in utero) [Dog]
  - (live vaccine)
- Cerebellitis
  - FIP Coronavirus [Cat]
  - Canine distemper virus [Dog]
  - Toxoplasma sp.
  - Neospora sp. [Dog]
  - Cryptococcus sp. [Cat]
  - Granulomatous Meningoencephalitis (GME)
- Cerebellar/brain stem tumours/tumour metastasis
  - Medulloblastoma
  - Lymphosarcoma [esp Cat]
- Cerebellar degeneration
  - Cerebellar abiotrophy
  - Lysosomal storage disease
  - Neuroaxonal dystrophy
  - Dysmyelogenesis
  - White Dog Shaker Syndrome [Dog]
- Toxic causes
  - Hexachlorophen poisoning
  - Heavy metal poisoning
  - Organophosphate poisoning
- Traumatic brain injury
- Cerebellar circulatory disturbance
- Thiamine deficiency [Cat]

Spinal Disease

Traumatic Causes

- Prolapsed disc
- Vertebral fracture/luxation
- Haematoma/haemorrhage
- Fibrocartilaginous embolism
- Thromboembolism

Congenital Causes

- Cervical instability (Wobbler Syndrome) [Dog]
- Lumbosacral stenosis (Cauda equina syndrome)
- Atlantoaxial subluxation [Dog]
- Spinal deformations [esp Bulldog]

Infectious Causes

- Discospondylitis/Osteomyelitis
  - Staphylococcus sp.
  - Brucella sp. [Dog]
  - Streptococcus sp.
  - E. coli
  - Pasteurella sp.
  - Actinomyces sp.
  - Nocardia sp.
  - Mycobacterium sp.
  - Aspergillus sp.
- Myelitis
  - Canine distemper virus [Dog]
  - FeLV/FIV [Cat]
  - FIP Coronavirus [Cat]
  - Rabies virus
  - Staphylococcus sp.
  - Lyme Borreliosis sp. [Dog]
  - Cryptococcus sp. [Cat]
  - Toxoplasma sp.
  - Neospora sp. [Dog]

– Larva migrans
– (Ehrlichia sp. [Dog])

Immunoreactive Causes

• Granulomatous meningoencephalitis (GME)
• Eosinophilic meningoencephalitis (EME)

Degenerative Causes

• Demyelinisation diseases [German Shepherd Dog]
• Prolapsed disc
• Lumbosacral stenosis (Cauda equina syndrome)
• Spondylosis deformans
• Dura–mater ossification

Spinal tumour

• Osteosarcoma
• Chondrosarcoma
• Multiple myeloma
• Tumour metastasis

Other Causes

• Hypervitaminosis A [Cat]

Neuromuscular Causes

Polyneuropathy

• Infectious Causes
  – FeLV/FIV [Cat]
  – Toxoplasma sp.
  – Neospora sp. [Dog]
• Immunoreactive causes
  – Lupus erythematosus
• Metabolic Causes
  – Diabetes mellitus

– Hypercortisolism (Cushing's disease) [esp Dog]
– Hypothyroidism [Dog]
• Toxic Causes
  – Organophosphate poisoning (chronic)
  – Lead poisoning
  – Cytostatics
  – Lindane
  – Botulinum toxin
  – Tick toxin (Tick paralysis)
• Congenital Causes
  – Axonopathy
  – Demyelinisation diseases
  – Lysosomal storage disease
  – Spinal muscular atrophy
• Other Causes
  – Nerve root compression syndrome
  – Feline dysautonomia [esp Cat]
  – Polyneuritis/ Polyradiculoneuritis [Dog]
  – Tetanus

Junctionopathy (Neuromuscular Endplate)

• Myasthenia gravis
  – acquired
  – congenital

Polymyopathy

• Infectious Causes
  – Toxoplasma sp.
  – Neospora sp. [Dog]
  – Lyme Borrelia sp. [Dog]
  – Leptospira sp. [Dog]
• Immunoreactive Causes
  – Lupus erythematosus
  – Eosinophilic myositis [Dog]

- Metabolic Causes
  - Hypokalaemia [esp Cat]
  - Hypercortisolism (Cushing's Disease) [esp Dog]
  - Hypothyroidism [Dog]
  - Hypoglycaemia
  - Vitamin E/Selenium deficiency
- Congenital Causes
  - Muscular dystrophy
  - Dermatomyositis [Collie]
  - Glycogen storage disease

Other Causes of Ataxia

- Feline aortic thromboembolism [Cat]
- Organ failure
  - Heart failure
  - Hepatic failure
  - Renal failure
  - Respiratory disease
- Metabolic Causes
  - Hypoglycaemia
  - Uraemia
  - Hepatoencephalopathy
  - Hypokalaemia
  - Hypocalcaemia
  - Metabolic acidosis
  - (Thiamine deficiency [Cat])
- Anaemia
- Bone/Joint disease
- Drugs
  - Sedatives/Narcotics
  - Antihistamines
  - Anticonvulsants

Diagnostic Approach

Ataxia

1. Case History

2. General Examination

3. Neurological Examination
- Awareness/Behaviour
- Body and limb posture/ stance
- Locomotion
- Muscle tone/strength
- Cranial nerves
  - Facial symmetry (VII)
  - Facial sensation (V)
  - Menace reflex (II, VII)
  - Blink reflex (V, VII)
  - Corneal reflex/ Eye movement (V, VI, VII/III, IV, VI)
  - Pupillary reflex (III, Sympathetic nerve)
  - Sight test (II)
  - Swallowing reflex/Glossal motor function (X, XI, XII/ XII)
  - Sense of smell/taste/hearing (I/V/VIII)
  - Cervical and shoulder muscles/(XI)
- Spinal reflexes
  - Bicipital reflex (C6–C8)
  - Triceps reflex (C7–T1)
  - Patellar reflex (L4–L6)
  - Withdrawal reflex (C6–T1 and L6–S1)

- Cutaneous trunci reflex (C7–T1)
- Anal sphincter reflex (S1–S3)
- Bladder – can it be expressed?
- Positional and postural reaction
  - Correction reaction
  - Hopping reaction
  - Side stepping reaction
  - Wheelbarrowing reaction
  - Righting reaction (hind limb)/Extensor postural thrust reaction
  - Righting reaction (fore limb)
  - Table edge reaction (visual/ tactile)

4. Examination of the Ear
- Otoscopy

5. Blood Tests
- Hct, Ery, Leuc, Hb
- Na, K, Ca
- TP, Alb, Glob
- GPT, AP, Urea, Crea, BG
- FIP Profile [Cat]
  - TP
  - Alb/Glob ratio
  - Bili
  - GOT
  - Serum electrophoresis
- Diff BC
- Thrombocytes
- Insulin (Insulin/Glucose ratio)

MICROBIAL SEROLOGY
- FeLV-/FIV Antigen [Cat]
- Toxoplasma Antibodies
- Ehrlichia Antibodies [Dog]
- Neospora Antibodies [Dog]

FUNCTION TESTS
- T_4
- TSH-/TRH Stimulation test [Dog]

6. Urinalysis
- Urinary output/volume
- Urine dip stick
- Specific gravity
- Urine sediment
  - Bacteria
  - Erythrocytes, Leucocytes
  - Epithelial cells
  - Casts
  - Crystals
  - Tumour cytology
- Bacterial culture (Cystocentesis)

7. X-Ray Study
- Skull (Tympanic bulla)
- Spine ± Myelography

8. Liquor Examination
- Chemistry
  - TP, Glucose, CK
  - Globulin (Pandy and Nonne-Apelt reaction)
- Electrophoresis
- Cytology
- Bacterial/Fungal culture
- Canine distemper antibodies [Dog]
- Liquor pressure

9. Further Tests
- Skull CT/MRT
- Electromyography (EMG)
- Muscle biopsy
- Canine distemper virus antigen [Dog] (Conjunctival smear)

Hearing Loss/Deafness

Surdity

Common Causes	
Dog	**Cat**
+++ Geriatric hearing loss	+++ Geriatric hearing loss
++ Otitis media/interna	++ Otitis media/interna
++ Congenital deafness	++ Congenital deafness

Hearing Loss

Otitis Media/Interna

- Parasitic Otitis
  - Otodectes sp.
  - Notoedres sp. [Cat]
  - Demodex sp.
  - Sarcoptes sp.
- Bacterial Otitis
  - Staphylococcus sp.
  - Proteus sp.
  - Pseudomonas sp.
  - Lyme Borrelia sp. [Dog]
- Mycotic Otitis
  - Malassezia sp.
  - Candida sp.
  - Aspergillus sp.
- Viral Otitis
  - Canine distemper virus [Dog]
  - FeLV/FIV [Cat]
  - FIP Coronavirus [Cat]
  - Herpes virus
- Immunoreactive Otitis
  - Atopy/Inhalation allergy
  - Ear mite allergy
  - Bacterial allergy
  - Fungal allergy
  - Drug allergy (Neomycin ear ointment)
- Toxic Causes
  - Aminoglycosides
  - Polymyxin B
  - Chloramphenicol
  - Diuretics
  - Cytostatics
  - Heavy metal poisoning
- Other Causes
  - Foreign body
  - Trauma
  - Polyps [Cat]
  - Rhinitis

Middle Ear Tumours

- Middle ear polyps [Cat]
- Osteosarcoma
- Chondrosarcoma
- Fibrosarcoma
- Squamous cell carcinoma
- Vestibular Schwannoma
- Cholesteatoma
- Vestibulocochlearis neurinoma

Congenital Causes

- Hydrocephalus
- Blue eyed cats with white fur
- Congenital deafness in Dalmatians

Other Causes

- Geriatric hearing loss
- Traumatic brain injury
- Encephalitis/ Meningoencephalitis

Diagnostic Approach

Hearing Loss/Deafness

1. Case History

2. General Examination

3. Neurological Examination
- Awareness/Behaviour
- Body and limb position/ posture
- Locomotion
- Cranial nerves
  - Facial symmetry (VII)
  - Facial sensation
  - Menace reflex (II, VII)
  - Blink reflex (V, VII)
  - Corneal reflex/ Eye movement (V, VI, VII/III, IV, VI)
  - Pupillary reflex (III, Sympathetic nerve)
  - Sight test (II)
  - Swallowing reflex/glossal motor function (X, XI, XII/ XII)
  - Sense of smell/taste and hearing (I/V/VIII)
  - Cervical and shoulder muscles (XI)

4. Examination of the Ear
- Otoscopy
- Hearing Test

5. Blood Tests
- Hct, Ery, Leuc, Hb
- FIP Profile [Cat]
  - TP
  - Alb/Glob Ratio
  - Bili
  - GOT
  - Serum electrophoresis

MICROBIAL SEROLOGY
- FeLV-/FIV Antigen [Cat]

6. X-Ray Study
- Skull (Tympanic bulla)

7. Further Tests
- Brain auditor evoked response Audiometry (BAERA)
- Canine distemper virus antigen (Conjunctival smear) [Dog]

Coma

Deep unconsciousness: Patient cannot be awoken by external stimuli

Common Causes		
Dog		**Cat**
+++ Metabolic causes	+++	Metabolic causes
++ Traumatic brain injury	++	Traumatic brain injury
++ Poisoning	++	Poisoning
+ Encephalitis/ meningoencephalitis	+	Encephalitis/ meningoencephalitis
+ Brain tumour	+	Brain tumour

Cerebral Causes

Traumatic Causes

- Intracerebral haemorrhage/ haematoma (subdural/epidural)
- Cerebral contusion
- Cerebral oedema
- Thromboembolism (Hemispheral infarction)

Congenital Causes

- Hydrocephalus
- Lissencephaly
- Lysosomal storage disease

Brain Tumours/Tumour Metastasis

- Lymphosarcoma [esp Cat]
- Meningeoma
- Neurinoma
- Glioma
- Medulloblastoma
- Plexus chorioideus papilloma
- Neuroblastoma

Other Causes

- Seizures (postictal coma)
- Heat stroke
- Cerebral circulatory disturbance (hypoxia)
- Thiamine deficiency [Cat]

Encephalitis/ Meningoencephalitis

- Viral encephalitis
  - (Rabies virus)
  - Pseudorabies Herpes virus
  - Canine distemper virus [Dog]
  - CAV-1 (Hepatitis c. c.) [Dog]
  - Canine/feline Herpes virus
  - Canine/feline Parvovirus
  - FeLV/FIV [Cat]
  - FIP Coronavirus [Cat]
  - TBE Virus [Dog]

- Bacterial encephalitis
  - Lyme Borrelia sp. [Dog]
  - Listeria sp. [Dog]
  - Aerobes + Anaerobes (peripheral source of infection)
- Parasitic encephalitis
  - Toxoplasma sp.
  - Neospora sp. [Dog]
  - (Encephalitozoon sp. [Dog])
  - Larva migrans
  - Toxocara sp.
  - Ancylostoma sp.
  - (Dirofilaria sp.)
- Immunoreactive encephalitis
  - Granulomatous meningoencephalitis (GME)
  - Eosinophilic meningoencephalitis (EME)
- Rickettsial encephalitis
  - (Ehrlichia sp. [Dog])
  - (Rickettsia sp. [Dog])
- Mycotic encephalitis
  - Cryptococcus sp. [Cat]
  - Aspergillus sp. [Dog]
  - (Histoplasma sp.)
  - (Blastomyces sp.)
  - (Coccidioides sp.)
- Other causes
  - Feline spongiform encephalopathy [Cat]
  - Feline polioencephalomyelitis [Cat]
  - Foreign body/abscess

Extracerebral Causes

Metabolic Causes

- Hypoglycaemia (Insulinoma)
- Hyperglycaemia (Diabetes mellitus)
- Uraemia
- Hepatoencephalopathy (liver cirrhosis, portocaval shunt)
- Acidosis/Alkalosis
- Hypoxia
- Hypernatriaemia
- Hyperosmolality/ Hyperviscosity syndrome
- Hypocortisolism (Addison's Disease) [Dog]
- Hypothyroidism [Dog]
- Hyperlipidaemia

Toxic Causes

- Narcotics
- Antiectoparasitics
  - Ivermectin
  - Amitraz
- Theophylline
- Phenytoin/Phenobarbital
- Paracetamol
- Metaldehyde poisoning (slug pellets)
- Heavy metal poisoning
- Household agents
- Toxic plants

Other Causes

- Anaemia/ Methaemoglobinaemia
- Shock
- Anaesthetic incident (hypoxia)
- Cardiac/respiratory disease (hypoxia)
- Hypertension/Hypotension
- Hyperthermia/Hypothermia
- Haemorrhage

Diagnostic Approach

Coma

1. Case History

2. General Examination

3. Neurological Examination
- Arousal
- Body/limb position
- Muscle tone
- Cranial nerves
  - Corneal reflex/ eye movement (V, VI, VII/III, IV, VI)
  - Pupillary reflex (III, Sympathetic nerve)
  - Swallowing reflex/glossal motor function (X, XI, XII/XII)
- Spinal reflexes
  - Bicipital reflex (C6–C8)
  - Triceps reflex (C7–T1)
  - Patellar reflex (L4–L6)
  - Withdrawal reflex (C6–T1 and L6–S1)
  - Cutaneous trunci reflex (C7–T1)
  - Anal sphincter reflex (S1–S3)
  - Bladder – can it be expressed?

4. ECG

5. Blood Tests
- Hct, Ery, Leuc, Hb
- Thrombocytes
- Na, K, Ca
- TP, Alb, Glob
- GPT, AP, Urea, Crea
- BG, Insulin (Insulin/Glucose)
- Ammonium
- Blood gas analysis (BGA)

- FIP Profile [Cat]
  - TP
  - Alb/Glob ratio
  - Bili
  - GOT
  - Serum electrophoresis
- Diff BC

MICROBIAL SEROLOGY
- FeLV-/FIV Antigen [Cat]
- Coronavirus Antibodies/PCR [Cat]
- Toxoplasma Antibodies
- Ehrlichia Antibodies [Dog]
- Cryptococcus Antibodies [Cat]
- Lyme Borrelia Antibodies [Dog]
- Neospora Antibodies [Dog]

FUNCTION TESTS
- T_4, fT_4

COAGULATION
- Bleeding time
- Prothrombin time (PT/Quick)
- (Activated) partial Thromboplastin time (PTT/aPTT)
- Fibrin Degradation product (FDP)

6. Urinalysis
- Urinary output/volume
- Urine dip stick
- Specific gravity
- Urine sediment
  - Bacteria
  - Erythrocytes, Leucocytes
  - Epithelial cells
  - Casts

- – Crystals
- – Tumour cytology
- Bacterial culture (Cystocentesis)

7. X-Ray Study
- Skull
- Thorax
- Abdomen

8. Liquor Examination (After Exclusion of Trauma/ Haemorrhage)
- Chemistry
  - – TP, Glucose, CK

- – Globulin (Pandy and Nonne-Apelt reaction)
- Electrophoresis
- Cytology
- Bacterial/fungal culture
- Canine distemper antibodies [Dog]
- (Liquor pressure)

9. Further Tests
- Skull MRT
- EEG
- Canine distemper virus antigen (conjunctival smear) [Dog]

Head Tilt

Often indicates a balance disorder (vestibular disturbance) ± nystagmus
Head tilt usually towards the affected side

Common Causes	
Dog	Cat
+++ Peripheral vestibular disturbance	+++ Peripheral vestibular disturbance
++ Central vestibular disturbance	++ Central vestibular disturbance

Peripheral Vestibular Disturbance

Otitis Media/Interna

- Parasitic otitis
  - – Otodectes sp.
  - – Notoedres sp. [Cat]
  - – Demodex sp.
  - – Sarcoptes sp.
- Bacterial otitis
  - – Staphylococcus sp.
  - – Proteus sp.
  - – Pseudomonas sp.

  - – Lyme Borrelia sp. [Dog]
- Mycotic otitis
  - – Malassezia sp.
  - – Candida sp.
  - – Aspergillus sp.
- Viral otitis
  - – Canine distemper virus [Dog]
  - – FeLV/FIV [Cat]
  - – FIP Coronavirus [Cat]
  - – Herpes virus
- Immunoreactive otitis
  - – Atopy/Inhalation allergy

- Ear mite allergy
- Bacterial allergy
- Fungal allergy
- Drug allergy (Neomycin ear ointment)
- Toxic Causes
  - Aminoglycosides
  - Polymyxin B
  - Chloramphenicol
  - Diuretics
  - Cytostatics
  - Heavy metal poisoning
- Other causes
  - Foreign body
  - Trauma
  - Polyps [Cat]
  - Rhinitis

Middle Ear Tumours

- Middle ear polyps [Cat]
- Osteosarcoma
- Chondrosarcoma
- Fibrosarcoma
- Squamous cell carcinoma
- Vestibular Schwannoma
- Cholesteatoma
- Vestibulocochlear neurinoma

Other Causes

- Vestibular circulatory disturbance
- Geriatric vestibular syndrome
- Traumatic causes
  - Fracture of the petrous bone
  - Contusion of the labyrinth
- Polyneuropathy
  - Esp hypothyroidism [Dog]

Central Vestibular Disturbance

Congenital Causes

- Hydrocephalus
- Lissencephaly
- Lysosomal storage disease
- Degenerative encephalopathies
  - Dysmyelogenesis

Encephalitis/ Meningoencephalitis

- Viral encephalitis
  - (Rabies virus)
  - Pseudo rabies Herpes virus
  - Canine distemper virus [Dog]
  - CAV-1 (Hepatitis c. c.) [Dog]
  - Canine/feline Herpes virus
  - Canine/feline Parvovirus
  - FeLV/FIV [Cat]
  - FIP Coronavirus [Cat]
  - TBE Virus [Dog]
- Bacterial encephalitis
  - Lyme Borrelia sp. [Dog]
  - Listeria sp. [Dog]
  - Aerobes + Anaerobes (peripheral source of infection)
- Immunoreactive encephalitis
  - Granulomatous meningoencephalitis (GME)
  - Eosinophilic meningoencephalitis (EME)
- Rickettsial encephalitis
  - (Ehrlichia sp. [Dog])
  - (Rickettsia sp. [Dog])
- Mycotic encephalitis
  - Cryptococcus sp. [Cat]
  - Aspergillus sp. [Dog]

- (Histoplasma sp.)
- (Blastomyces sp.)
- (Coccidioides sp.)
- Parasitic encephalitis
  - Toxoplasma sp.
  - Neospora sp. [Dog]
  - (Encephalitozoon sp. [Dog])
  - Larva migrans
  - Toxocara sp.
  - Ancylostoma sp.
  - (Dirofilaria sp.)
- Other Causes
  - Feline spongiform encephalopathy [Cat]
  - Feline polioencephalomyelitis [Cat]
  - Foreign body/abscess

Brain Tumours/Tumour Metastasis

- Lymphosarcoma [esp Cat]
- Meningeoma
- Neurinoma
- Glioma
- Medulloblastoma
- Plexus chorioideus papilloma
- Neuroblastoma

Other Causes

- Idiopathic vestibular syndrome
- Traumatic brain injury
- Cerebral circulatory disorder
- Thiamine deficiency [Cat]

Diagnostic Approach

Head Tilt

1. **Case History**

2. **General Examination**

3. **Neurological Examination**
   - Awareness/behaviour
   - Body/limb position and posture
   - Locomotion
   - Cranial nerves
     - Facial symmetry (VII)
     - Facial sensation
     - Menace reflex (II, VII)
     - Blink reflex (V, VII)
     - Corneal reflex/ Eye movements (V, VI, VII/III, IV, VI)
     - Pupillary reflex (III, Sympathetic nerve)
     - Sight test (II)
   - Swallowing reflex/glossal motor function (X, XI, XII/XII)
   - Sense of smell/taste/hearing (I/V/VIII)
   - Cervical and shoulder muscles (XI)

4. **Examination of the Ear**
   - Otoscopy
     ± Analysis of the aural discharge
     - Bacterial/fungal culture

5. **Blood Tests**
   - Hct, Ery, Leuc, Hb
   - Na, K, Ca
   - TP, Alb, Glob
   - GPT, AP, Urea, Crea, BG
   - FIP Profile [Cat]

- TP
- Alb/Glob ratio
- Bili
- GOT
- Serum electrophoresis
- Diff BC
- Thrombocytes
- Insulin (Insulin/Glucose ratio)

MICROBIAL SEROLOGY
- FeLV-/FIV Antigen [Cat]
- Toxoplasma Antibodies
- Ehrlichia Antibodies [Dog]

FUNCTION TESTS
- T_4
- TSH-/TRH Stimulation test [Dog]

6. X-Ray Study
- Skull (Tympanic bulla)
- Spine ± Myelography

7. Liquor Examination
- Chemistry
  - TP, Glucose, CK
  - Globulin (Pandy and Nonne–Apelt reaction)
- Electrophoresis
- Cytology
- Bacterial/fungal culture
- Canine distemper antibodies
- [Dog] (Liquor pressure)

8. Further Tests
Skull MRT

Differentiation Parameters of the Pathological Nystagmus

Spontaneous Nystagmus	Peripheral vestibular disturbance	Central vestibular disturbance
Horizontal Nystagmus – fast phase:	+ Often towards the unaffected/ healthy side Rarely towards affected/ diseased side (irritative nystagmus)	+
Rotating Nystagmus	+	+
Vertical Nystagmus		+
Periodic alternating Nystagmus		+
Positional Nystagmus (exhaustible and reproducible)	+	

Seizures

Seizure Phases
1. Prodromal phase (early stage): often associated with unrest and clinginess
2. Ictus (main stage)
3. Postictal phase (late stage): often associated with unrest, disorientation, hunger/thirst, sleep

Common Causes	
Dog	**Cat**
Age: < 1 Year	
+++ Congenital Disease 　– Hydrocephalus 　– Portosystemic shunt ++ Meningoencephalitis 　– Canine distemper virus 　– Bacterial ++ Hypoglycaemia + Trauma + Poisoning	+++ Congenital Disease 　– Hydrocephalus 　– Portosystemic shunt ++ Meningoencephalitis 　– FIP Coronavirus 　– Toxoplasma sp. 　– (Cryptococcus sp.) 　– Bacterial ++ Hypoglycaemia + Trauma
Age: 1–5 Years	
+++ Idiopathic epilepsy ++ Poisoning ++ Meningoencephalitis 　– Canine distemper virus 　– Bacterial 　– Granulomatous 　　meningoencephalitis (GME) ++ Hypoglycaemia ++ Uraemia + Trauma + Portosystemic shunt	++ Meningoencephalitis 　– FIP Coronavirus 　– Toxoplasma sp. 　– (Cryptococcus sp.) 　– Bacterial 　– Granulomatous 　　meningoencephalitis (GME) ++ Hypokalaemia ++ Uraemia ++ Idiopathic epilepsy ++ Poisoning + Hypoglycaemia + Trauma

Common Causes	
Dog	**Cat**
Age: > 5 Years	
+++ Brain tumour/tumour metastasis	+++ Brain tumour/tumour metastasis
++ Hypoglycaemia/insulinoma	++ Uraemia
++ Uraemia	++ Hepatoencephalopathy
++ Hepatoencephalopathy	+ Meningoencephalitis
+ Meningoencephalitis	– FIP Coronavirus
– Canine distemper virus	– Bacterial
– Bacterial	– Granulomatous
– Granulomatous meningoencephalitis (GME)	meningoencephalitis (GME)
+ Hypoxia	+ Hypoxia
– Heart failure	– Heart failure
– Respiratory disease	– Feline asthma
– Anaemia	– Anaemia

Cerebral Causes

Encephalitis/ Meningoencephalitis

- Viral encephalitis
  - Canine distemper virus [Dog]
  - CAV-1 (Hepatitis c. c.) [Dog]
  - Canine/feline Herpes virus
  - Canine/feline Parvovirus
  - FeLV/FIV [Cat]
  - FIP Coronavirus [Cat]
  - FSME Virus [Dog]
- Bacterial encephalitis
  - Lyme Borrelia sp. [Dog]
  - Listeria sp. [Dog]
  - Aerobes + Anaerobes (peripheral source of infection)
- Immunoreactive encephalitis
  - Granulomatous meningoencephalitis (GME)
  - Eosinophilic meningoencephalitis (EME)
- Rickettsial encephalitis
  - (Ehrlichia sp. [Dog])
  - (Rickettsia sp. [Dog])
- Mycotic encephalitis
  - Cryptococcus sp. [Cat]
  - Aspergillus sp. [Dog]
  - (Histoplasma sp.)
  - (Blastomyces sp.)
  - (Coccidioides sp.)
- Parasitic encephalitis
  - Toxoplasma sp.
  - Neospora sp. [Dog]
  - (Encephalitozoon sp. [Dog])
  - Larva migrans
  - Toxocara sp.
  - Ancylostoma sp.
  - (Dirofilaria sp.)

- Other Causes
  - Feline spongiform encephalopathy [Cat]
  - Feline polioencephalo-myelitis [Cat]
  - Foreign body/abscess

Traumatic Causes

- Intracerebral haemorrhage/haematoma (subdural/epidural)
- Cerebral contusion
- Cerebral oedema
- Thromboembolism
- (Hemispheral infarction)

Congenital Causes

- Hydrocephalus
- Lissencephaly
- Lysosomal storage disease

Brain Tumours/Tumour Metastasis

- Lymphosarcoma [esp Cat]
- Meningeoma
- Neurinoma
- Glioma
- Medulloblastoma
- Corioidal plexus papilloma
- Neuroblastoma

Other Causes

- Cerebral circulatory disturbances
  - Hypoxia (esp heart/respiratory tract disease)
  - Anaemia
  - Thrombo-/fat-/tumour embolism
  - Atherosclerosis
  - Feline ischaemic encephalopathy [Cat]
- Heat stroke

Extracerebral Causes

Metabolic Causes

- Hypoglycaemia
- Uraemia
- Hepatoencephalopathy (esp hepatic cirrhosis, portosystemic shunt)
- Diabetic ketoacidosis
- Hypocalcaemia (eclampsia)
- Hypokalaemia [esp Cat]
- Hyperviscosity syndrome
- Hyper-/Hyponatriaemia
- Thiamine deficiency [Cat]

Toxic Causes

- Drugs
  - Ketamine
  - Lidocaine
  - Pentetrazol
  - Caffeine [Cat]
  - Theophylline/Theobromine
  - Acetylsalicylic acid [Cat]
  - Paracetamol [Cat]
  - Tricyclic antidepressants
  - Cytostatics
  - Antiparasitics
- Poisonings
  - Organophosphates (insecticides)
  - Metaldehyde (slug pellets)
  - Strychnine
  - Ethylene glycol (antifreeze)
  - Phenol (Household detergents)
  - Heavy metals
  - Toxic plants

Diagnostic Approach

Seizures

1. Case History

2. General Examination

3. Neurological Examination

(changes possible in postictal phase or during anticonvulsant therapy)

- Awareness/behaviour
- Body/limb position and posture
- Locomotion
- Muscle tone
- Cranial nerves
  - Facial symmetry (VII)
  - Facial sensation (V)
  - Menace reflex (II, VII)
  - Blink reflex (V, VII)
  - Corneal reflex/ eye movement
    (V, VI, VII/III, IV, VI)
  - Pupillary reflex
    (III, Sympathetic system)
  - Sight test (II)
  - Swallowing reflex/glossal motor function
    (X, XI, XII/XII)
  - Sense of smell/taste/hearing
    (I/V/VIII)
  - Cervical/shoulder muscles
    (XI)
- Spinal reflexes
  - Bicipital reflex (C6–C8)
  - Triceps reflex (C7–T1)
  - Patellar reflex (L4–L6)
  - Withdrawal reflex (C6–T1 and L6–S1)
  - Cutaneous trunci reflex
    (C7–T1)

- Anal sphincter reflex
  (S1–S3)
- Bladder – can it be expressed?
- Positional and postural reaction
  - Correction reaction
  - Hopping reaction
  - Side stepping reaction
  - Wheelbarrowing reaction
  - Righting reaction (hind limb)/ Extensor postural thrust reaction
  - Righting reaction (fore limb)
  - Table edge reaction(visual/ tactile)

4. Ocular Examination
- Ophthalmoscopy (Ocular fundus)

5. Blood Tests
- Hct, Ery, Leuc, Hb
- Na, K, Ca
- TP, Alb, Glob
- GPT, AP, Urea, Crea, BG
- Ammonium
- FIP Profile [Cat]
  - TP
  - Alb/Glob ratio
  - Bili
  - GOT
  - Serum electrophoresis
- Therapeutic control
  - Phenobarbital
  - Potassium bromide
- Diff BC
- Thrombocytes
- Insulin (Insulin/Glucose ratio)

MICROBIAL SEROLOGY
- FeLV-/FIV Antigen [Cat]
- Toxoplasma Antibodies
- Ehrlichia Antibodies [Dog]
- Neospora Antibodies [Dog]
- Lyme Borrelia Antibodies [Dog]
- Cryptococcus Antibodies [Cat]

FURTHER SEROLOGY
- Serum led
- Serum acetylcholinesterase

6. Urinalysis
- Urinary output/volume
- Urine dip stick
- Specific gravity
- Urine sediment
  - Bacteria
  - Erythrocytes, leucocytes
  - Epithelial cells
  - Casts
  - Crystals
  - Tumour cytology
- Bacterial culture (Cystocentesis)

7. X-Ray Study
- Thorax
- Abdomen
- Skull

8. Liquor Examination
(postictal changes possible)
- Chemistry
  - TP, Glucose, CK
  - Globulin (Pandy and Nonne-Apelt reaction)
- Electrophoresis
- Cytology
- Bacterial/fungal culture
- Canine distemper Antibodies [Dog]
- (Liquor pressure)

9. Further Tests
- Skull MRT
- Electroencephalography (EEG)
- Canine distemper virus antigen [Dog] (conjunctival smear)

Paralysis

Paresis: Incomplete loss of muscle function
Paralysis/Paraplegia: Complete loss of muscle function

Monoparesis (One Fore Limb)
LMN signs (Flaccid Paresis)
- Muscle tone: flaccid
- Muscle strength: ↓
- Muscle fasciculations: present
- Muscle atrophy: early
- Bicipital reflex: ↓
- Triceps reflex: ↓
- Withdrawal reflex: ↓

Causes
- Ventral nerve root lesion
  - Incarceration (compression syndrome)
  - Trauma

- – Tumours
- – Abscess/haematoma
- Brachial plexus lesion
  - – Trauma (avulsion)
  - – Tumours
  - – Abscess/haematoma
- Peripheral nerve lesion

Monoparesis (One Hind Limb)

LMN Signs (flaccid paresis)

- Muscle tone: flaccid
- Muscle strength: ↓
- Muscle fasciculations: present
- Muscle atrophy: early
- Patellar reflex: ↓
- Withdrawal reflex: ↓

Causes

- Lumbosacral spinal lesion (L4–S3)
  - – Lateral disc prolapse
  - – Fibrocartilaginous embolism
- Ventral nerve root lesion
  - – Incarceration (compression syndrome)
  - – Trauma
  - – Tumours
  - – Abscess/haematoma
- Thromboembolism of the femoral artery
- Peripheral nerve lesion

Paraparesis (Both Hind Limbs)

UMN Signs (Spastic Paresis)

- Muscle tone: spastic
- Muscle strength: normal to ↑
- Muscle fasciculations: absent
- Muscle atrophy: late

- Patellar reflex: normal to ↑
- Withdrawal reflex: normal to ↑
- Anal sphincter reflex: normal to ↑
- Tail wagging: normal to ↑ Bladder – can it be expressed? Usually difficult
- Cutaneous trunci reflex: Absent caudal of the lesion

Causes

- Thoracolumbar spinal chord lesion (L4–S3)
  Traumatic causes
  - – Disc prolapse
  - – Vertebral fracture/luxation
  - – Haemorrhage/haematoma
  - – Fibrocartilaginous embolism
  - – Thromboembolism
  Congenital Causes
  - – Deformations of the vertebral spine
  - – Meningocele
  - – Globoid cells Leucodystrophy (Terrier)
  Infectious Causes
  - – Discospondylitis/ Osteomyelitis
  - – Abscess
  - – Myelitis
  Immunoreactive Causes
  - – Granulomatous meningoencephalitis
  Degenerative Causes
  - – Spondylosis deformans
  - – Lumbosacral stenosis (Cauda equina syndrome) [Dog]
  - – Dura-mater ossification

Tumours/Tumour metastasis

- Lymphosarcoma [esp Cat]
- Osteosarcoma
- Chondrosarcoma
- Multiple myeloma

Other Causes

- Hypervitaminosis A [Cat]

LMN Signs (Flaccid Paresis)

- Muscle tone: flaccid
- Muscle strength: ↓
- Muscle fasciculations: present
- Muscle atrophy: early
- Patellar reflex: ↓
- Withdrawal reflex: ↓
- Anal sphincter reflex: ↓
- Tail wagging: ↓
- Bladder – can it be expressed? Usually easily

Causes

- Lumbosacral spinal lesion (L4–S3)

  ### Traumatic Causes
  - Disc prolapse
  - Vertebral fracture/luxation
  - Haemorrhage/haematoma
  - Fibrocartilaginous embolism
  - Thromboembolism

  ### Congenital Causes
  - Deformations of the vertebral spine
  - Meningocele

  ### Infectious Causes
  - Discospondylitis/ osteomyelitis
  - Abscess
  - Myelitis

Immunoreactive Causes
  - Granulomatous meningoencephalitis

Degenerative Causes
  - Spondylosis deformans
  - Lumbosacral stenosis (Cauda equina syndrome) [Dog]
  - Dura-mater ossification

Tumours/Tumour metastasis
  - Lymphosarcoma [esp Cat]
  - Osteosarcoma
  - Chondrosarcoma
  - Multiple myeloma

Other Causes
  - Hypervitaminosis A [Cat]

- Feline aortic thromboembolism [Cat]
- Polyneuropathy
- Polymyopathy

Schiff-Sherrington Phenomenon

- Muscle tone: Fore limb/ neck: Hyperextension Hind limb: spastic (UMN) to flaccid (LMN) paresis

Causes

- Thoracolumbar spinal lesion (T2–L2)

  ### Traumatic Causes
  - Vertebral fracture/luxation
  - Disc prolapse

Tetraparesis (Both Fore Limbs/ Both Hind Limbs)

UMN Signs (Spastic Paresis)

- Muscle tone: spastic

- Muscle strength: normal to ↑
- Muscle fasciculations: absent
- Muscle atrophy: late
- Bicipital reflex: normal to ↑
- Triceps reflex: normal to ↑
- Patellar reflex: normal to ↑
- Withdrawal reflex: normal to ↑
- Anal sphincter reflex:
- normal to ↑
- Tail wagging: normal to ↑
- Bladder – can it be expressed? Usually easily
- Cranial nerve absence: variable

Causes

- Cerebral lesion
  - Traumatic brain injury
  - Hydrocephalus
  - Encephalitis/ Meningoencephalitis
  - Granulomatous meningoencephalitis (GME)
  - Brain tumours
- Brain stem lesion
- Cranial cervical spinal lesion (C1–C5)

  Traumatic Causes
  - Disc prolapse
  - Vertebral fracture/ luxation
  - Haemorrhage/haematoma
  - Fibrocartilaginous embolism
  - Thromboembolism

  Congenital Causes
  - Atlantoaxial subluxation [Dog]
  - Cervical instability [Dog] (Wobbler syndrome)
  - Meningocele

Infectious Causes
- Discospondylitis/ Osteomyelitis
- Abscess
- Myelitis

Immunoreactive Causes
- Granulomatous meningoencephalitis

Degenerative Causes
- Spondylosis deformans
- Dura-mater ossification

Tumours/Tumour metastasis
- Lymphosarcoma [esp Cat]
- Osteosarcoma
- Chondrosarcoma
- Multiple myeloma

Other Causes
- Hypervitaminosis A [Cat]

LMN Signs (Flaccid Paresis)

- Muscle tone: flaccid
- Muscle strength:↓
- Muscle fasciculations: present
- Muscle atrophy: early
- Bicipital reflex: ↓
- Triceps reflex: ↓
- Patellar reflex: ↓
- Withdrawal reflex: ↓
- Anal sphincter reflex: ↓
- Tail wagging: ↓
- Bladder – can it be expressed? Usually easily

Causes

- Polyneuropathy
- Junctionopathy
- Polymyopathy

LMN Sign (Fore limbs) + UMN Signs (Hind limbs)

- Muscle tone: front: flaccid
  hind: spastic
- Muscle strength:
  front: ↓
  hind: ↑
- Muscle fasciculations:
  front: present
  hind: absent
- Muscle atrophy:
  front: early
  hind: late
- Patellar reflex: normal to ↑
- Anal sphincter reflex:
  normal to ↑
- Tail wagging: normal to ↑
- Bladder – can it be expressed?
  Usually with difficulty

Causes

- Caudal cervical spinal lesion
  (C6–T2)
  Traumatic Causes
  - Disc prolapse
  - Vertebral fracture/luxation
  - Haemorrhage/haematoma
  - Fibrocartilaginous embolism
  - Thromboembolism
  Congenital Causes
  - Deformations of the
    vertebral spine
  - Meningocele
  Infectious Causes
  - Discospondylitis/
    Osteomyelitis
  - Abscess
  - Myelitis

Immunoreactive Causes
- Granulomatous
  meningoencephalitis
Degenerative Causes
- Spondylosis deformans
- Dura-mater ossification
Tumours/Tumour metastasis
- Lymphosarcoma[esp Cat]
- Osteosarcoma
- Chondrosarcoma
- Multiple myeloma
Other Causes
- Hypervitaminosis A [Cat]

Hemiparesis (One Fore Limb and One Hind Limb Ipsilateral)

UMN Signs (Spastic Paresis)

- Muscle tone: spastic
- Muscle strength: normal to ↑
- Muscle fasciculations: absent
- Muscle atrophy: late
- Bicipital reflex: normal to ↑
- Triceps reflex: normal to ↑
- Patellar reflex: normal to ↑
- Withdrawal reflex: normal to ↑
- Anal sphincter reflex:
  normal to ↑
- Tail wagging: normal to ↑
- Bladder – can it be expressed?
  Usually with difficulty
- Cranial nerve function
  absences

Causes

- Cerebral lesion (contralateral to
  the paralysis)
  - Traumatic brain injury

- Cerebral contusion
- Intracerebral haemorrhage
- Haematoma (subdural, epidural)
- Fibrocartilaginous embolism
- Thromboembolism (hemispheral infarction)
- Cerebral abscess
- Brain tumour/ tumour metastasis
- Lymphosarcoma [esp Cat]
- Neurinoma
- Glioma
- Medulloblastoma
- Chorioidal plexus papilloma
- Neuroblastoma
• Brain stem lesion (Causes as above)

Diagnostic Approach

Paralysis

1. Case History

2. General Examination (Incl. Femoral Arterial Pulse)

3. Neurological Examination

• Awareness/behaviour
• Body/limb position and posture
• Muscle tone/strength
• Cranial nerves
  - Facial symmetry (VII)
  - Facial sensation (V)
  - Menace reflex (II, VII)
  - Blink reflex (V, VII)
  - Corneal reflex/ eye movements (V, VI, VII/III, IV, VI)
  - Pupillary reflex (III, Sympathetic system)
  - Sight test (II)
  - Swallowing reflex/glossal motor function (X, XI, XII/ XII)
  - Sense of smell/taste/hearing (I/V/VIII)
  - Cervical/shoulder muscles (XI)
• Spinal reflexes
  - Bicipital reflexes (C6–C8)
  - Triceps reflex (C7–T1)
  - Patellar reflex (L4–L6)
  - Withdrawal reflex (C6–T1 and L6–S1)
  - Cutaneous trunci reflex (C7–T1)
  - Anal sphincter reflex (S1–S3)
  - Bladder – can it be expressed?
• Postural Responses
  - Correction response
  - Hopping response
  - Side stepping response
  - Wheelbarrowing response
  - Righting response (hind limb)
  - Righting response (fore limb)
  - Table edge response (visual/ tactile)

4. X-Ray Study

• Vertebral spine ± Myelography

5. Blood Tests

• Hct, Ery, Leuc, Hb

- Na, K, Ca
- TP, Alb, Glob
- BG, CK, Aldolase
- FIP Profile [Cat]
  - TP
  - Alb/Glob ratio
  - Bili
  - GOT
  - Serum electrophoresis
- Diff BC
- Insulin (Insulin/Glucose ratio)
- Serum electrophoresis

MICROBIAL SEROLOGY
- FeLV-/FIV Antigen [Cat]
- Coronavirus Antibodies [Cat]
- Toxoplasma Antibodies
- Ehrlichia Antibodies [Dog]
- Neospora Antibodies [Dog]
- Canine Distemper antibodies [Dog]

FUNCTION TESTS
- T_4, fT_4
- TSH-/TRH stimulation test [Dog]

6. Urinalysis
- Urinary output/volume
- Urinalysis

- Specific gravity
- Urine sediment
  - Bacteria
  - Erythrocytes, leucocytes
  - Epithelial cells
  - Casts
  - Crystals
  - Tumour cytology
- Bacterial culture (Cystocentesis)

7. Liquor Examination
- Chemistry
  - TP, Glucose, CK
  - Globulin (Pandy and Nonne-Apelt reaction)
- Electrophoresis
- Cytology
- Bacterial/fungal culture
- Canine distemper antibodies [Dog]
- (Liquor pressure)

8. Further Tests
- Skull/spinal MRT/(CT)
- Electrodiagnostics
  - Electromyography (EMG)
  - Measurement of impulse conduction
- Muscle biopsy
- Angiography

Principal symptoms/findings with cerebral and spinal lesions (presenting individually or combined)

Cerebral lesion	• Altered awareness • Circling movements (ipsilateral) • Head pressing • Loss of eye sight (contralateral) • Seizures • Hemiparesis: contralateral UMN signs • Tetraparesis: UMN signs
Thalamic/Hypothalamic lesion	• Altered awareness • Loss of eye sight (bilateral) • Sleeping/eating/drinking/body temperature disturbances • (Cardiac arrhythmias) • Dyspnoea • Electrolyte disturbances • Endocrine disturbances • Seizures • Opisthotonus • Hemiparesis: contralateral UMN signs • Tetraparesis: UMN signs

Brain stem lesion	• Altered awareness
	• Ataxia
	• Circling movements (ipsilateral)
	• Opisthotonus
	• Hemiparesis: ipsilateral UMN signs
	• Tetraparesis: UMN signs
	• Cranial nerve disorders:
	  − N. oculomotorius (III)
	  − N. trochlearis (IV)
	  − N. trigeminus (V)
	  − N. abducens (VI)
	  − N. facialis (VII)
	  − N. vestibulocochlearis (VIII)
	  − N. glossopharyngeus (IX)
	  − N. vagus (X)
	  − N. hypoglossus (XII)

Principal symptoms/findings with cerebral and spinal lesions (presenting individually or combined)	
Cerebral lesion	• Ataxia • Dysmetria/Hypermetria • Tremor (Head/Intention tremor) • Absent menace response • Opisthotonus

Cranial Cervical (C1 – C5)	• Tetraparesis
	  – Fore limb: UMN signs
	  – Hind limb: UMN signs

Caudal cervical (C6 – T2)	• Tetraparesis
	  – Fore limb: LMN signs
	  – Hind limb: UMN signs

Thoracolumbar spinal lesion (T3 – L3)	• Paraparesis
	  – Fore limb: normal
	  – Hind limb: UMN signs

Lumbosacral spinal (L4 – S3)	• Paraparesis
	  – Fore limb: normal
	  – Hind limb: LMN signs

Sacral spinal lesion (S1 – S3)	• Tail Paralysis
	• Bladder paralysis (Detrusor)
	• Anal sphincter paralysis
	  – Fore limb: normal
	  – Hind limb: normal
	  – Tail/Anus/Bladder LMN signs

Tremor

Trembling: Involuntary rhythmic muscle contractions of antagonising muscles (continuous tremor/intention tremor)

Common Causes	
Dog	Cat
+++ Distemper	+++ FIP
++ Poisoning	++ Poisoning
++ Metabolic causes	++ Metabolic causes
++ Cerebellar hypoplasia	++ Cerebellar hypoplasia

Tremor

Physiological Causes

- Excitement/fear
- Exhaustion
- Coldness

Cerebellar/Brain Stem Diseases

- Cerebellar hypoplasia
  - Feline parvovirus (in utero) [Cat]
  - Canine Herpes virus (in utero) [Dog]
  - Live vaccine (in utero)
- Cerebellar degeneration
  - Cerebellar abiotrophy
  - Lysosomal storage disease
  - Neuroaxonal dystrophy
  - Dysmyelogenesis
  - White Dog Shaker Syndrome [Dog]
- Cerebellitis
  - FIP Coronavirus [Cat]
  - Canine distemper virus [Dog]
  - Toxoplasma sp.
  - Neospora sp. [Dog]
  - Cryptococcus sp. [Cat]
  - Granulomatous meningoencephalitis (GME)
- Cerebellar/brain stem tumours/tumour metastasis
  - ie medulloblastoma
  - Lymphosarcoma [esp Cat]
- Traumatic brain injury
- Cerebellar circulatory disorder
- Thiamine deficiency [Cat]

Metabolic Causes

- Hypoglycaemia
- Hypocalcaemia
- Hyperkalaemia/Hypokalaemia
- Hypercortisolism (Cushing's disease) [esp Dog]
- Hyperthyroidism [Cat]

Toxic Causes

- Drugs
  - Lidocaine
  - Ivermectin
  - Amitraz
  - Pyrethroids
  - Lindane
  - β_2 Agonists
  - Tricyclic antidepressants
  - Cytostatics
  - Theophylline
  - Ephedrine
  - Metoclopramide
  - Diphenhydramide

- Poisons
  - Pyrethrin/Pyrethroids
    (Insecticides)
  - Nicotine sulfate (Insecticide)
  - Organophosphates/
    Carbamate (Insecticide)
  - Metaldehyde (slug
    pellets)
  - Phenoxyacetate (Herbicide)
  - Toxic plants
  - Household detergents

Other Causes

- Pain
- Spinal disease

Diagnostic Approach

Tremor

1. **Case History**

2. **General Examination**

3. **Neurological Examination**
- Awareness/behaviour
- Body/limb position and posture
- Locomotion
- Cranial nerves
  - Facial symmetry (VII)
  - Facial sensation (V)
  - Menace reflex (II, VII)
  - Blink reflex (V, VII)
  - Corneal reflex/ eye
    movements
    (V, VI, VII/III, IV, VI)
  - Pupillary reflex (III,
    Sympathetic system)
  - Sight test (II)
  - Swallowing reflex/glossal
    motor function (X, XI, XII/
    XII)
  - Sense of smell/taste/hearing
    (I/V/VIII)
  - Cervical and shoulder
    muscles (XI)
- Spinal reflexes
  - Bicipital reflex (C6–C8)
  - Triceps reflex (C7–T1)
  - Patellar reflex (L4–L6)
  - Withdrawal reflex
    (C6–T1 and L6–S1)
  - Cutaneous trunci reflex
    (C7–T1)
  - Anal sphincter reflex
    (S1–S3)
  - Bladder – can it be
    expressed?
- Postural responses
  - Correction response
  - Hopping response
  - Side stepping response
  - Wheelbarrowing response
  - Righting response (fore
    limb)
  - Righting response (hind
    limb)
  - Table edge response
    (visual/tactile)

4. **Blood Tests**
- Hct, Ery, Leuc, Hb
- Na, K, Ca
- TP, Alb, Glob
- GPT, AP, Urea, Crea, BG
- FIP Profile [Cat]

- TP
- Alb/Glob ratio
- Bili
- GOT
- Serum electrophoresis
- Diff BC
- Thrombocyte
- Insulin (Insulin/Glucose ratio)

MICROBIAL SEROLOGY
- FeLV-/FIV Antigen [Cat]
- Toxoplasma Antibodies
- Ehrlichia Antibodies [Dog]
- Neospora Antibodies [Dog]

FUNCTION TESTS
- T_4
- TSH/TRH-Stimulation test [Dog]

5. Urinalysis
- Urinary output/volume
- Urine dip stick
- Specific gravity
- Urine sediment
  - Bacteria
  - Erythrocytes, Leucocytes
  - Epithelial cells
  - Casts
  - Crystals
  - Tumour cytology
- Bacterial culture (Cystocentesis)

6. X-Ray Study
- Skull (Tympanic bulla)
- Spine ± Myelography

7. Liquor Examination
- Chemistry
  - TP, Glucose, CK
  - Globulin (Pandy and Nonne-Apelt reaction)
- Electrophoresis
- Cytology
- Bacterial-/fungal culture
- Canine distemper Antibodies [Dog]
- (Liquor pressure)

8. Further Tests
- Skull MRT
- Electrodiagnostics

8 Orthopaedic Principal Symptoms

Further Relevant Principal Symptoms

Lameness of the fore limb

Common Causes		
Large Dog Breeds		Small Dog Breeds
Growing Dogs < 1 Year		
+++	Trauma (Distortion)	+++ Trauma (Distortion)
++	Panosteitis	+ Atlantoaxial Instability
+	Fragmented medial coronoid process	+ Distractio cubiti
		+ Congenital luxations (Shoulder/Elbow)
+	Isolated anconeal process	+ Short radius/ulna syndrome
+	Osteochondrosis dissecans (OCD) (shoulder/elbow)	++ Cardiac Arrhythmias
Adult Dogs > 1 Year		
+++	Trauma	+++ Trauma
++	Arthrosis	++ Arthrosis
+	Biceps tendovaginitis	++ Cervical spine disease
+	Bone tumours	++ Luxations (Elbow/Shoulder)

Common Causes
Cats
Growing Cats < 1 Year
+++ Trauma
Adult Cats > 1 Year
+++ Trauma

Shoulder

Joint Disease

- Traumatic Causes
  - (Sub-)Luxation
  - Torn ligaments/Capsular injury
  - Contusion
  - Distortion
  - Epiphyseal fracture
  - Perforating wounds
  - Brachial plexus/Nerve damage as a result of a fracture
- Tumours/Synovial cysts
- Inflammatory Causes
  - Infectious arthritis
  - Non-infectious arthritis
  - Arthrosis
- Other Causes
  - Coagulopathy (Haemarthros)

Bone Disease

- Traumatic Causes
  - Traumatic fractures
  - Pathological fractures
- Bone tumours (humerus)
- Osteomyelitis
- Metabolic Causes
  - Osteoporosis
  - Osteopetrosis
  - Rickets/osteomalacia
  - Secondary hyperparathyroidism
  - Hypervitaminosis A [Cat]
- Other Causes
  - Hypertrophic pulmonary osteopathy

Muscle/Tendon Disease

- Traumatic Causes
  - Ruptured bicipital tendon
  - Strained muscle/haematoma
- Inflammatory Causes
  - Myositis
  - Tendovaginitis/Bursitis (Bicipital tendon)
- Tumours
- Other Causes
  - M. supraspinatus/infraspinatus contraction

Growth Disturbances

- Panosteitis
- Osteochondrosis dissecans (OCD) [Dog]
- Shoulder joint dysplasia
- Epiphyseal damage/premature closure of the epiphyseal plate

- Epiphyseal fracture
- Congenital shoulder luxation
- Hypertrophic osteodystrophy [Dog]
- Juvenile bone cysts
- Dwarfism/Chondrodysplasia

Neurological Disease

- Spinal Disease
- Compression syndrome
- Brachial plexus lesion/tumour
- Peripheral nerve lesion

Elbow
Joint Disease

- Traumatic Causes
  - (Sub-)Luxation
  - Rupture of the collateral ligaments
  - Contusion/distortion
  - Epiphyseal fracture
  - Perforating wounds
- Inflammatory Causes
  - Infectious arthritis
  - Non-infectious arthritis
  - Arthrosis
- Tumours/Synovial cysts
- Other Causes
  - Coagulopathy (Haemarthros)

Bone Disease

- Traumatic Causes
  - Traumatic fractures
  - Pathological fractures
- Inflammatory Causes
  - Osteomyelitis
- Bone tumours
- Metabolic Causes

  - Osteoporosis
  - Osteopetrosis
  - Rickets/osteomalacia
  - Secondary hyperparathyroidism
  - Hypervitaminosis A [Cat]
- Other Causes
  - Hypertrophic pulmonary osteopathy

Muscle/Tendon Disease

- Traumatic Causes
  - Rupture of the triceps tendon
  - Strained muscle/haematoma
- Inflammatory Causes
  - Myositis
  - Tendovaginitis/bursitis
- Tumours
- Hygroma [Dog]

Growth Disturbances

- Panosteitis
- Osteochondrosis dissecans (OCD) [Dog]
- Isolated anconaeal process [Dog]
- Fragmented medial coronoid process [Dog]
- Short radius/ulna syndrome
- Epiphyseal fracture
- Hypertrophic osteodystrophy [Dog]
- Luxation/Subluxation
- Juvenile bone cysts

Neurological Disease

- Spinal Disease
- Compression syndrome

- Brachial plexus lesion/tumour
- Peripheral nerve lesion

Carpus

Joint Disease

- Traumatic Causes
  - (Sub-)Luxation
  - Contusion
  - Distortion
  - Perforating wounds
  - Hyperextension syndrome
- Inflammatory Causes
  - Infectious arthritis
  - Non-infectious arthritis
  - Arthrosis
- Tumours/Synovial cysts
- Other Causes
  - Coagulopathy

Bone Disease

- Traumatic Causes
  - Traumatic fractures
  - Pathological fractures
- Inflammatory Causes
  - Osteomyelitis
- Bone tumours

Muscle/Tendon Dsiease

- Traumatic Causes
  - Rupture of the ligamentous apparatus (hyperflexion)
  - Flexor muscle rupture
  - Strained muscle
  - Haematoma
- Inflammatory Causes
  - Myositis
  - Tendovaginitis/Bursitis
- Tumours

Growth Disturbances

- Hypertrophic osteodystrophy [Dog]
- Weakness of the flexor tendon (hyperextension syndrome)
- Epiphyseal damage/ premature closure of the epiphyseal plate
- Epiphyseal fracture
- Osteochondrosis dissecans (OCD) [Dog]

Neurological Disease

- Spinal Disease
- Compression syndrome
- Brachial plexus lesion/tumour
- Peripheral nerve lesion

Fore Foot

Joint Disease

- Traumatic Causes
  - (Sub-)Luxation
  - Rupture of the collateral ligaments
  - Contusion
  - Distortion
  - Perforating Wounds
- Inflammatory Causes
  - Infectious arthritis
  - Non-infectious arthritis
  - Arthrosis
- Tumours/Synovial cysts

Bone Disease

- Traumatic Causes
  - Traumatic fractures
  - Pathological fractures
  - Sesamoid fracture (esp Rottweiler)

- Inflammatory Causes
  - Osteomyelitis
- Bone tumours

Muscle/Tendon Disease

- Traumatic Causes
  - Flexor muscle rupture
  - Strained muscle
  - Haematoma
- Inflammatory Causes
  - Myositis
  - Tendovaginitis/bursitis

Growth Disturbances

- Epiphyseal damage/premature closure of the epiphyseal plate
- Epiphyseal fracture

Disease of the Paw

- Pulled out claw/fracture
- Interdigital foreign body
- Cut pad/granula
- Paronychia
- Bone fracture
- Luxation
- Tendon rupture
- Tumours

Neurological Disease

- Spinal Disease
- Compression syndrome
- Brachial plexus lesion/tumour
- Peripheral nerve lesion

Diagnostic Approach

Lameness

1. Case History

2. General Examination

3. Orthopaedic Examination
- Position/posture (body and limbs)
- Gait
- Muscle tone
- Comparative limb palpation (distal proximal)
  - pain
  - (joint) swelling
  - crepitus
  - extension/flexion/rotation
  - joint stability
  - Patella – mobility?
  - Drawer test (cruciate ligament stability)
  - Ortolani test (hip joint stability)
- Spinal palpation

4. Neurological Examination
- Cutaneous sensation test
- Spinal reflexes
  - Bicipital reflex (C6–C8)
  - Triceps reflex (C7–T1)
  - Patellar reflex (L4–L6)
  - Withdrawal reflex (C6–T1 and L6–S1)
  - Cutaneous trunci reflex (C7–T1)
  - Anal sphincter reflex (S1–S3)
  - Bladder – can it be expressed?

- Postural Responses
  - Correction response
  - Hopping response
  - Sidestepping response
  - Wheelbarrowing response
  - Righting response (fore limb)
  - Righting response (hind limb)
  - Table edge response (visual/tactile)

5. X-Ray Study
- Bones
- Joints
- Spine

6. Urinalysis
- Urine dip stick
- Specific gravity
- Urine sediment

7. Blood Tests
- Hct, Ery, Leuc, Hb
- Na, K, Ca
- TP
- BG
- CK

MICROBIAL SEROLOGY
- FeLV-/FIV Antigen [Cat]
- Lyme Borrelia Antibodies [Dog]

8. Arthrocentesis
- Synovial Analysis
  - colour, transparency, viscosity
  - mucin precipitation cytology
  - bacterial culture,
  - fungal culture
  - TP
  - Electrophoresis Glucose Rheumatoid factor

9. Further Tests
- Diagnostic joint anaesthesia
- Bone scintigraphy
- Contrast arthrography/Arthroscopy
- Joint capsule biopsy/Bone biopsy
- Muscle biopsy

Lameness of the Hind Limb

Common Causes	
Large Dog Breeds	Small Dog Breeds
Growing Dogs < 1 Year	
+++ Hip dysplasia (HD) ++ Panosteitis ++ Trauma + Hypertrophic osteodystrophy	+++ Trauma ++ Aseptic femoral head necrosis (Legg-Calvé-Perthes disease) + Patellar luxation
Adult Dogs > 1 Year	
+++ Trauma	+++ Trauma

	− Fractures		− Fractures
	− Luxations		− Luxations
	− Ligament ruptures (esp	++	Arthrosis
	cruciates ± Meniscal rupture)	++	Patellar luxation
++	Hip joint arthrosis/HD (Coxarthrosis)		
++	Lumbar spinal disease		
+	Bone tumours		

Cats

Growing Cats < 1 Year

+++	Trauma	+	Patellar luxation
++	Lumbar spine disease		

Adult Cats > 1 Year

+++	Trauma
	Fractures
	Luxations

Hip

Joint Disease

- Traumatic Causes
  - (Sub-)Luxation
  - Torn ligament
  - Contusion
  - Distortion
  - Epiphyseal fracture
  - Perforating wounds
- Tumours/Synovial cysts
- Inflammatory Causes
  - Infectious arthritis
  - Non-infectious arthritis
  - Arthrosis (Coxarthrosis)

Bone Disease

- Traumatic Causes
  - Traumatic fractures

  - Pathological fractures
- Metabolic Causes
  - Osteoporosis
  - Osteopetrosis
  - Rickets/osteomalacia
  - Secondary hyperparathyroidism
  - Hypervitaminosis A [Cat]
- Bone tumours
- Inflammatory Causes
  - Osteomyelitis
- Other Causes
  - Hypertrophic pulmonary osteopathy

Muscle/Tendon Disease

- Traumatic Causes
  - M. gracilis rupture
  - Sprained muscle
  - Haematoma

- Inflammatory Causes
  - Myositis
  - Tendovaginitis/Bursitis
- Tumours
- Other Causes
  - M. quadriceps contraction
  - M. gracilis contraction
  - M. semitendinosus contraction
  - Polymyopathy

Growth Disturbances

- Panosteitis
- Hip dysplasia (HD) [esp Dog]
- Legg-Calvé-Perthes disease [small dog breeds)
- Epiphyseal damage/premature closure of the epiphyseal plate
- Epiphyseal fracture
- Congenital luxation
- Juvenile bone cysts
- Hypertrophic osteodystrophy [Dog]

Neurological Disease

- Spinal disease (Cauda equina syndrome)
- Compression syndrome
- Sciatic nerve lesion
- Peripheral nerve lesion

Knee

Joint Disease

- Traumatic Causes (Sub-)Luxation
  - Cranial (caudal) cruciate ligament rupture
  - Rupture of the collateral ligaments

  - Meniscal damage
  - Patellar luxation
  - Contusion/distortion
  - Epiphyseal fracture
  - Perforating wounds
- Inflammatory Causes
  - Arthrosis
  - Infectious arthritis
  - Non-infectious arthritis
- Tumours/Synovial cysts

Bone Disease

- Traumatic Causes
  - Traumatic fractures
  - Pathological fractures
- Inflammatory Causes
  - Osteomyelitis
- Metabolic Causes
  - Osteoporosis
  - Osteopetrosis
  - Rickets/Osteomalacia
  - Secondary hyperparathyroidism
- Bone tumours

Muscle/Tendon Disease

- Traumatic Causes
  - Rupture of the patellar tendon/ patellar fracture
  - M. popliteus rupture (tendon of origin)
  - M. gastrocnemius rupture (tendon of origin)
  - Muscle sprain/haematoma
- Inflammatory Causes
  - Myositis
- Tumours
- Other Causes
  - M. quadriceps contraction

Growth Disturbances

- Panosteitis
- Congenital lateral patellar luxation
- Congenital medial patellar luxation
- Osteochondrosis dissecans (OCD) [Dog]
- Epiphyseal damage/ premature closure of the epiphyseal plate
- Epiphyseal fracture
- Hypertrophic osteodystrophy [Dog]
- Juvenile bone cysts

Neurological Disease

- Spinal disease (Cauda equina syndrome)
- Compression syndrome
- Sciatic nerve lesion
- Peripheral nerve lesion

Tarsal Joint

Joint Disease

- Traumatic Causes
  - (Sub-)Luxation
  - Rupture of the collateral ligaments
  - Contusion
  - Distortion
  - Perforating wounds
- Inflammatory Causes
  - Arthrosis
  - Infectious arthritis
  - Non-infectious arthritis
- Tumours/Synovial cysts

Bone Disease

- Traumatic Causes
  - Traumatic fractures
  - Pathological fractures
- Inflammatory Causes
- Osteomyelitis
- Bone tumours

Muscle/Tendon Disease

- Traumatic causes
  - Achilles tendon rupture
  - Muscle strain
  - Haematoma
- Inflammatory Causes
  - Myositis
  - Tendovaginitis/Bursitis
- Other Causes
  - Tendon displacement of the Superficial flexor digitalis muscle

Growth Disturbances

- Panosteitis
- Osteochondrosis dissecans (OCD) [Dog]
- Weakness of the flexor tendon (hyperextension syndrome) [esp Rottweiler]
- Epiphyseal plate damage/ premature closure of the epiphyseal plate
- Epiphyseal fracture
- Tibial dysplasia

Neurological Disease

- Spinal disease (Cauda equine syndrome)
- Compression syndrome

- Psiatic nerve lesion
- Peripheral nerve lesion

Hind Foot
Joint Disease

- Traumatic Causes
  - (Sub-)luxation
  - Rupture of the collateral ligaments
  - Contusion
  - Distortion
  - Perforating wounds
- Inflammatory Causes
  - Infectious arthritis
  - Non-infectious arthritis
  - Arthrosis
- Tumours/Synovial cysts

Bone Disease

- Traumatic Causes
  - Traumatic fractures
  - Pathological fractures
- Inflammatory Causes
  - Osteomyelitis
- Bone tumours

Muscle/Tendon Disease

- Traumatic Causes
  - Flexor rupture

  - Muscle sprain
  - Haematoma
- Inflammatory Causes
  - Myositis
  - Tendovaginitis/Bursitis

Growth Disturbances

- Epiphyseal plate damage/ premature closure of the epiphyseal plate
- Epiphyseal fracture

Diseases of the Paw

- Pulled out claw/fracture
- Interdigital foreign body
- Cut pad/Granuloma
- Paronychia
- Bone fracture
- Luxation
- Ligament rupture
- Tumours

Neurological Disease

- Spinal disease (Cauda equina syndrome)
- Compression syndrome
- Sciatic nerve lesion
- Peripheral nerve lesion

Lameness of multiple limbs

Common Causes	
Dog	Cat
+++ Spinal disease	+++ Polymyopathy
++ Panosteitis	++ Polyarthritis

+	Polyarthritis	++	Spinal disease
+	Polymyopathy	+	Polyneuropathy
+	Polyneuropathy		

Spinal disease

Traumatic Causes

- Disc prolapse
- Vertebral fracture/luxation
- Haematoma/haemorrhage
- Fibrocartilaginous embolism
- Thromboembolism

Congenital Causes

- Atlantoaxial subluxation [Dog]
- Cervical instability (Wobbler syndrome) [Dog]
- Spinal deformations [esp bull dog]

Infectious Causes

- Discospondylitis/Osteomyelitis
  - Staphylococcus sp.
  - Brucella sp. [Dog]
  - Streptococcus sp.
  - E. coli
  - Pasteurella sp.
  - Actinomyces sp.
  - Nocardia sp.
  - Mycobacterium sp.
  - Aspergillus sp.
- Myelitis
  - Canine Distemper virus [Dog]
  - FeLV/FIV [Cat]
  - FIP Coronavirus [Cat]
  - (Rabies virus)
  - Staphylococcus sp.
  - Lyme Borrelia sp. [Dog]
  - Cryptococcus sp. [Cat]
  - Toxoplasma sp.
  - Neospora sp. [Dog]
  - Larva migrans
  - (Ehrlichia sp. [Dog])

Immunoreactive Causes

- Granulomatous meningoencephalitis (GME)
- Eosinophilic meningoencephalitis (EME)

Degenerative Causes

- Lumbosacral stenosis (Cauda equina syndrome)
- Disc prolapse
- Spondylosis deformans
- Demyelinisation disease [German shepherd Dog]
- (Dura-mater ossification)

Spinal Tumours

- Osteosarcoma
- Chondrosarcoma
- Multiple myeloma
- Tumour metastasis

Other Causes

- Hypervitaminosis A [Cat]

Bone Disease

Traumatic Causes

- Traumatic fractures

- Pathological fractures

Inflammatory Causes

- Osteomyelitis
  Bacterial Osteomyelitis
  - Staphylococcus sp.
  - Streptococcus sp.
  - Proteus sp.
  - E. coli
  - Klebsiella sp.
  - Pseudomonas sp.
  - Actinomyces sp.
  - Clostridium sp.
  - Peptostreptococcus sp.
  - Bacteroides sp.
  - Fusobacterium sp.
  Mycotic Osteomyelitis
  - Cryptococcus sp.

Growth Disturbances

- Panosteitis

Metabolic Causes

- Hypertrophic osteodystrophy [Dog]
  - Malnutrition (Ca : P)
  - Vitamin C deficiency?
- Osteoporosis
  - Congenital osteoporosis (Osteogenesis imperfecta)
  - Senile osteoporosis
  - Inactivity osteoporosis
  - Hyperparathyroidism
  - Hypoalbuminaemia
  - Hypercortisolism (Cushing's disease) [Dog]
  - Diabetes mellitus
  - Hyperthyroidism [Cat]
  - Multiple myeloma [esp Dog]

- Heparin long term therapy
- Rickets/Osteomalacia
  - Vitamin D deficiency
  - Calcium deficiency
  - Malnutrition (Ca : P)
- Mucopolysaccharidosis Type I, VI [Cat]

Bone Tumours

- Osteoma/Osteosarcoma
- Chondroma/Chondrosarcoma
- Multiple myeloma [esp Dog]
- Lymphosarcoma [esp Cat]
- Fibrosarcoma
- Bone metastasis

Joint Disease

Traumatic Causes

- Multiple joint trauma
- Multiple ligament ruptures/ meniscal damage

Inflammatory Causes

- Infectious polyarthritis
  Viral polyarthritis
  - Feline calici virus [Cat]
  Bacterial polyarthritis
  - Lyme Borrelia sp. [Dog]
  - Mycoplasma sp. [esp Cat]
  - Staphylococcus sp.
  - Streptococcus sp.
  - E. coli
  - Pasteurella sp.
  - Fusobacterium sp.
  - Peptostreptococcus sp.
  - Bacteroides sp.
  Rickettsial polyarthritis
  - (Ehrlichia sp. [Dog])
  - (Rickettsia sp. [Dog])

Mycotic polyarthritis
- Cryptococcus sp. [Cat]
- (Blastomyces sp.)
- (Coccidioides sp.)
- Non-infectious polyarthritis
Immunoreactive polyarthritis
- Lupus erythematosus
- Rheumatoid arthritis
- Lymphoplasmacellular synovitis
- Feline chronic progressive polyarthritis [Cat]
- Immune complex disease
- Drug allergy (Sulfonamides, Erythromycin, Lincomycin, Cephalosporines, Penicillins)
- Coagulopathy (Haemarthros)
- Arthrosis
- Degenerative Causes
- Unequal load distribution/ overload (obesity)
- Posture anomalies
- Gout (Dalmatian)

Growth Disorders

- Osteochondrosis dissecans (OCD) [Dog]
- Hip dysplasia (HD) [esp Dog]
- Aseptic femoral head necrosis [Dog] (Legg-Calvé-Perthes disease)

Neuromuscular Disease

Polyneuropathy

- Congenital Causes
- Axonopathy
- Demyelinisation disease
- Lysosomal storage disease
- Spinal muscular atrophy

[Dog]
- Inflammatory Causes
- Polyradiculoneuritis [Dog]
- Polyneuritis
- FeLV/FIV [Cat]
- Toxoplasma sp.
- Neospora sp. [Dog]
- Immunoreactive Causes
- Lupus erythematosus
- Myasthenia gravis
- Metabolic Causes
- Hypothyroidism [Dog]
- Diabetes mellitus
- Paraneoplastic syndrome (insulinoma)
- Toxic Causes
- Organophosphate poisoning (chronic)
- Lead poisoning
- Thallium poisoning
- Cytostatics
- Lindane
- Botulism
- Tick paralysis
- Other Causes
- Nerve root compression syndrome
- Feline dysautonomia [esp Cat]

Polymyopathy

- Congenital Causes
- Muscular dystrophy
- Dermatomyositis [Dog]
- Glycogen storage disease
- Inflammatory Causes
- Toxoplasma sp.
- Neospora sp. [Dog]
- Lyme Borrelia sp. [Dog]
- Leptospira sp. [Dog]

- Immunoreactive Causes
  - Eosinophilic myositis [Dog]
- Metabolic Causes
  - Vitamin E/Selenium deficiency
  - Hypokalaemia [esp Cat]
  - Hypercortisolism (Cushing's disease) [Dog]
  - Glucocorticoid long term therapy
  - Hypothyroidism [Dog]
- Other Causes
  - Feline aortic thromboembolism [esp Cat]

Tendon Disease

- Tendon weakness (Hyperextension syndrome)
  - Malnutrition (Protein overload, Ca : P, Vitamin C deficiency?)
- Bilateral patellar luxation
- Tendovaginitis/Bursitis
- Hygroma [Dog]

9 Ophthalmological Principal Symptoms

Further Relevant Principal Symptoms

Anisocoria

Uneven pupillary size

Common Causes			
Dog		**Cat**	
+++	Traumatic brain injury	+++	FeLV/FIV, FIP Coronavirus
++	Spinal trauma	++	Traumatic brain injury
++	Encephalitis/ Meningoencephalitis	++	Encephalitis/ Meningoencephalitis
++	Tumours	++	Tumours
++	Eye disease	++	Eye disease

Unilateral Miosis

Ocular Disease

- Uveitis anterior/synechia
- Ulcerative keratitis
- Foreign body
- Keratoconjunctivitis sicca
- Pupillary spasm (FeLV) [Cat]

Sympathetic Nerve Lesion

- Horner syndrome (miosis, ptosis, enophthalmos, prolapse of the nictitating membrane)
  - Brain stem lesion
  - Cervical spinal lesion
  - Thoracic spinal lesion (T1–T3)
  - Nerve root compression syndrome (T1–T3)
  - Brachial plexus lesion
  - Mediastinal disease
  - Middle ear lesion
  - Retrobulbar lesion
- Traumatic brain injury
- Encephalitis/ Meningoencephalitis
- Brain tumours
- Spinal trauma
- Otitis media/interna

- Brachial plexus avulsion/ tumours/abscess
- Mediastinitis/ Mediastinal tumours
- Middle ear tumours
- Retrobulbar abscess/tumours

Unilateral Mydriasis

Ocular Disease

- Glaucoma
- Lens luxation
- Progressive retinal atrophy
- Eye tumours
- Iridal atrophy/hypoplasia
- Drugs
  - Atropine

Parasympathetic Nerve Lesion

- Optic nerve (I) lesion (lesion ipsilateral)
- Optic tract lesion (lesion contralateral)
- Oculomotor nerve (III) lesion (lesion ipsilateral)
- Traumatic brain injury
- Tonometry
- Gonioscopy
- Conjunctival smear

Diagnostic Approach

Anisocoria

1. **Case History**

2. **General Examination**

3. **Ocular Examination**
- Inspection
- Sight test

- Reflex responses
  - Sight test (II)
  - Menace reflex (II, VII)
  - Blink reflex (V, VII)
  - Corneal reflex (V, VI, VII)

- Pupillary reflex (III, Sympathetic nerve)
- Pupillary symmetry/size
- Eye movements (III, IV, VI)
- Facial symmetry (VII)
- Schirmer tear test
- Eversion of the nictitating membrane
- Fluorescein test
- Direct/indirect ophthalmoscopy
- Neuritis
  - FeLV/FIV [Cat]
  - FIP Coronavirus [Cat]
- Encephalitis/ Meningoencephalitis
- Brain tumours
- Retrobulbar abscess/tumours
- Peripheral nerve tumours (Neurinoma)
  - Chlamydia sp.
  - Canine distemper virus antigen
  - Feline Herpes virus antigen
  - Cytology
  - Bacterial culture
- Flushing of the tear duct
- Ultrasound
- Puncture of the vitreous body
  - Tumour cytology
  - Bacterial/fungal culture
- Electroretinogram (ERG)

4. Blood Tests
- Hct, Ery, Leuc
- FIP Profile [Cat]
  - TP
  - Alb/Glob ratio
- Bili
- GOT
- Serum electrophoresis
- Diff BC

MICROBIAL SEROLOGY
- FeLV-/FIV Antigen [Cat]

5. Pharmacological Function Tests
- Sympathetic nerve
  - Phenylephrine (1%) test
  - Hydroxyamphetamine test
- Parasympathetic nerve
  - Pilocarpine (1%) test
  - Physostigmine test

6. X-Ray Study
- Thorax
- Skull
- Spine ± Myelography

7. Ultrasound
- Orbit
- Thorax

8. Further Tests
- Liquor puncture/analysis
  - Liquor pressure
  - Leucocyte number + Diff
  - TP, Glucose, CK
  - Globulin (Pandy and Nonne-Apelt reaction)
  - Bacterial/fungal culture
  - Tumour cytology
  - Electrophoresis
  - Canine distemper antibodies [Dog]
- Skull CT/MRT

Ocular Discharge

Epiphora: Overflow of tears above the edge of the lid

Common Causes	
Dog	Cat
+++ Keratoconjunctivitis	+++ Cat flu
++ Foreign body	+ Keratoconjunctivitis
++ Entropium/ectropium	++ Foreign body
++ Conjunctivitis follicularis	++ Ulcerative conjunctivitis
++ Ulcerative keratitis	++ Eosinophilic keratoconjunctivitis
+ Nasolacrimal stenosis	++ Nasolacrimal stenosis

↑ Tear Production

Mechanical Irritation

- Trauma
- Entropium/ectropium
- Distichiasis/Trichiasis
- Foreign body
- Eye lid tumours
- Dermoid cysts
- Eyelid coloboma
- Hordeolum (stye)
- Chalazion
- High nasolabial fold (Pekingese)

Infectious Causes

- Viral keratoconjunctivitis
  - Feline Herpes virus [Cat]
  - Canine distemper virus [Dog]
- Bacterial keratoconjunctivitis
  - Staphylococcus spp.
  - Mycoplasma sp. [esp Cat]
  - Chlamydia sp. [Cat]

Immunoreactive Causes

- Feline eosinophilic keratoconjunctivitis [Cat]
- Plasmacell keratoconjunctivitis (esp German Shepherd Dog)
- Lymphofollicular hyperplasia (conjunctivitis follicularis) [Dog]
- Dust/Pollen allergy

Other Causes

- Rhinitis [esp Cat]
- Blepharitis
- Ulcerative keratitis
- Endonasal foreign body
- Endonasal tumours
- Uveitis anterior

Tear Flow Disturbances

Congenital Causes

- Tear duct stenosis/absent lacrimal punctum
- Nasolacrimal atresia

- Symblepharon [esp Cat]
- Eyelid agenesis
- Foreign body
- Tumours
- Entropium/ectropium

Acquired Causes

- Rhinitis/Sinusitis
- Trauma

Diagnostic Approach

Ocular Discharge

1. **Case History**

2. **General Examination**

3. **Ocular Examination**
- Inspection
- Sight test
- Schirmer tear test
- Eversion of the nictitating membrane
- Conjunctival smear
  - Chlamydia sp.
  - Canine distemper virus antigen
  - Feline Herpes virus antigen

  - Cytology
  - Bacterial culture
- Fluorescein test
- Flushing of the tear duct
- Direct/indirect ophthalmoscopy
- Reflex responses
- Tonometry
- Gonioscopy

4. **Further Tests**
- Ultrasound
- Puncture of the vitreous body + analysis
  - Tumour cytology
  - Bacterial/fungal culture

Reddening of the Eye

Often in combination with blepharospasm (tight closure of the eye lids) as a result of painful ocular disease

Common Causes	
Dog	Cat
+++ Conjunctivitis	+++ Conjunctivitis
++ Blepharitis	++ Blepharitis
++ Glaucoma	++ Glaucoma
++ Uveitis anterior	++ Uveitis anterior

Reddening of the Eyelids

Blepharitis

- Traumatic blepharitis
  - abrasion/scratch/bite wounds/foreign body
- Bacterial blepharitis
  - Staphylococcal pyoderma
  - Hordeolum (stye)
- Mycotic blepharitis
  - Microsporum sp.
  - Trichophyton sp.
- Parasitic blepharitis
  - Demodex sp.
  - Sarcoptes sp.
  - Notoedres sp. [Cat]
- Immunoreactive blepharitis
  - Atopy/inhalation allergy
  - Contact allergy
  - Drug allergy
  - Feline eosinophilic granuloma [Cat]
  - Lupus erythematosus
  - Pemphigus complex
- Eyelid tumours
  - Meibomian gland adenoma/carcinoma
  - Squamous cell carcinoma
  - Melanoma
  - Warts
- Other Causes
  - Collie dermatomyositis [Dog]
  - Hypothyroidism [Dog]
  - Hypercortisolism (Cushing's disease) [Dog]
  - Diabetes mellitus
  - Zinc deficiency dermatosis [Dog]

Conjunctival Reddening

Conjunctivitis

- Traumatic conjunctivitis
  - abrasion/scratch/bite wounds/foreign body
- Mechanical irritation
  - Entropium/ectropium
  - Eyelid tumours
  - Distichiasis/trichiasis
  - Nasolacrimal stenosis/agenesis
  - Foreign body
  - Draught
  - Hyperplasia of the nictitating gland
  - Eversion of the cartilage of the nictitating membrane [Dog]
- Viral conjunctivitis
  - Canine distemper virus [Dog]
  - Feline herpes virus [Cat]
  - Feline calici virus [Cat]
- Bacterial conjunctivitis
  - Staphylococcus sp.
  - Streptococcus sp.
  - Chlamydia sp. [Cat]
  - Mycoplasma sp. [esp Cat]
- Immunoreactive conjunctivitis
  - Atopy/inhalation allergy
  - Contact allergy
  - Drug allergy (Neomycin eye ointment)
  - Feline eosinophilic conjunctivitis [Cat]
  - Plasmacell keratoconjunctivitis [Dog]

- Lymphofollicular
  hyperplasia (Conjunctivitis
  follicularis) [Dog]
  - Lupus erythematosus
- Toxic conjunctivitis
  - Irritant gases/Chemicals
- Conjunctival tumours
  - Melanoma
  - Lymphosarcoma [esp Cat]
  - Haemangioma/
    Haemangiosarcoma
  - Mast cell tumour [esp Dog]
  - Papilloma
  - Histiocytoma

Scleral Reddening

Episcleritis

- Immunoreactive Episcleritis
  - Atopy/Inhalation allergy
  - Drug allergy (Neomycin eye
    ointment)
  - Feline eosinophilic
    conjunctivitis [Cat]
  - Plasmacell
    keratoconjunctivitis [Dog]
  - Lupus erythematosus

Glaucoma

Primary Glaucoma

- Wide iridocorneal angle
- Narrow iridocorneal
  angle
- Goniodysplasia

Secondary Glaucoma

- Lens luxation
- Uveitis anterior
- Hypermature cataract

- Hyphaema
- Neoplasia

Uveitis anterior

- Trauma
- Viral uveitis
  - FeLV/FIV [Cat]
  - FIP Coronavirus [Cat]
  - Canine distemper virus
    [Dog]
  - CAV-1 (Hepatitis c. c.)
    [Dog]
- Bacterial uveitis
  - Brucella sp. [Dog]
  - Lyme Borrelia sp. [Dog]
  - Leptospira sp. [Dog]
  - Mycobacterium sp.
- Rickettsial uveitis
  - (Ehrlichia sp. [Dog])
  - (Rickettsia sp. [Dog])
- Mycotic uveitis
  - Candida sp.
  - Cryptococcus sp. [Cat]
  - (Histoplasma sp.)
  - (Blastomyces sp.)
  - (Coccidioides sp.)
- Parasitic uveitis
  - Toxoplasma sp.
  - (Dirofilaria sp. [esp Dog])
  - (Leishmania sp. [esp Dog])
  - Larva migrans
- Immunoreactive uveitis
  - After rupture of the lens
    capsule
  - Vasculitis
  - Periarteritis nodosa
- Tumours
  - Melanoma
  - Lymphosarcoma [esp Cat]
- Arterial hypertension

Other Causes

- Lens luxation
- Retrobulbar abscess/tumours
- Trauma

Corneal Reddening

Secondary Vascularisation

- Chronic corneal injury
- Chronic ulcerative keratitis
- Chronic keratoconjunctivitis sicca
- Chronic glaucoma
- Corneal acid burn (esp household agents)

Reddening of the Ocular Chamber

Anterior Chamber (Hyphaema)

- Trauma
- Coagulopathy
- Lens luxation
- Tumours

- — Haemangioma/ Haemangiosarcoma
  - — Melanoma
  - — Lymphosarcoma [esp Cat]
- Haemorrhagic uveitis anterior
  - — FeLV/FIV [Cat]
  - — FIP Coronavirus [Cat]
  - — Larva migrans
  - — (Ehrlichia sp. [Dog])
- Vasculitis
- Hypertension
  - — Renal failure
  - — Hyperthyroidism [Cat]

Posterior Chamber (Fundal Haemorrhage)

- Hyphaema
- Retinal detachment
- Progressive retinal atrophy
- Granulomatous meningoencephalitis (GME)
- Ocular anomaly in the collie [Dog]

Diagnostic Approach

Reddening of the Eye

1. **Case History**

2. **General Examination**

3. **Ocular Examination**
- Inspection
- Sight test
- Schirmer tear test
- Eversion of the nictitating membrane
- Conjunctival smear

  - — Chlamydia sp.
  - — Canine distemper virus antigen
  - — Feline Herpes virus antigen
  - — Cytology
  - — Bacterial culture
- Fluorescein test
- Direct/indirect ophthalmoscopy
- Tonometry
- Gonioscopy

- Reflex responses
- Flushing of the tear ducts
- Ultrasound
- Puncture of the vitreous body
  - Tumour cytology
  - Bacterial/fungal culture

4. Blood Tests
- Hct, Ery, Leuc
- TP, Alb, Glob
- FIP Profile [Cat]
  - TP
  - Alb/Glob ratio
  - Bili
  - GOT
  - Serum electrophoresis
- Urea, Crea
- Diff BC

Microbial Serology
- FeLV-/FIV Antigen [Cat]
- Toxoplasma Antibodies

- Ehrlichia Antibodies [Dog]
- Leptospira Antibodies [Dog]
- Lyme Borrelia Antibodies [Dog]
- Brucella Antibodies [Dog]
- Leishmania Antibodies [Dog]

Immunoserology
- ANA Test

Coagulation
- Bleeding time
- Prothrombin time (PT/Quick)
- (Activated) partial Thromboplastin time (PTT/aPTT)
- Fibrin degradation products (FDP)
- Thrombocyte number

5. Further Tests
- Blood pressure measurement (indirect/direct

Cataract

Cloudiness of the cornea, lens or aqueous fluid

Common Causes	
Dog	Cat
+++ Cataract	+++ Cataract
++ Ulcerative keratitis	++ Ulcerative keratitis
++ Corneal oedema	++ Corneal oedema

Cataract of the Cornea

Corneal Oedema

- Mechanical Irritation
  - Entropium
  - Distichiasis
  - Trauma
  - High nasal fold (Pekingese)
- Glaucoma
- Drugs
  - Dimethylsulfoxide (DMSO)

- Idiopathic in Manx cats
- Endothelial dystrophy

Keratitis

- Trauma
- Mechanical Irritation
  - Foreign body
  - Entropium/Ectropium
  - Distichiasis/Trichiasis
- Viral Keratitis
  - Canine distemper virus [Dog]
  - Feline Herpes virus [Cat]
  - CAV-1 (Hepatitis c. c.) [Dog]
- Immunoreactive Keratitis
  - Keratoconjunctivitis sicca [esp Dog]
  - Sjögren syndrome [Dog]
  - Drug allergy (Neomycin eye ointment)
  - Feline eosinophilic keratitis [Cat]
  - Plasmacell keratoconjunctivitis [Dog]
- Ulcerative keratitis
- Toxic conjunctivitis
  - Irritant gases/chemicals
- Other Causes
  - Feline corneal sequestrum [Cat]
  - Dermoid

Infiltrative Corneal Disease

- Lipid deposits
  - Hypothyroidism [Dog]
  - Corneal dystrophy
- Immunecomplex disease
- Mucopolysaccharidosis [Cat]
- Gangliosidosis
- Mannosidosis

Cataract of the Anterior Chamber

Hyphaema (Haemorrhage)

- Trauma
- Coagulopathy
- Lens luxation
- Haemorrhagic uveitis anterior
  - FeLV/FIV [Cat]
  - FIP Coronavirus [Cat]
  - Larva migrans
  - (Ehrlichia sp. [Dog])
- Arterial hypertension
  - Renal failure
  - Hyperthyroidism [Cat]
- Tumours
  - Haemangioma/ Haemangiosarcoma
  - Melanoma
  - Lymphosarcoma [esp Cat]
- Vasculitis

Hypopyon (Pus)

- Bacterial uveitis
  - Brucella sp. [Dog]
  - Lyme Borrelia sp. [Dog]
  - Leptospira sp. [Dog]
  - Mycobacterium sp.
- Rickettsial Uveitis
  - (Ehrlichia sp. [Dog])
  - (Rickettsia sp. [Dog])
- Mycotic Uveitis
  - Candida sp.
  - Cryptococcus sp. [Cat]
  - (Histoplasma sp.)
  - (Blastomyces sp.)
  - (Coccidioides sp.)
- Parasitic uveitis
  - Toxoplasma sp.
  - (Dirofilaria sp. [esp Dog])

- (Leishmania sp. [esp Dog])
- Larva migrans

Fibrin

- Chronic inflammation

Cataract of the Lens

Cataract

- Senile cataract (senile sclerosis)

- Acquired cataract
  - Diabetes mellitus
  - Chronic uveitis
  - Progressive retinal atrophy
  - Hypocalcaemia
  - Electrical accident
  - Radiation
  - Dinitrophenole
  - Dimethylsulfoxide (DMSO)
  - Selenium deficiency
- Congenital/juvenile cataract

Diagnostic Approach

Cataract

1. Case History

2. General Examination

3. Ocular Examination

- Inspection
- Sight test
- Schirmer tear test
- Eversion of the nictitating membrane
- Conjunctival smear
  - Chlamydia sp.
  - Canine distemper virus antigen
  - Feline herpes virus antigen
  - Cytology
  - Bacterial culture
- Fluorescein test
- Direct/indirect ophthalmoscopy
- Tonometry
- Gonioscopy
- Reflex responses
- Flushing of the tear ducts
- Ultrasound

- Puncture of the vitreous body
  - Tumour cytology
  - Bacterial/fungal culture

4. Blood Tests

- Hct, Ery, Leuc
- TP, Alb, Glob
- FIP Profile [Cat]
  - TP
  - Alb/Glob ratio
  - Bili
  - GOT
  - Serum electrophoresis
- Diff BC
- Urea, Crea

MICROBIAL SEROLOGY

- FeLV-/FIV antigen [Cat]
- Toxoplasma antibodies
- Ehrlichia antibodies [Dog]
- Leptospira antibodies [Dog]
- Lyme Borrelia antibodies [Dog]
- Brucella antibodies [Dog]
- Leishmania antibodies [Dog]

IMMUNE SEROLOGY
- ANA Test
- Coagulation
- Bleeding time
- Prothrombin time (PT/Quick)
- (Activated) partial Thromboplastin time (PTT/aPTT)

- Fibrin degradation product (FDP)
- Thrombocyte number

5. Further Tests
- Blood pressure measurement (indirect/direct)

Enophthalmos/Exophthalmos

Enophthalmos: Posterior displacement of the bulbus into the orbit
Exophthalmos: Protrusion of the bulbus out of the orbit

Common Causes	
Dog	**Cat**
Enophthalmos	
+++ Chronic painful ocular disease	+++ Chronic painful ocular disease
++ Orbital fracture	++ Orbital fracture
Exophthalmos	
+ Retrobulbar abscess	++ Retrobulbar abscess
+ Retrobulbar tumours	+ Retrobulbar tumours

Enophthalmos

Chronic Painful Ocular Disease

- Infectious keratoconjunctivitis
- Ulcerative keratitis
- Keratoconjunctivitis sicca [esp Dog]
- Entropium/Ectropium
- Distichiasis
- Iridocyclitis
- Chorioretinitis
- Lens luxation

Other Causes

- Orbital fracture

- Horner syndrome (Sympathetic nerve lesion)
  - Brain stem lesion
  - Cervical spine lesion
  - Thoracic spinal lesion (T1–T3)
  - Nerve root compression syndrome (T1–T3)
  - Brachial plexus lesion
  - Mediastinal disease
  - Middle ear lesion
  - Retrobulbar lesion
- Microphthalmus
  - congenital
  - chronic panophthalmia

- Bulbal rupture
- Orbital fat atrophy (cachexia)

Exophthalmos

Bulbar Causes

- Glaucoma
- Bulbar prolapse
  - Trauma
  - Brachycephalic dog breeds[Dog]

Retrobulbar Causes

- Retrobulbar abscess
  - Foreign body
  - Dental abscess
  - Mycotic granuloma
  - Cryptococcus sp. [Cat]
  - Aspergillus sp. [Dog]
  - Sialoadenitis (Gl. zygomatica)
- Retrobulbar/Orbital tumours
  - Fibrosarcoma
  - Lymphosarcoma
  - Osteosarcoma
  - Squamous cell carcinoma
  - Adenocarcinoma
  - Rhabdomyosarcoma
- Orbital trauma/haemorrhage
- Eosinophilic myositis [Dog]
- Sialocele (Gl. zygomatica)

Diagnostic Approach

Enophthalmos/Exophthalmos

1. **Case History**

2. **General Examination**

3. **Examination of the Oral and Oropharyngeal Cavity**

4. **Ocular Examination**
- Inspection
- Sight test
- Reflex responses
- Schirmer tear test
- Eversion of the nictitating membrane
- Fluorescein test
- Direct/indirect ophthalmoscopy
- Tonometry
- Gonioscopy
- Ultrasound
- Puncture of the vitreous body

5. **X-Ray Study**
- Skull (Orbit)

6. **Ultrasound**
- Orbit

7. **Blood Tests**
- FIP Profile [Cat]
  - TP
  - Alb/Glob ratio
  - Bili
  - GOT
  - Serum electrophoresis

MICROBIAL SEROLOGY
- FeLV-/FIV Antigen [Cat]

Prolapse of the Nictitating Membrane

Protrusion of the third eyelid (Membrana nictitans) across the eye

Common Causes	
Dog	Cat
+++ Painful ocular disease	+++ Painful ocular disease
++ Pyrexic systemic disease	++ Pyrexic systemic disease
++ Sedatives/Anticonvulsants	++ Sedatives/Anticonvulsants

Unilateral prolapse

- Blepharospasm
  - Foreign body
  - Ulcerative keratitis
  - Uveitis anterior
  - Glaucoma
  - Distichiasis/Trichiasis
  - Lens luxation
  - Entropium/Ectropium
- Exophthalmos
  - Retrobulbar abscess/tumours
- Enophthalmos
  - Chronic painful ocular disease
- Horner syndrome (Sympathetic lesion)
  - Brain stem lesion
  - Cervical spinal lesion
  - Thoracic spinal lesion (T1–T3)
  - Nerve root compression syndrome (T1–T3)
  - Brachial plexus lesion
  - Mediastinal disease
  - Middle ear disease
  - Retrobulbar lesion
- Hyperplasia/tumour/prolapse of the nictitating gland
- Eversion of the cartilage of the nictitating membrane [Dog]
- Symblepharon [esp Cat]
  - Congenital
  - Chronic inflammation

Bilateral Prolapse

- Blepharospasm
  - Conjunctivitis
  - Keratoconjunctivitis sicca [esp Dog]
  - Lymphofollicular hyperplasia (Conjunctivitis follicularis) [Dog]
  - Uveitis anterior
  - Glaucoma
  - Distichiasis/Trichiasis
  - Entropium/Ectropium
- Pyrexic systemic disease
- Sedatives

- Acepromazine
- Anticonvulsants
- Exophthalmos
  - Eosinophilic myositis [Dog]
- Enophthalmos

- Chronic painful ocular disease
- Feline dysautonomia [esp Cat]
- Tetanus [Dog]
- (Intestinal parasites)

Diagnostic Approach

Prolapsed Nictitating Membrane

1. Case History

2. General Examination

3. Ocular Examination
- Inspection
- Sight test
- Reflex responses
- Schirmer tear test
- Eversion of the nictitating membrane
- Conjunctival smear
  - Chlamydia sp.
  - Canine distemper virus antigen
  - Feline Herpes virus antigen
  - Cytology
  - Bacterial culture
- Fluorescein test
- Direct/indirect ophthalmoscopy
- Tonometry
- Gonioscopy

- Ultrasound
- Puncture of the vitreous body
  - Tumour cytology
  - Bacterial/fungal culture

4. Blood Tests
- Hct, Ery, Leuc
- Na, K, Ca
- TP, Alb, Glob
- GPT, AP, Urea, Crea, BG
- Diff BC
- FIP Profile [Cat]
  - TP
  - Alb/Glob ratio
  - Bili
  - GOT
  - Serum electrophoresis

MICROBIAL SEROLOGY
- FeLV-/FIV Antigen [Cat]

FAECAL EXAMINATION
- Flotation

Loss of Eyesight/Blindness

Reduced to complete lack of vision (Amaurosis)

Common Causes	
Dog	**Cat**
+++ Cataract	+++ Optic neuritis
++ Retinal detachment/atrophy	(FeLV/FIV, FIP Coronavirus)
++ Glaucoma	++ Encephalitis/
++ Uveitis	meningoencephalitis
++ Tumours	++ Tumours
++ Granulomatous meningo-	++ Cataract
encephalitis	++ Arterial hypertension
	++ Retinal detachment/atrophy
	++ Glaucoma

Unilateral Loss of Eyesight

Acute Causes

- Acute trauma
- Hyphaema
- Acute glaucoma
- Lens luxation
- Traumatic cataract
- Sudden acute retinal detachment/atrophy (SARD)
- Optical nerve (HN-II) lesion
  - Bulbus prolapse
  - Head trauma
- Central nervous lesions (Occipital cortex)
  - Traumatic brain injury
  - Cerebral haemorrhage
  - Cerebral abscess
  - Brain tumours

Chronic Causes

  - Keratitis
  - Corneal oedema
- Clouding of the anterior chamber
  - Hyphaema

- Hypopyon (Uveitis anterior)
- Fibrin/synechia
- Cataract
  - Traumatic cataract
  - Cataract as a result of uveitis
- Retinal detachment/atrophy
  - Glaucoma
  - Fundal haemorrhage
  - Chorioretinitis
  - Collie eye anomaly [Dog]
  - Progressive retinal atrophy
- Optical nerve lesion (HN-II)
  - Tumours
  - Retrobulbar abscess/ tumour
  - Congenital hypoplasia/ aplasia

Bilateral Loss of Eyesight

Acute Causes

- Traumatic Brain Injury
- Acute glaucoma
- Cataract
  - Traumatic cataract
  - Diabetic cataract

- Lens luxation
- Sudden acute retinal detachment/atrophy (SARD)
- Optical nerve (HN-II) lesion
  - Bulbus prolapse
  - Head trauma
- Central nervous lesions (Occipital cortex)
  - Traumatic brain injury
  - Cerebral haemorrhage
  - Cerebral abscess
  - Brain tumours
- Hypoxia
  - Anaesthetic incident
  - Drowning
- Poisoning
  - Lead
  - Organophosphates
  - Ethylene glycol
  - Toxic plants

Chronic Causes

- Chronic glaucoma
- Corneal opacity
  - Keratitis
  - Corneal oedema
  - Infiltrative disease
- Cataract
  - Congenital cataract
  - Senile cataract
  - Diabetic cataract
  - Cataract as a result of uveitis
  - Cataract as a result of progressive retinal atrophy
  - Cataract as a result of hypocalcaemia

- Retinal detachment/atrophy
  - Canine distemper virus [Dog]
  - FeLV/FIV [Cat]
  - FIP Coronavirus [Cat]
  - Cryptococcus sp. [Cat]
  - (Blastomyces sp.)
  - (Coccidioides sp.)
  - (Ehrlichia sp. [Dog])
  - Brucella sp. [Dog]
  - Lyme Borrelia sp. [Dog]
  - Immunoreactive chorioretinitis
  - Tumours
  - Arterial hypertension [esp Cat]
  - Hypercortisolism (Cushing's disease) [Dog]
  - Collie eye anomaly [Dog]
  - Progressive retinal atrophy
  - Taurine deficiency [Cat]
  - Vitamin A/E deficiency
  - Fundal haemorrhage
- Optical nerve neuritis
  - Canine distemper virus [Dog]
  - FIP Coronavirus [Cat]
  - Cryptococcus sp. [Cat]
  - Toxoplasma sp.
  - Neospora sp. [Dog]
  - Granulomatous meningoencephalitis (GME)
  - Lead poisoning
  - Tumours
  - Congenital hypoplasia
- Central nervous disturbances

– Granulomatous
  meningoencephalitis (GME)
– Hydrocephalus
– Encephalitis
– Endocrine encephalopathy
– Chronic lead poisoning
– Brain tumours
– Hypoxia

Diagnostic Approach

Loss of Eyesight/Blindness

1. **Case History**

2. **General Examination**

3. **Ocular Examination**
- Inspection
- Sight test
- Reflex responses
  - Sight test (II)
  - Menace response (II, VII)
  - Blink reflex (V, VII)
  - Corneal reflex (V, VII)
  - Pupillary reflex (II, III)
  - Pupillary symmetry/width
  - Eye movements (III, IV, VI)
  - Facial symmetry (VII)
- Schirmer tear test
- Eversion of the nictitating
  membrane
- Fluorescein test
- Direct/indirect ophthalmoscopy
- Tonometry
- Gonioscopy
- Ultrasound
- Electroretinography (ERG)
- Conjunctival smear
  - Chlamydia sp.
  - Canine distemper virus
    antigen
  - Feline Herpes virus antigen
  - Cytology
  - Bacterial culture

- Flushing of the tear duct
- Puncture of the vitreous body
  - Tumour cytology
  - Bacterial/fungal culture

4. **Blood Tests**
- Hct, Ery, Leuc, Hb
- Na, K, Ca, P
- TP, Alb, Glob
- GPT, AP, Urea, Crea, BG
- FIP Profile [Cat]
  - TP
  - Alb/Glob ratio
  - Bili
  - GOT
  - Serum electrophoresis
- Diff BC

MICROBIAL SEROLOGY
- FeLV-/FIV antigen [Cat]
- Toxoplasma antibodies
- Dirofilaria antigen [Dog]
- Lyme Borrelia antibodies
  [Dog]
- Ehrlichia antibodies [Dog]

FUNCTION TESTS
- Adrenal gland function tests
  [Dog]
  - Dexamethasone Suppression
    test
  - ACTH Stimulation test

- – Cortisol/Creatinine Ratio
- T_4, fT_4
- TSH/TRH Stimulation test [Dog]
- T_3 Suppression test [Cat]

5. Further Tests

- Liquor puncture/analysis
  - – Liquor pressure
  - – Leucocyte number + Diff
  - – TP, Glucose, CK
  - – Globulin (Pandy and Nonne-Apelt Reaction)
  - – Bacterial/fungal culture
  - – Tumour cytology
  - – Electrophoresis
  - – Canine distemper antibodies [Dog]
- Skull CT/MRT
- X-Ray Study
- (skull, thorax)
- (Doppler) Echocardiography
- Measure of blood pressure (indirect/direct)

Strabismus

Common Causes		
Dog		**Cat**
+++ Retrobulbar abscess/tumours		+++ Physiological in Siamese
++ Traumatic causes		++ Retrobulbar abscess/tumours
++ Cerebral causes		++ Traumatic causes
		++ Cerebral causes

Unilateral Strabismus

Towards medial

- Abducens nerve (CN VI) paralysis

Towards ventrolateral

- Oculomotor nerve (CN-III) paralysis

- Facial nerve (CN-VII) paralysis

Multidirectional

- Retrobulbar abscess/tumours/ haemorrhage
- Orbital fracture
- Bulbus prolapse
- Trochlear (CN-IV) paralysis

Bilateral Strabismus

Towards medial

- Congenital defect in Siamese cats

Towards ventrolateral

- Hydrocephalus

Multidirectional

- Otitis interna
- Encephalitis
- Brain tumours

Diagnostic Approach

Strabismus

1. Case History

2. General Examination

3. Ocular Examination

- Inspection
- Sight test
- Reflex responses
  - Sight test (II)
  - Menace reflex (II, VII)
  - Blink reflex (V, VII)
  - Corneal reflex (V, VII)
  - Pupillary reflex (II, III)
  - Pupillary symmetry/width
  - Eye movements (III, IV, VI)
  - Facial symmetry (VII)
- Direct/indirect ophthalmoscopy
- Ultrasound (Orbit)

4. X-Ray Study

- Skull

5. Blood Tests

  Hct, Ery, Leuc FIP Profile [Cat]

  - TP
  - Alb/Glob ratio
  - Bili
  - GOT
  - Serum electrophoresis
- Diff BC

MICROBIAL SEROLOGY

- FeLV-/FIV Antigen [Cat]

6. Further Tests

- Liquor puncture/analysis
  - (Liquor pressure)
  - Leucocyte number + Diff
  - TP, Glucose, CK
  - Globulin (Pandy and Nonne-Apelt Reaction)
  - Bacterial/Fungal culture
  - Tumour cytology
  - Electrophoresis
  - Canine distemper antibodies [Dog]
- Skull CT/MRT

10 Otological Principal Symptoms

Further Relevant Principal Symptoms

Aural Discharge

Otorrhoea	
Common Causes	
Dog	Cat
+++ Bacterial Otitis	+++ Ear mite Otitis
++ Ear mite Otitis	++ Bacterial Otitis
++ Immunoreactive Otitis	++ Mycotic Otitis
++ Foreign body Otitis	++ Immunoreactive Otitis
++ Mycotic Otitis	+ Foreign body Otitis

Ceruminal Discharge

Otitis Externa

- Congenital Causes
  - Floppy ears
  - Anomalies of the ear canal
- Foreign body Otitis
  - Grass seeds
  - Hair
- Bacterial Otitis
  - Staphylococcus sp.
  - Pseudomonas sp.
- Mycotic Otitis
  - Malassezia sp.

- Candida sp.
- Aspergillus sp.
- Parasitic Otitis
  - Otodectes sp.
  - Notoedres sp. [Cat]
  - Demodex sp.
  - Sarcoptes sp.
  - Fly larvae
- Immunoreactive Otitis
  - Atopy
  - Ear mite allergy
  - Bacterial/fungal allergy
  - Drug allergy (topical aural medication)
- Tumours of the external ear canal
  - Polyp
  - Ceruminal adenoma/ carcinoma
  - Squamous cell carcinoma
  - Papilloma
  - Fibroma/Fibrosarcoma
- Seborrhoea

Purulent Discharge
Otitis Externa/Media

- Foreign body Otitis
  - Grass seeds
  - Hair
- Bacterial Otitis
  - Staphylococcus sp.

- Proteus sp.
- Pseudomonas sp.
- Parasitic Otitis
  - Otodectes sp.
  - Notoedres sp. [Cat]
  - Demodex sp.
  - Sarcoptes sp.
  - Fly larvae
- Tumours of the external ear canal
  - Polyp
  - Ceruminal adenoma/ carcinoma
  - Squamous cell carcinoma
  - Papilloma
  - Fibroma/Fibrosarcoma

Haemorrhagic Discharge

- Traumatic Causes
  - Head injury
  - Foreign body
- Chronic bacterial Otitis
- Tumours of the external ear canal
  - Polyp
  - Ceruminal adenoma/ carcinoma
  - Squamous cell carcinoma
  - Papilloma
  - Fibroma/Fibrosarcoma

Diagnostic Approach

Aural Discharge

1. **Case History**

2. **General Examination**

3. **Otoscopic Examination**

4. **Examination of the Ear Secretion**
   - Cytology
   - Ear mites
   - Bacterial/fungal culture

5. **Pharyngeal Examination**

6. **X-Ray Study**
   - Skull (Tympanic bulla)

7. **Blood Tests**
   - Hct, Ery, Leuc
   - Diff BC
   - TP
   - FC Receptor test

11 Dermatological Principal Symptoms

Hair Loss

Alopecia	
Common Causes	
Dog	**Cat**
Hair Loss with Pruritus	
+++ Ectoparasitosis	+++ Ectoparasitosis
+++ Pyoderma	+++ Allergy
++ Pyotraumatic Dermatitis	+ Dermatophytosis
++ Allergy	
+ Autoimmune Disease	
+ Dermatophytosis	
Hair Loss without Pruritus	
+++ Endocrine Causes	++ Psychogenic Causes
+++ Psychogenic Causes	+ Endocrine Causes
+ Toxic Causes	+ Toxic Causes

Hair Loss with Pruritus

Infectious Causes

• Parasitic Dermatitis

Ticks
– Ixodes sp.
– Rhipicephalus sp.

Mites
- Demodex sp.
- Sarcoptes sp.
- Cheyletiella sp.
- Notoedres sp. [Cats]
- Neotrombicula sp.
- Dermanyssus sp.
- Otodectes sp.

Fleas
- Ctenocephalides sp.
- Pulex sp.
- Archaeopsylla sp.
- Ceratophyllus sp.

Lice
- Linognathus sp. [Dog]

Biting Lice
- Trichodectes sp. [Dog]
- Felicola sp. [Cat]

Protozoa
- (Leishmania sp. [esp Dog])

Nematodes (Larva migrans)
- Ancylostoma sp.
- Uncinaria sp.
- Pelodera sp.
- Strongyloides sp.
- Trichobilharzia sp.
- (Dirofilaria sp.)
- (Dracunculus sp.)
- Mycotic Dermatitis
  - Microsporum sp.
  - Trichophyton sp.
  - Sporothrix sp.
  - Candida sp.
  - Mallassezia sp.
- Bacterial Dermatitis/ Pyoderma
  - Staphylococcus sp.
  - Streptococcus sp.

- E. coli
- Proteus sp.
- Pseudomonas sp.
- Lyme Borrelia sp. [Dog]
- Rickettsial Dermatitis
  - (Ehrlichia sp. [esp Dog])
  - (Rickettsia sp.)

Immunoreactive Causes

- Atopy/Inhalation allergy
  - House dust, House dust mites
  - Epithelium (Dog, Cat, Human)
  - Feathers
  - Mould fungus
  - Pollen
- Parasitic allergy
  - Fleas/Ticks/Mites
  - Round-/Tapeworms
  - (Dirofilaria Microfilaria)
- Bacterial allergy
  - Staphylococcus sp.
- Food allergy
  - Soya/Maize/Oat meal
  - Peanuts
  - Animal Protein
  - Mould fungus
  - Food mites
  - Food additives
- Contact allergy
  - Plants
  - Local medication
  - Shampoo
  - Flea/Tick collars
  - Cat litter
  - Washing agents
  - Fertilizer
  - Household detergents

- Hormonal allergy
  - Endogenous progesterone
  - Endogenous oestrogens
- Fungal allergy
  - Microsporum sp.
  - Candida sp.
  - Malassezia sp.
- Autoimmune disease
  - Systemic Lupus erythematosus
  - Discoid Lupus erythematosus
  - Pemphigus foliaceus
  - Pemphigus vulgaris
  - Pemphigus erythematosus
  - (Pemphigus vegetans)
  - Bullous Pemphigoid [Dog]

Other Causes

- Pyotraumatic dermatitis (hot spots)
- Keratinisation disturbances
  - Primary idiopathic Seborrhoea
  - Secondary keratinisation disturbances
- Skin tumours
  - Mast cell tumour
  - Basal cell tumour
  - Squamous cell carcinoma
  - Mycosis fungoides
  - Epitheliotrophic lymphoma

Hair Loss Without Pruritus

Congenital Causes

- Feline generalised alopecia [Sphinx cat]
- Alopecia of colour mutants
- Follicular dysplasia of the black hair
- Hairless dog breeds
- Feline hypotrichosis [Siamese Cat]
- Ectodermal defects (Ehlers-Danlos syndrome)
- Epidermal dysplasia [West Highland White Terrier]
- Lichenoid psoriasiform
- Dermatosis [Springer Spaniel]
- Hypophyseal dwarfism [German Shepherd Dog]
- Dermatomyositis [Collie]

Endocrine Causes

- Hypercortisolism (Cushing's disease) [esp Dog]
- Hypothyroidism [Dog]
- Hypophyseal dwarfism (STH deficiency) [Dog]
- Hyperoestrogenism
  - Sertoli cell tumour [Dog]
  - Cryptorchism
  - Ovarian cysts
  - Granulosa cell ovarian tumour
- Hypoestrogenism [esp Dog] Ovariectomy
- Hypoandrogenism [esp Dog]
- Hyperthyroidism [Cat]
- Diabetes mellitus

Nutritional Causes

- Deficiency of essential fatty acids
- Vitamin A deficiency
- Vitamin E deficiency
- Biotin deficiency
- Zinc deficiency

Psychogenic Causes

- Acral lick dermatitis [esp Dog]
- Feline neurodermatitis? [Cat]
- Feline psychogenic alopecia [Cat]
- Telogen/anagen defluvium [esp Cat]

Toxic Causes

- Thallium poisoning

Traumatic Causes

- Abrasive/bite/lick wounds
- Burns
- Chemical burns
- Solar dermatitis

Other Causes

- Eosinophilic Granuloma [Cat]
- Paraneoplastic syndrome (Pancreatic tumour) [Cat]
- Pattern baldness [Dachshund]
- Yorkshire Terrier alopecia
- Acanthosis nigricans [Dachshund]

Diagnostic Approach

Hair Loss

1. Case History

2. General Examination

3. Skin/Hair Examination
- Characterisation of the lesions
- Distribution
- Pattern of the lesions
- Flea comb examination
- Wood lamp
- Multiple Skin scrapes
  +/– Bacterial/fungal culture
  +   Parasitological Examination
  +   Cytological Examination
- Trichogram
- Skin biopsy
- Intracutaneous Allergy test (Prick Test)

4. Blood Tests
- Hct, Ery, Leuc
- Diff BC
- TP, Alb, Glob
- Cholesterol
- GPT, AP, Urea, Crea, BG
- Serum electrophoresis
- Zinc, copper
- Thallium

MICROBIAL SEROLOGY
- Sarcoptes antibodies [Dog]
- FeLV-/FIV Antigen [Cat]

- Leishmania antibodies [Dog]

IMMUNOSEROLOGY
- FC Receptor test
- Monoclonal antibodies Allergy test
- ANA-Test

FUNCTION TESTS
- T_4, fT_4 [Dog]
- Thyroglobulin antibodies [Dog]

- TRH/TSH Stimulation test [Dog]
- Adrenal gland function tests [Dog]
  - Dexamethasone Suppression test
  - ACTH Stimulation test
  - Cortisol Creatinine Ratio
- STH Stimulation test [Dog]
- Oestradiol

FAECAL EXAMINATION
- Flotation

Dermal Efflorescences

Morphological classification of skin lesions

Primary Efflorescences	
Patch (Macula):	Area of different colour, but with the same consistency and skin level
Pimple (Papula):	Up to pea sized, solid, non-mobile matter in the epidermis/dermis
Plaque:	Slab-like expansion of papules
Nodule (Nodus):	Larger than pea-sized, circumscribed, dermal/subcutaneous matter
Wheal (Urtica):	Circumscribed oedema of the upper dermis
Vesicle (Vesicula):	Fluid-filled intraepidermal/subepidermal cavity
Pustule (Pustula):	Pus-filled epidermal hollow
Atrophy:	Thinning of the skin (Ehlers-Danlos Syndrome)
Scales (Squama):	Loose epidermal components (exfoliation)
Secondary Efflorescences	
Scales (Squama):	Loose epidermal components (exfoliation)
Scab (Crusta):	Dried secretion, blood, pus, cells and scales
Scar (Cicatrix):	Replacement tissue built of connective tissues after deep skin lesions have healed

Erosion (Erosio):	Superficial skin defect reaching the lower epidermal border (heals without scar)
Ulcer (Ulcus):	Deep skin defect reaching under the epidermal border (heals with scar formation)
Excoriation (Excoriatio):	Superficial separation of the epidermis by abrasion/licking or scratching

Secondary Efflorescences

Rhagade/Fissure (Fissura):	Stab-like tearing of skin
Atrophy:	Thinning of the skin
Lichenification:	Areal skin thickening with hyperpigmentation
Hyper-/Hypopigmentation:	Patch-like colour changes of the skin
Necrosis:	dead tissue

Primary Efflorescences

Patch (Macula)

- Hyperpigmentation
  - Lentigo
  - (Melanoma)
- Hypopigmentation
  - Albinism
  - Alopecia of the colour mutants
  - Tyrosinase deficiency [Chow Chow]
  - Chediak-Higashi syndrome [Persian cats]
  - Cyclic neutropenia [Grey Collie]
  - Vitiligo

Nodule (Nodus)

- Skin tumours
  - Squamous cell carcinoma
  - Basalioma
  - Mast cell tumour
  - Histiocytoma
  - Cutaneous lymphosarcoma
  - Lipoma/Liposarcoma
  - Fibroma/Fibrosarcoma
  - Melanoma
  - Papilloma
  - Trichoepithelioma
  - Adenoma/adenocarcinoma (sebaceous/sweat/hepatoid gland, anal sac)
  - Haemangioma/Haemangiosarcoma
  - Intracutaneous cornifying epithelioma
- Dermal cysts
  - Sweat gland cyst
  - Sebaceous gland retention cyst [esp Dog]
  - Hair follicle cyst
  - Dermoid cyst [Dog]
- Granulomata
  - Bacterial granuloma
  - Actinomycosis
  - Callus/hygroma

- Eosinophilic granuloma [esp Cat]
- Foreign body granuloma
- Lick granuloma
- Mycobacterial granuloma [esp Cat]
- Sterile pyogranuloma
- Systemic mycosis
- Inflamed sebaceous gland [esp Dog]
- Larva migrans
• Other skin nodules
  - Nodular panniculitis [Dog]
  - Abscess
  - Haematoma
  - Furunculosis
  - Insect sting
  - Calcinosis cutis (Cushing's disease) [esp Dog]

Pimple (Papula)

• Parasitic dermatitis
  - Ticks
  - Larva migrans
• Acne

Wheal (Urtica)

• Allergic dermatitis
  - Food allergy
  - Contact allergy
  - Insect bite/sting allergy
  - Drug allergy
  - Intracutaneous allergy test

Small Vesicle/Vesicle (Vesicula/ Bulla)

• Allergic dermatitis
  - Contact allergy
• Autoimmune dermatitis

- Pemphigus vulgaris
- Bullous Pemphigoid [Dog]
• Viral dermatitis
  - Feline pox [Cat]
• Burn

Pustule (Pustula)

• Bacterial dermatitis/ Pyoderma [esp Dog]

Scales (Squama)

Primary Keratinisation Disorders
• Primary idiopathic seborrhoea
• Follicular dystrophy
• Vitamin A deficiency dermatosis
• Zinc deficiency dermatosis [Dog]
• Epidermal dysplasia [West Highland White Terrier]
• Lichenoid psoriasiform dermatosis [Springer Spaniel]
• Schnauzer comedo syndrome [Dog]
• Canine ichthyosis [Dog]
• Idiopathic nasodigital hyperkeratosis [Dog]
• Canine seborrhoea of the ear edges [Dog]

Secondary Efflorescences

Scales (Squama)

Secondary Keratinisation Disorder
• Ectoparasitic dermatitis
• Bacterial dermatitis/ pyoderma [esp Dog]

- Allergic dermatitis
- Autoimmune dermatitis
- Endocrine dermatosis
- Supracaudal gland (Violet gland) dermatosis
- Inflamed sebaceous gland [esp Dog]
- (Leishmania sp. [esp Dog])

Scab (Crusta)

- Bacterial dermatitis/Pyoderma [esp Dog]
- Parasitic dermatitis
  - Mites
- Autoimmune dermatitis
  - Pemphigus complex
  - Lupus erythematosus

Ulcer (Ulcus)
- Bacterial dermatitis [esp Dog]
  - Folliculitis/Furunculosis
  - Pyotraumatic dermatitis (Hot spots)
- Parasitic dermatitis
  - Mites
- Viral dermatitis
  - Feline pox [Cat]
- Allergic dermatitis
  - Drug allergy
  - Flea allergy
- Autoimmune dermatitis
  - Pemphigus complex
- Skin tumours
- Granulomata
- Burns
- Toxic epidermal necrolysis
- Acral lick dermatitis

Erosion (Erosio)
- Scratched/burst pustules, small vesicles, vesicles

Rhagade/Fissure (Fissura)

- Dermatosis of the edge of the ear
- Pododermatitis
- Hyperkeratosis

Excoriation (Excoriatio)
- Traumatic skin lesions
- Scratch wounds with pruritus

Scar (Cicatrix)
- Traumatic skin lesion
- Deep pyoderma
- Secondary with Ehlers-Danlos syndrome
- Ulcers

Atrophy
- Hypercortisolism (Cushing's disease) [esp Dog]
- Glucocorticoid long term therapy
- Lupus erythematosus

Necrosis
- Traumatic skin lesions
- Burn/chemical burn
- Solar dermatitis
- Contact allergy dermatitis
- Toxic epidermal necrolysis
- Lupus erythematosus
- Deep pyoderma
- Vasculitis/Thromboembolism
- Gangrene

Lichenification
- Chronic inflammation
- Acanthosis nigricans [Dog]
- Acral lick dermatitis
- Atopy/Inhalation allergy
- Flea allergy
- Sertoli cell tumour [Dog]

Hyperpigmentation
- Chronic demodicosis [esp Dog]

- Chronic sarcoptic mange
- Chronic dermatophytosis
- Chronic pyoderma [esp Dog]
- Acanthosis nigricans [Dog]
- Hypercortisolism (Cushing's disease) [esp Dog]
- Sertoli cell tumour [Dog]
- Hypothyroidism [Dog]
- Hyperoestrogenism [esp Dog]

Topographic Distribution Pattern of Skin Disease

Head Region

- Parasitic dermatitis
  - Demodex sp. [esp Dog]
  - Notoedres sp. [Cat]
- Bacterial dermatitis
  - Pyoderma [esp Dog]
  - Pyotraumatic dermatitis (Hot spots) [Dog]
  - Feline Leprosy [Cat]
- Mycotic dermatitis
  - Microsporum sp.
  - Trichophyton sp.
  - Malassezia sp.
  - Sporothrix sp.
- Immunoreactive dermatitis
  - Atopy/inhalation allergy
  - Contact allergy
  - Food allergy
  - Pemphigus foliaceus
  - Pemphigus erythematosus
  - Discoid lupus erythematosus
- Skin tumours
  - Papilloma
  - Mast cell tumour
  - Histiocytoma [esp Dog]
  - Fibrosarcoma [esp Cat]
  - Melanoma [esp Dog]
  - Basal cell tumour [esp Dog]
- Nutrionally caused dermatosis
  - Zinc deficiency [Dog]
- Other skin disease
  - Trauma

Auricular Region

- Parasitic dermatitis
  - Sarcoptes sp.
  - Notoedres sp. [Cat]
  - (Leishmania sp. [esp Dog])
- Skin tumours
  - Squamous cell carcinoma
  - Adenoma
- Autoimmune dermatitis
  - Pemphigus foliaceus
  - Pemphigus erythematosus
  - Lupus erythematosus
- Other skin diseases
  - Burn
  - Frost bite
  - Yorkshire Terrier alopecia
  - Otitis externa
  - Solar dermatitis
  - Dermatosis of the ear edge
  - Othaematoma
  - Local seborrhoea

Ocular Region

- Parasitic dermatitis
  - Demodex sp. [esp Dog]
- Bacterial dermatitis/ Blepharitis/Folliculitis
- Mycotic dermatitis/ Blepharitis

- Microsporum sp.
- Trichophyton sp.
- Malassezia sp.
- Sporothrix sp.
- Candida sp.
• Immunoreactive dermatitis
  - Contact allergy
  - Pemphigus foliaceus
  - Pemphigus erythematosus
  - Lupus erythematosus
• Skin tumours
  - Sebaceous gland adenoma
  - Melanoma
• Other skin diseases
  - Conjunctivitis
  - Skin tumours
  - Chalazion/hordeolum
  - Seborrhoea

Nasal Region

• Parasitic dermatitis
  - Demodex sp. [esp Dog]
  - Notoedres sp. [Cat]
  - (Leishmania sp. [Dog])
• Bacterial dermatitis
  - Pyoderma [esp Dog]
  - Folliculitis/furunculosis [esp Dog]
• Mycotic dermatitis
  - Microsporum sp.
  - Trichophyton sp.
  - Malassezia sp.
  - Sporothrix sp.
  - Candida sp.
• Immunoreactive dermatitis
  - Contact allergy
  - Insect sting/bite allergy
  - Pemphigus foliaceus
  - Pemphigus erythematosus

- Discoid Lupus erythematosus
• Skin tumours
  - Squamous cell carcinoma
  - Papilloma [esp Dog]

Mucocutaneous Junctions

• Immunoreactive dermatitis
  - Contact allergy
  - Drug allergy
  - Pemphigus vulgaris
  - Bullous Pemphigoid [Dog]
  - Systemic Lupus erythematosus
  - Eosinophilic granuloma [esp Cat]
• Other skin diseases
  - Thallium poisoning
  - Skin tumours
• Skin tumours
  - Melanoma
  - Sarcoma

Chin Region

• Parasitic dermatitis
  - Demodex sp. [esp Dog]
• Bacterial dermatitis/ Pyoderma [esp Dog]
• Other skin diseases
  - Acne

Throat/Neck Region

• Immunoreactive dermatitis
  - Contact allergy (collar)
  - Flea allergy
  - Food allergy
• Bacterial dermatitis/ Pyoderma [esp Dog]
• Skin Tumours

- Basal cell tumour
- Fibroma/sarcoma [esp Cat]
- Cutaneous lymphosarcoma
- Epithelioma
- Dermal cysts
  - Dermoid cysts [esp Rhodesian Ridgeback]

Axillar Region

- Immunoreactive dermatitis
  - Contact allergy
  - Atopy/Inhalation allergy
  - Pemphigus vulgaris
  - Bullous pemphigoid [Dog]
- Other skin diseases
  - Automutilation in case of pruritus
  - Acanthosis nigricans

Sternal Region

- Immunoreactive dermatitis
  - Contact allergy
- Other skin diseases
  - Pressure sores (Callus) [Dog]

Abdominal Region

- Immunoreactive dermatitis
  - Contact allergy
  - Food allergy
  - Drug allergy
  - Atopy/Inhalation allergy
  - Flea allergy
  - Eosinophilic granuloma/Plaque [Cat]
  - Bullous pemphigoid [Dog]
- Bacterial dermatitis
  - Pyoderma [esp Dog]
  - Feline leprosy [Cat]

- Psychogenic Causes
  - Lick dermatitis [esp Cat]
- Endocrine dermatosis
  - Hypercortisolism (Cushing's disease) [esp Dog]
  - Symmetric alopecia [Cat]
- Parasitic dermatitis
  - Larva migrans
- Other skin diseases
  - Skin tumours (carcinoma, melanoma)

Flank Region

- Endocrine dermatosis
  - Hypercortisolism (Cushing's disease) [esp Dog]
  - Hypothyroidism [Dog]
  - Hypophyseal dwarfism (STH deficiency) [Dog]
  - Hyperoestrogenism
  - Sertoli cell tumour [Dog]
  - Cryptorchism
  - Ovarian cysts
  - Granulosa cell ovarian tumour
  - Hypoestrogenism [esp Dog]
  - Hypoandrogenism [esp Dog]

Dorsal Region

- Parasitic dermatitis
  - Fleas/Ticks/Mites/ Lice/ Biting lice
- Immunoreactive dermatitis
  - Flea allergy
  - Food allergy
  - Atopy/Inhalation allergy
- Psychogenic Causes

- Lick dermatitis [Cat]
- Mycotic dermatitis
  - Microsporum sp.
  - Trichophyton sp.
  - Malassezia sp.
  - Sporothrix sp.
- Bacterial dermatitis
  - Pyoderma/Folliculitis [esp Dog]
- Skin tumours
  - Cutaneous lymphosarcoma
  - Epithelioma
  - Mast cell tumour
  - Haemangioma [esp Dog]
  - Adenoma [esp Dog]
  - Fibrosarcoma [esp Cat]
  - Lipoma
- Other skin diseases
  - Seborrhoea
  - Dermal cysts/atheroma
  - Abscesses

Tail Region

- Parasitic dermatitis
  - Fleas, intestinal parasites (esp Trichuris sp.)
- Bacterial dermatitis
  - Pyotraumatic dermatitis (Hot spots)
- Immunoreactive dermatitis
  - Flea allergy
  - Cold agglutination
- Psychogenic dermatosis
  - Lick dermatitis
- Other skin diseases
  - Tail tip necrosis
  - Hyperplasia of the supracaudal gland (Violet gland)
  - Perianal diseases

Anal Region

- Anal sac abscess
- Perianal fistula [Dog]
- Perianal adenoma [Dog]
- Immunoreactive dermatitis
  - Bullous pemphigoid [Dog]
- Other diseases
  - Lick dermatitis
  - Chronic diarrhoea

Limbs

- Psychogenic dermatosis
  - Acral lick dermatitis
- Other skin disease
  - Pressure sores (decubitus)
  - Hygroma
  - Haematoma
  - Phlegmon/abscess/foreign body
- Parasitic dermatitis
  - Demodex sp. [esp Dog]
  - Sarcoptes sp. [esp Dog]
  - Larva migrans
  - (Leishmania sp. [esp Dog])
- Bacterial dermatitis
  - Pyoderma/Folliculitis [esp Dog]
  - Pyotraumatic dermatitis (Hot spots)
  - Feline leprosy [Cat]
- Immunoreactive dermatitis
  - Contact allergy
  - Food allergy
  - Linear granuloma [Cat]
  - Pemphigus foliaceus
- Skin tumours
  - Squamous cell carcinoma
  - Melanoma

- Fibrosarcoma
- Lipoma

Pads

- Hyperkeratosis
  - Canine distemper virus [Dog]
  - (Leishmania sp. [Dog])
- Pododermatitis [esp Cat]

Claws

- Bacterial Paronychia
- Onychomycosis
  - Trichophyton sp.
  - Microsporum sp.
  - Candida sp.
- Onychorrhexis (brittle claws)
- Nutrional causes
- Microangiopathy (esp Diabetes mellitus, Autoimmune diseases, lymphatic leukaemia)
- Onychomadesis (shedding of the claws)
  - Autoimmune disease
  - Trauma
  - Bacterial/mycotic infection
- Hyperkeratosis
  - Hyperthyroidism [Cat]
  - Zinc deficiency [Dog]
  - Acromegaly [Dog]
  - (Leishmania sp. [esp Dog])
- Claw tumours
  - Squamous cell carcinoma
  - Melanoma

12 Toxicological Principal Symptoms

Symptoms of Poisoning

Common Causes	
Dog	Cat
+++ Medicines	+++ Medicines
+++ Dicoumarin derivatives (rat poison)	+++ Organophosphates (insecticides)
++ Metaldehyde (slug pellets)	++ Phenols (household cleaners)
++ Organophosphates (insecticides)	++ (Organic) chlorinated hydrocarbons
++ Heavy metals	++ Thallium (rat poisons)
++ Ethylene glycol (antifreeze)	++ Dicoumarin derivatives (rat poison)
+ Methanol (Alcohol)	+ Toxic plants
+ Toxic plants	

Miscarriage

Medicines

- Ergotamine
- Prostaglandins
- Cytostatics
- Bromocriptine
- Glucocorticoids
- Oestrogens
- Cabergoline
- Chloramphenicol

Household Agents

- Fertilizers (Nitrites, Nitrates)

Toxic Plants/Animals

- Ergot (Secale alkaloids)
- Parsley (Petroselinum spp.)
- Spanish Fly (Cantharidin sp.)
- Nutmeg (Myristica sp.)
- Juniper (Juniperus spp.)

- Toxic fungi (Amanita spp., Clitocybe spp.)

Other Poisons

- Heavy metals
  - Lead
  - Mercury
- Rodenticides
  - Thallium
  - Dicoumarin derivatives
- Toxic gases
  - CO_2
  - NO_2
- Nitrites/Nitrates

Anaemia, Aplastic

Medicines

- Antibiotics
  - Chloramphenicol
  - Tetracyclines
  - (Sulfonamides)

- NSAID
  - Phenylbutazone
  - Metamizole
  - Acetylsalicylic acid
- Cytostatics
- Ionising radiation
- Other medicines
  - Primidone
  - Oestrogens
  - Arsenic derivatives
  - Griseofulvin [esp Cat]

Other Toxins

- Heavy metals
  - Lead
  - Aluminium
  - Cadmium

Anaemia, Haemolytic

Medicines

- NSAID
  - Acetylsalicylic acid
  - Paracetamol
- Other medicines
  - Zinc
  - Benzocaine
  - Methionine [Cat]
  - Water enema [Cat]
  - Propylene glycol
  - Antiarrhythmics
  - Anticonvulsants
  - Cimetidine
  - Levamisole
  - Metronidazole
  - Griseofulvin [Cat]
  - Phenothiazine
  - Methylene blue
  - Vitamin K

Household Agents

- Paint solvent (turpentine)
- Moth powder (naphthalene)
- Matches (potassium chlorate)
- Anionic detergents (quaternary ammonium cations)
- Furniture/Shoe polish
- Coins (Cu, Zn, Ni)

Toxic Plants/Animals

- Snake venom
  - Common european viper (Vipera sp.)
  - Horn-nosed viper (Vipera sp.)
- Onions/Garlic/Broccoli
- Soft Maple (Acer sp.)
- Red Sage (Lantana sp.)
- Oleander (Nerium sp.)

Other Poisons

- Heavy metals
  - Lead
  - Copper
  - Zinc
- Total herbicides
  - Sodium chlorate
  - Potassium chlorate

Anaemia/ Methaemoglobinaemia

Medicines

- Paracetamol
- Methylene blue
- Toluidine blue
- Local anaesthetics
  - Benzocaine
  - Lidocaine

Household Agents

- Fertilizer (Nitrates, Nitrites)
- Photo developer (p-Methylphenol)
- Shoe polish (Phenols)
- Household cleaners (Phenols)
- Matches (Potassium chlorate)
- Cured products (Nitrites)

Toxic Plants/Animals

- Solanum (Solanum sp.)
- Fool's Parsley (Aethusa sp.)

Other Poisons

- Heavy metals
  - Copper
- Herbicides
  - Sodium chlorate
  - Potassium chlorate
- Aniline/Aniline dyes
- Nitrites/Nitrates

Anaphylaxis

Medicines

- Antibiotics
- Medicines
  - Penicillins
  - Cephalosporins
  - Sulfonamides
  - Local anaesthetics
  - Iron preparations
  - Dextranes
  - Organ extracts
  - Vaccines
  - Iodine preparations
  - Vitamin K_1 (i. v.)
  - Radiographic contrast medium
  - Hyposensibilisation antigens

Household Agents

- Disinfection agents
- Household cleaner (Phenols)

Toxic Plants/Animals

- Insect toxins
  - Wasp venom (Vespa sp.)
  - Bee venom (Apis sp.)
- Snake venom (Vipera sp.)
- Brown tail larva (Euproctis sp.)

Ataxia

Medicines

- Antibiotics/ Chemotherapeutic drugs
  - Metronidazole
  - Aminoglycosides
- Antiparasitic drugs
  - Praziquantel
  - Amitraz
  - Pyrethroids
  - Ivermectin
- NSAID
  - Acetylsalicylic acid
- Anticonvulsants
- Antihistamines
- Sedatives/Narcotics
- Other Medicines
  - Theophylline
  - Lidocaine
  - Tricyclic antidepressants
  - Dextromethorphan
  - Propylene glycol
  - H_1 Antagonists
  - Sodium phosphate [Cat]

Household Agents

- Coffee/Tea (Caffeine)
- Chocolate (Theobromine)
- Tobacco (Nicotine)
- Drugs
  (Cannabis, LSD, Heroine)
- Moth Powder (Naphthalene)
- Alcohol
- Insect repellent
  (Diethyltoluamide, DEET)
- Furniture polish/Paint solvent
  (Turpentine)
- Fuel (petrol)
- Antifreeze
  (Ethylene glycol)
- Deodorant (p-Dichlorbenzole)
- Fertiliser (Nitrites/Nitrates)
- Disinfection agents (Phenols)
- Coins (Cu, Zi, Ni)

Toxic Plants/Animals

- Chestnuts (Aesculus sp.)
- Lobelia (Lobelia sp.)
- Black Bindweed (Tamus sp.)
- Hemp (Cannabis sp.)
- Fool's Parsley (Aethusa sp.)
- Mistletoe (Viscum sp.)
- Corn lilies (Veratrum sp.)
- Spurge (Euphorbia sp.)
- Snake venoms (Vipera sp.)
- Spider venoms
  (esp Loxosceles spp.)
- Ochratoxins
- Botulism toxins

Other Toxins

- Insecticides
  - Organophosphates
  - Carbamates
  - Nicotine sulphates
  - Pyrethrins/Pyrethroids
- Rodenticides
  - Thallium
  - Crimidine
  - ANTU
  - Sodium fluoroacetate
- Herbicides
  - Arsenic preparations
  - Diazine
- Heavy metals
  - Lead
  - Cadmium
  - Paraquat
  - Phenoxyacetate
  - Copper
- Toxic Gases
  - CO
  - NO/NO_2
  - H_2S

Dyspnoea/Respiratory distress

Medicines

- Antiparasitics
  - Ivermectin
  - Amitraz
  - Pyrethroids
  - Levamisol
- NSAID
  - Acetylsalicylic acid
  - Paracetamol
- Beta blockers
  (esp propranolol, metoprolol)
- $Beta_2$ Agonists
- Barbiturates
- Morphine/Morphine
  derivatives
- Curare/Succinylcholine

Household Agents

- Fuel (petrol)
- Alcohols
- Sun screen products (Phenylbenzimidazoles)
- Fertiliser (Nitrates/Nitrites)
- Lamp/engine oils (Petrol distillates)
- Fire extinguisher (Chlorobromomethane)
- Sprays (Dichlormethane)
- Drain unblockers (NaOH, KOH)
- Furniture/Shoe polish (Turpentines)
- Firelighters (Metaldehyde)
- Matches (Potassium chlorate)

Toxic Plants/Animals

- Lupines (Lupinus sp.)
- Yew tree (Taxus sp.)
- Hemp (Cannabis sp.)
- Golden chain (Laburnum sp.)
- Ground ivy (Glechoma sp.)
- Bitter almond tree (Prunus sp.)
- Fool's parsley (Aethusa sp.)
- Further high nitrate/ nitrite containing plants
- Snake venoms (Vipera sp.)
- Spider venoms (esp Loxosceles sp.)

Other Toxins

- Insecticides
  - Organophosphates
  - Carbamates
  - Nicotine sulphate
  - Pyrethrin/Pyrethroids
  - Rotenone

- Rodenticides
  - Dicoumarin derivatives
  - Strychnine
  - Phosphorus
  - Alpha-naphthylthiourea (ANTU)
  - Sodiumfluoroacetate
- Herbicides
  - Paraquat
  - Sodiumchlorate/Potassium chlorate
  - Nitrophenols
- Toxic gases
  - CO/CO_2
  - H_2S
  - HCN
  - Smoke
- Molluscicides
  - Metaldehyde
- Nitrates/Nitrites (Drinking water)

Coagulopathies

Medicines

- NSAID
  - Acetylsalicylic acid
- Heparin
- Warfarin/further coumarins/ indandiones
- Further medicines
  - oestrogens
  - sulfonamides

Toxic Plants/Animals

- Box wood (Buxus sp.)

Other Toxins

- Rodenticides

- Dicoumarin derivatives
- Indandione derivatives

Intestinal Spasms
Medicines

- Theophylline
- Acetylcysteine

Household Agents

- Coffee/Tea (Caffeine)
- Chocolate (Theobromine)
- Tobacco (Nicotine)
- Sun screen products
  (Phenylbenzimidazoles)
- Alcohols
- Detergents (cationic)
- Furniture polish/paint solvents
  (Turpentine)
- Glues (Acetone)
- Antifreeze
  (Ethylene glycol)
- Descaling agents
  (formic/acetic/oxalic acid)
- Bleaching agents
  (Hyperchloride)
- Metaldehyde
- Coins (Cu, Zi, Ni)
- Fireworks
  (Heavy metals, Salts)

Toxic Plants/Animals

- Crown imperial (Gloriosa sp.)
- Wisteria (Wisteria sp.)
- Pokeweed (Phytolacca sp.)
- Elder (Sambucus sp.)
- Meadow Saffron
  (Colchicum sp.)
- Oleander (Nerium sp.)
- Irises (Iris sp.)

- Mistletoe (Viscum sp.)
- Privet (Ligustrum sp.)
- Corn lilies (Veratrum sp.)
- Cedars (Thuja sp.)
- Tulips (Tulipa sp.)
- Ricinus (Ricinus sp.)
- Solanum (Solanum sp.)
- Fruit pips/stones

Other Toxins

- Insecticides
  - Organophosphates
  - Carbamates
  - Nicotine sulphate
- Rodenticides
  - Thallium
  - Zinc phosphide
- Herbicides
  - Paraquat
  - Nachlorate
- Heavy metals
  - Lead
  - Copper
- Molluscicides
  - Metaldehyde

Vomitus
Medicines

- Antibiotics
  - Tetracyclines
  - Chloramphenicol [Cat]
- Antiparasitics
- NSAID
  - Acetylsalicylic acid
  - Paracetamol
  - Ibuprofen
  - Indomethacin
- Cytostatics
- Beta$_2$ Agonists

- Apomorphine [Dog]
- Xylazine
- Syrup of Ipecac [Cat]
- Ephedrine
- Local anaesthetics
- Tricyclic Antidepressants
- Loperamide
- Bromocriptine
- Digitalis glycosides
- Ephedrine

Household Agents

- Firelighters (Metaldehyde)
- Drain unblocking agents (NaOH, KOH)
- Spray solvents (Tetra)
- De-icing salts (NaCl, CaCl$_2$)
- Denture cleaners (Perborate)
- Fireworks (Heavy metals, Salts)
- Antifreeze (Ethylene glycol)

Toxic Plants/Animals

- European/English yew (Taxus sp.)
- Crown imperial (Gloriosa sp.)
- Daphne (Daphne sp.)
- Wild sage (Lantana sp.)

Other Toxins

- Molluscicides
  - Metaldehyde
- Insecticides
  - Organophosphates
  - Carbamates

Vomitus and Diarrhoea

Medicines

- Antibiotics

- Antiparasitics
- NSAID/Glucocorticoids
- Cytostatics
- Theophylline
- Digitalis

Household Agents

- Coffee/Tea (Caffeine)
- Chocolate (Theobromine)
- Tobacco (Nicotine)
- Moth balls (Naphthalene)
- Alcohols
- Insect repellent (Diethyltoluamide)
- Furniture polish/Paint solvent (Turpentine)
- Engine oils/fuels (Petrol distillates + Benzines)
- Antifreeze (Ethylene glycol)
- Detergents (anionic)
- Matches (Potassium chlorate)
- Glues (Acetone)
- Coins (Cu, Zi, Ni)
- Fertiliser (Nitrites, Nitrates)
- Photo developer (Boric acid, p-Methylphenol)

Toxic Plants/Animals

- Aflatoxins
- Holly (Ilex sp.)
- Crab's Eye (Abrusus sp.)
- Nightshade family (Solanum sp.)
- Hortensia (Hydrangea sp.)
- Sheep laurel (Kalmia sp.)
- Chestnuts (Aesculus sp.)
- Rhododendron (Rhododendron sp.)
- Ranunculus (Ranunculus sp.)

- Manchineel tree
  (Hippomane sp.)
- Primroses (Primula sp.)
- Crown imperial (Gloriosa sp.)
- Wisteria (Wisteria sp.)
- Pokeweed (Phytolacca sp.)
- Elder (Sambucus sp.)
- Meadow saffron
  (Colchicum sp.)
- Iris (Iris sp.)
- Mistletoe (Viscum sp.)
- Privet (Ligustrum sp.)
- Boxwood (Buxus sp.)
- Tetterwort (Chelidonium sp.)
- Red bryony (Bryonia sp.)
- Hemp (Cannabis sp.)
- Lily of the Valley
  (Convallaria sp.)
- Cedars (Thuja sp.)
- Tulips (Tulipa sp.)
- Onions/Garlic (Allium sp.)
- Fruit pips/stones

Other Toxins

- Insecticides
  - Organophosphates
  - Carbamates
  - Pyrethrin/Pyrethroids
  - Rotenone
  - Scilliroside
  - Bromethalin
- Rodenticides
  - Thallium
  - Zinc phosphide
  - Cholecalciferol
  - ANTU
  - Sodium fluoroacetate
- Herbicides
  - Arsenic preparations
  - Phenoxyacetate/carbonate

  - Nitrophenols
- Heavy metals
  - Lead
  - Copper
  - Zinc
- Fertilisers
  - NaCl
  - Nitrite
- Toxic gases
  - CO/CO_2
  - H_2S
  - HCN
  - Smoke
- Molluscicides
  - Metaldehyde

Hair Loss

Household Agents

- Household cleaners
  (Phenols)

Other Toxins

- Rodenticides
  - Thallium
- Semimetals
  - Arsenic
  - Selenium
- Heavy metals
  - Copper
  - Zinc

Skin Reactions, Allergic

Medicines

- Antibiotics
- Local anaesthetics
  (esp Benzocaine)
- Propylene glycol

Household Agents

- Glues (Acetones)
- Furniture polish/Paint solvent (Turpentine)
- Fuels (petrols)
- Deodorants (p-Dichlorbenzole)
- Detergents (cationic)
- Disinfection agents (Phenols, Formaldehyde)
- Paint strippers (Phenols)
- Household cleaners (Phenols)
- Sprays (Xylol)

Toxic Plants/Animals

- Ivy (Toxicodendron sp.)
- Calla lily (Zantedeschia sp.)
- Alocaisa (Alocasia sp.)
- Elephant ear (Caladium sp.)
- Woolflowers (Colocasia sp.)
- Dumb canes (Dieffenbachia sp.)
- Philodendron (Philodendron sp.)
- Epipremnum (Epipremnum sp.)
- Chrysanthemum (Chrysanthemum sp.)
- Ranunculus (Ranunculus sp.)
- Machineel tree (Hippomane sp.)
- Primroses (Primula sp.)
- Amaryllis (Hippeastrum sp.)
- Brown tail caterpillar (Euproctis sp.)

Other Toxins

- Anilin/Anilin dyes

Cardiac Arrhythmias, Bradycardic

Medicines

- Sedatives/Narcotics
  - Xylazine
  - Acepromazine
  - Halothane
  - Diazepam
- Atropine (paradoxic reaction)
- Butylscopolamine [Cat]
- Beta blockers
  - Propranolol/Metoprolol
- Lidocaine
- Phenytoin
- Procainamide
- Potassium chloride

Household Agents

- Spray propellent gases (Propane, Butane)
- Spray solvents (Tri, Tetra)

Toxic Plants/Animals

- Rhododendron (Rhododendron sp.)
- Bog Rosemary (Kalmia sp.)
- Monk's hood (Aconitum sp.)
- Calycanthus sp.
- Oleander (Nerium sp.)
- Corn Lilies (Veratrum sp.)
- Ground ivy (Glechoma sp.)
- Vipera sp.

Cardiac Arrhythmias, Tachycardic

Medicines

- Atropine
- Adrenalin
- Theophylline
- Calcium chloride
- Digitalis
- Beta$_2$ Agonists
- Tricyclic Antidepressants
- Antiectoparasitics (Pyrethroids)

Household Agents

- Coffee/Tea (Caffeine)
- Chocolate (Theobromine)
- Tobacco (Nicotine)
- Antifreeze (Ethylene glycol)
- Fire Lighters (Metaldehyde)

Toxic Plants/Animals

- Belladonna (Atropa sp.)
- Fools' Parsley (Aethusa sp.)
- Jimson weed (Datura sp.)
- Oleander (Nerium sp.)
- Lily of the valley (Convallaria sp.)
- Tulips (Tulipa sp.)
- Crown imperial (Gloriosa sp.)
- Helleborus (Helleborus sp.)
- Red bryony (Bryonia sp.)
- Sea onion (Urginea sp.)
- Adder venom (Vipera sp.)
- Nose horned viper venom (Vipera sp.)
- Wasp venom (Vespa sp.)
- Toad venom (Bufo sp.)

Other Toxins

- Rodenticides
  - Thallium
  - Scilliroside
- Molluscicides
  - Metaldehyde

Hypersalivation

Medicines

- Antiparasitics
  - Arecolin
  - Ivermectin
  - Pyrethrin/Pyrethroids

Household Agents

- Insect repellent (Diethyltoluamide)
- Furniture polish/Paint solvent (Turpentine)
- Fuels (Petrol)
- Household cleaners (NaOH, KOH)
- Denture cleaners (Perborate)
- Sprays (Dichlormethane)
- Glass fibre wool
- Cured products (Nitrites)

Toxic Plants/Animals

- Aflatoxins
- Rhododendrons (Rhododendron sp.)
- Bog Rosemary (Kalmia sp.)
- Monk's hood (Aconitum sp.)
- Dumb canes (Dieffenbachia sp.)
- Daphne (Daphne sp.)
- Larkspur (Delphinium sp.)

- Philodendrons (Philodendron sp.)
- Fungi (Amanita sp.)
- Rhubarb (Rheum sp.)
- Oleander (Nerium sp.)
- Fool's parsley (Aethusa sp.)
- Hemp (Cannabis sp.)
- Cedars (Thuja sp.)
- Tulips (Tulipa sp.)
- Monstera (Monstera sp.)
- Corn lilies (Veratrum sp.)
- Brown tail larvae (Euproctis sp.)

Other Toxins

- Avicides
  - Aminopyridine
- Insecticides
  - Nicotine sulphate
  - Organophosphates
  - Carbamates
  - Pyrethroids
- Rodenticides
  - ANTU
  - Crimidine
- Molluscicides
  - Metaldehyde
- Herbicides
  - Phenoxyacetate
- Heavy metals
  - Copper (acute)

Coma

Medicines

- Narcotics
  - Barbiturates
- Antiectoparasitics
  - Ivermectin
  - Amitraz

- Theophylline
- Phenytoin
- Paracetamol

Household Agents

- Coffee/Tea (Caffeine)
- Chocolate (Theobromine)
- Alcohols
- Furniture polish/Paint solvents (Turpentines)
- Engine oils (Petrol distillates)
- Fuels (petrols)
- Antifreeze (Ethylene glycol)
- Firelighters (Metaldehyde)
- Fire extinguisher (Chlorobromomethane)

Toxic Plants/ Animals

- Rhododendrons (Rhododendron sp.)
- Belladonna (Atropa sp.)
- Helleborus (Helleborus sp.)
- Spider venoms

Other Toxins

- Toxic Gases
  - H_2S
  - CO/CO_2
- Rodenticides
  - Zinc phosphide
  - HCN Gas
- Molluscicides
  - Metaldehyde

Seizures

Medicines

- Sedatives/Narcotics
  - Ketamine

- Antiparasitics
  - Praziquantel
  - Organophosphates
  - Carbamates
- Methylxanthins [Cat]
  - Caffeine
  - Theophylline
  - Theobromine
- NSAID
  - Acetylsalicylic acid [Cat]
  - Paracetamol [Cat]
- Cytostatics
  - 5-Fluorouracil
- Local anaesthetics
  - Lidocaine
- Pentetrazole
- Tricyclic antidepressants

Household Agents

- Coffee/Tea (Caffeine)
- Chocolate (Theobromin)
- Tobacco (Nicotine)
- Moth balls (Naphthalene)
- Alcohols
- Insect repellent (Diethyltoluamide)
- Furniture polish/paint solvents (Turpentines)
- Engine oils (Petrol distillates)
- Fuels (petrols)
- Antifreeze (Ethylene glycol)
- Anti-rust agents (Oxalic acid, NaF)
- Detergents (cationic)
- Disinfecting agents (Phenols)
- De-icing salts (NaCl, $CaCl_2$)

Toxic Plants/Animals

- Rhododendrons (Rhododendron sp.)
- Lobelia (Lobelia sp.)
- Bog Rosemary (Kalmia sp.)
- Lupines (Lupinus sp.)
- Sweetshrub (Calycanthus sp.)
- Golden chain tree (Laburnum sp.)
- Oleander (Nerium sp.)
- Bitter almond tree (Prunus sp.)
- Cherry laurel (Prunus sp.)
- Helleborus (Helleborus sp.)
- Poinsettia plant (Euphorbia sp.)
- Dumb canes (Dieffenbachia sp.)
- Philodendron (Philodendron sp.)
- Monstera (Monstera sp.)

Other Toxins

- Avicides
  - Aminopyridine
  - Cyanide/hydrocyanic acid
- Insecticides
  - Organophosphates
  - Carbamates
  - Pyrethrins/Pyrethroids
  - Nicotine sulphate
  - Chlorinated hydrocarbons
- Rodenticides
  - Thallium
  - Zinc phosphide
  - Cholecalciferol
  - Strychnine
  - Sodium fluoroacetate
  - Bromethaline
  - Crimidine
- Herbicides
  - Paraquat
  - Sodium chlorate
  - Diazine
- Heavy metals

- Lead
- Copper
- Arsenic
- Toxic gases
  - CO
  - H_2S
  - NO/NO_2
- Molluscicides
  - Metaldehyde

Hepatic Damage

Medicines

- Antibiotics
  - Ampicillin
  - Erythromycin
  - Nitrofurantoin
  - Tetracyclines
  - Cyclosporin A [Cat]
- Antimycotics
  - Griseofulvin [Cats]
  - Ketoconazole
- Antiparasitics
  - Mebendazole
  - Oxibendazole
- NSAID
  - Paracetamol
  - Phenylbutazone
  - Naproxen
  - Acetylsalicylic acid
  - Ibuprofen
  - Indometacin
- Inhalation anaesthetics
  - Halothane
  - Methoxyflurane
- Anticonvulsants
  - Phenobarbitone [Dog]
  - Primidone

- Diazepam [Dog]
- Glucocorticoids
- Cytostatics
- Other medicines
  - Procainamide
  - Warfarin
  - Haloperidol
  - Phenothiazides
  - Cimetidine
  - Vitamin A
  - Megestrol acetate
  - Butylscopolamin [Cat]

Household Agents

- Paint solvents (Turpentines)
- Alcohols
- Fuels (Petrols)
- Dentures cleaners (Perborates)
- Sprays/Stain removers (Tetrachlorethylene)
- Coins (Cu, Zn)

Toxic Plants/Animals

- Death cap fungus (Amanita sp.)
- Blue-green Algae
- Aflatoxins
- Ricinus (Ricinus sp.)
- Wild sage (Lantana sp.)

Other Toxins

- Halogenated hydrocarbons
- Phosphorus
- Heavy metals
  - Iron
  - Copper
  - Zinc

Miosis

Medicines

- Pilocarpine
- Neostigmine
- Physostigmine
- Pyridostigmine
- Morphine/Morphine derivatives

Household Agents

- Tobacco (Nicotine)
- Recreational drugs (Heroin)

Toxic Plants/Animals

- Toadstool (Amanita sp.)
- Inocybe fungi (Inocybe sp.)
- Clitocybe mushroom (Clitocybe sp.)
- Panther cap (Amanita sp.)

Other Toxins

- Insecticides
  - Organophosphates
  - Carbamate

Mydriasis

Medicines

- Atropine
- Butylscopolamine
- Adrenalin
- Ephedrine/Pseudoephedrine
- Cyclic antidepressants

Toxic Plants/Animals

- Belladonna (Atropa sp.)
- Fungi (Amanita sp.)
- Fool's parsley (Aethusa sp.)

- Ground ivy (Glechoma sp.)
- Mistletoe (Viscum sp.)
- Jimson weed (Datura sp.)
- Solanum (Solanum sp.)

Renal Damage

Medicines

- Antibiotics
  - Ampicilline
  - Cephaloridine
  - Gentamicin
  - Kanamycin
  - Neomycin
  - Vancomycin
  - Bacitracin
  - Oxacillin
  - Penicillin
  - Polymyxin B
  - Sulfonamides
  - Tetracycline
- Antimycotics
  - Amphotericin B
- NSAID
  - Paracetamol
  - Phenylbutazone
  - Naproxen
  - Acetylsalicylic acid
  - Ketoprofen
  - Ibuprofen
- Methylxanthines
  - Caffeine
  - Theophylline
  - Theobromine
- Cytostatics
- Sodium phosphate [Cat]
- Other Medicines
  - Furosemide
  - Mannitol
  - Dextranes
  - Thiazide

- Captopril
- Penicillamin

Household Agents

- Furniture polish/Paint solvent (Turpentine)
- Antifreeze (ethylene glycol)
- Deodorant (p-Dichlorbenzol)
- Alcohols
- Sun screen (Phenylbenzimidazoles)
- Anti-rust agents (Oxalic acid, NaF)
- Dentures cleaners (Perborates)
- Matches (Potassium chlorate)

Toxic Plants/Animals

- Ochratoxins
- Crown Imperial (Gloriosa sp.)
- Dumb canes (Dieffenbachia sp.)
- Philodendron (Philodendron sp.)
- Flamingo plant (Anthurium sp.)
- Elephant ear (Alocasia sp.)
- Daphne (Daphne sp.)
- Ricinus (Ricinus sp.)
- Snake venom (Vipera sp.)

Other Toxins

- Rodenticides
  - Thallium
  - Cholecalciferol
- Herbicides
  - Arsenic preparations
  - Paraquat
  - Sodium chlorate
- Heavy metals

- Lead
- Cadmium

Paresis/Paralysis

Medicines

- Curare
- Antiectoparasitics
  - Organophosphates
  - Carbamates
  - Pyrethroids
  - Ivermectin

Toxic Plants/Animals

- Lupines (Lupinus sp.)
- Mistletoe (Viscum sp.)
- Snake venom (Vipera sp.)
- Tick venoms
- Botulism toxins

Other Toxins

- Insecticides
  - Organophosphates
  - Carbamates
  - Pyrethroids
  - Chlorinated hydrocarbons
- Rodenticides
  - Thallium
  - Strychnine
  - Bromethalin
- Herbicides
  - Arsenic preparations
  - Nitrophenols
- Tricresyl phosphate

Tremor

Medicines

- Local anaesthetics

- Lidocaine
- Antiparasitics
  - Amitraz
  - Ivermectin
  - Pyrethroids
  - Lindane
- Beta$_2$ Agonists
- Tricyclic antidepressants
- Cytostatics
  - 5-Fluorouracil
- Theophylline
- Metoclopramide
- Diphenhydramine
- Ephedrine

Household Agents

- Coffee/Tea (caffeine)
- Chocolate (Theobromine)
- Tobacco (Nicotine)
- Insect repellent (Diethyltoluamide)
- Paint solvent (Turpentine)
- Fuels (petrols)
- Moth balls (Naphthalene)
- Disinfection agents (Phenols)
- Spray propellent gas (propane, butane)

Toxic Plants/Animals

- Lobelia (Lobelia sp.)
- Hemp (Cannabis sp.)
- Rushfoil (Codiaeum sp.)
- Poinsettia plant (Euphorbia sp.)
- Jimson weed seeds (Datura sp.)

Other Toxins

- Insecticides
  - Pyrethrin/Pyrethroids
  - Nicotine sulphate
  - Organophosphates
  - Carbamates
- Molluscicides
  - Metaldehyde
- Herbicides
  - Phenoxyacetate
- Heavy metals
  - Lead

Central Nervous Depression

Medicines

- Sedatives/Narcotics
- Digitalis glycosides
- Loperamide
- Apomorphines
- Antihistamines
- Anticonvulsants

Household Agents

- Antifreeze (ethylene glycol)
- Alcohols
- Detergents (quarternated ammonium cations)
- Furniture/Shoe polish (Turpentine, Turpentine alcohols)
- Engine oils (Petrol distillates)
- Fire extinguisher (Chlorobromomethane)
- Sour dough starter (Ethanol)

Toxic Plants/Animals

- Black bryony (Tamus sp.)
- English yew (Taxus sp.)
- Japanese yew (Taxus sp.)

Other Toxins

- Rodenticides
  - Cholecalciferol
- Heavy metals
  - Zinc
  - Cadmium
- Toxic gases
  - CO/CO_2

Central Nervous Excitation

Medicines

- Paradox reactions
  - Acepromazine
  - Morphine [Cat]
- Methylxanthins
  - Caffeine
  - Theophylline
  - Theobromine
- Local anaesthetics

Household Agents

- Coffee/Tea (Caffeine)
- Chocolate (Theobromine)
- Tobacco (Nicotine)
- Drugs (Amphetamines, Cocaine)
- Fuel fumes (petrols)
- Alcohols
- Furniture/Shoe polish (Turpentine)
- Disinfection agents (Phenols)
- Paint stripper (Phenols)

Toxic Plants/Animals

- Lobelia (Lobelia sp.)
- Mistletoe (Viscum sp.)
- Cat mint (Nepeta sp.)

- Valerian (Valeriana sp.)
- Cat thyme (Teucrium sp.)
- Hemp (Cannabis sp.)

Other Toxins

- Insecticides
  - Nicotine sulphates
  - Chlorinated hydrocarbons
- Rodenticides
  - Strychnine
  - Sodium fluoroacetate
- Herbicides
  - Paraquat
  - Nitrophenols
- Heavy metals
  - Lead
  - Copper
- Toxic gases
  - H_2S

Cyanosis

Medicines

- Antiparasitics
  - Pyrethroids
- Paracetamol
- Barbiturates

Household Agents

- Antifreeze (ethylene glycol)
- Matches (Potassium chlorate)
- Cured meats (Nitrites)
- Fertiliser (Nitrates/Nitrites)

Toxic Plants/Animals

- Fool's parsley (Aethusa sp.)
- English yew (Taxus sp.)

Other Toxins

- Insecticides
  - Organophosphates
  - Carbamates
- Rodenticides
  - Dicoumarin derivatives
  - ANTU
  - Zinc phosphide
- Herbicides
  - Paraquat
  - Sodium/Potassium chlorate
- Toxic gases
  - CO
  - NO_2
  - H_2S

13 Behavioural Disorders

Behavioural Disorders

Aggression

Psychogenic Causes

- Territorial behaviour
- Dominance behaviour
- Protective behaviour
- Competitive behaviour
- Playfulness
- Fear
- Attention seeking
- Envy
- Conditioning/Training
- Frustration
- Antisocial behaviour

Organic Causes

- Pain
- Postictal seizure phase
- Encephalitis
  - Rabies
- Metabolic causes
  - Hypoglycaemia
- Toxic encephalopathy
  - Lead poisoning
  - Organophosphate poisoning
- Brain tumours
- Genetic/hormonal causes
  - Maternal protective instinct
  - Puppy's self-protective instinct
  - Breed predisposition?

Allotriophagia (Compulsive Ingestion of Foreign Bodies)

Psychogenic Causes

- Stress
- Playfulness

Organic Causes

- Exocrine pancreatic insufficiency
- Hypercortisolism (Cushing's disease) [Dog]
- Glucocorticoid therapy
- Enteral malabsorption
- Intestinal parasites
- Diabetes mellitus
- Hyperthyroidism [Cat]
- Crude fibre deficiency (Grass)
- Thiamine deficiency [Cat]
- Encephalitis
  - Rabies
- Brain tumours
- Neurotransmitter disturbances

Fearfulness

Psychogenic Causes

- Separation anxiety
- Understimulated/unsociable rearing
- Negative experiences [pain association]
- Phobias
  - Thunder/lightning phobia
  - Noise phobia
  - Stair/lift phobia

Organic Causes

- Painful disease
- Encephalitis
- Metabolic encephalopathy
  - Thiamine deficiency [Cat]
- Toxic encephalopathy
  - Lead poisoning
  - Organophosphate poisoning
- Hyperthyroidism [Cat]
- Brain tumours
- Respiratory distress/Dyspnoea
- Congestive heart failure

Automutilation

Psychogenic Causes

- Acral lick dermatitis [Dog]
- Feline neurodermatitis [Cat]
- Feline lick granuloma [Cat]

Organic Causes

- Pruritus
- Arthritis/Arthrosis
- Bone diseases
- Paronychia/Onychomycosis
- Neurotransmitter disturbances
  - Dopamine
  - Serotonin
  - Endorphines
- Sensibility disturbances
  - Feline neurodermatitis [Cat]
  - Polyneuropathy
  - Paresis

Barking, Continuous

Psychogenic Causes

- Separation anxiety
- Frustration/Boredom
- Territorial behaviour
- Fear
- Conditioning/Training
- Attention seeking

Organic Causes

- Deafness
- Toxic encephalopathy
  - Lead poisoning

Micturition Problems

Psychogenic Causes

- Insufficient toilet training
- Excitement
  - fear
  - joy
- Territorial marking behaviour
- Unsuitable cat litter tray [Cat]
  - dirty
  - disturbing factors
- Frustration

Organic Causes

- Urinary incontinence
- Polydipsia/Polyuria
- Painful muscular/ skeletal disease

Hypersexuality/Nymphomania

Psychogenic Causes

- Sexual frustration
- Bitch in season/queen on heat

Organic Causes

- Ovarian cysts

Infanticide (Killing and Ingestion of the Puppies/ Kittens)

Psychogenic Causes

- Overreactive nesting behaviour

- Overreactive protective instinct
- Environmental disturbances

Organic Causes

- Hormonal infantophobia
- Caesarian section
  - Ketamine anaesthesia

Personality Change

Psychogenic Causes

- Personality change in the attachment figure
- Stress
  - Household changes
  - New family member
  - Altered daily routine
  - Disturbing factors

Organic Causes

- Brain tumours
- Encephalitis
- Granulomatous meningoencephalitis (GME)
- Metabolic encephalopathy
- Toxic encephalopathy
- Degenerative encephalopathy
- Congenital encephalopathy
- Cerebral circulatory disorder
- Traumatic brain injury
- Systemic disease
- Seizures

14 Paediatrics

Paediatric Diseases

Important puppy/kitten diseases (from birth up to 6 months of age)

Common Causes			
Dog		Cat	
+++	Gastrointestinal foreign bodies	+++	Cat flu
		++	FeLV/FIV
++	Intestinal parasites	++	Gastrointestinal foreign bodies
++	Invagination		
++	Hernias	++	Intestinal parasites
++	Hypertrophic osteodystrophy	++	Invagination
++	Hip dysplasia (HD)	++	Hernias
++	Cleft palate	++	Infectious skin diseases
++	Congenital cardiac deformation	++	Portosystemic shunt
++	Infectious skin disease		

Common Causes	
Dog	Cat
++ Portosystemic shunt	
+ Tumours (Histiocytoma, Papilloma)	

Cardiac Diseases

Congenital Diseases

- Patent ductus arteriosus (PDA)
- Subaortic stenosis [Dog]
- Stenosis of the pulmonary arteries
- Atrial septal defect (ASD)
- Ventricular septal defect (VSD)
- Dysplastic valves
- Tetralogy of Fallot
- Persistent right aortic arch
- Endocardial fibroelastosis [Cat]
- Ebstein anomaly

Acquired Diseases

- Secondary cardiomyopathy
  - Parvovirus
  - Toxoplasma sp.
  - Electric shock
  - Trauma
  - Cor pulmonale
- Primary cardiomyopathy
  - Dilated cardiomyopathy
  - Hypertrophic cardiomyopathy

Respiratory Diseases

Congenital Diseases

- Tracheal hypoplasia [esp Dog]
- Diaphragmatic hernia
- Brachycephalic syndrome
  - Stenotic nares
  - Conchal anomalies
  - Short pharyngeal space
  - Mucosal hyperplasia
  - Overlong soft palate
  - Laryngeal collapse
  - Tracheal hypoplasia
- Tracheal collapse [Dog]
- Laryngeal paralysis
- Ciliar dyskinesia
- Laryngeal stenosis
- Laryngeal hypoplasia
- Bronchial collapse
- Pulmonary emphysema
- Pectus excavatum

Acquired Diseases

- Infectious rhinitis/sinusitis
- Trauma
- Foreign body rhinitis
- Infectious tracheobronchitis (Kennel cough) [Dog]
- Infectious pneumonia
- Aspiration pneumonia
- Pleuritis

Gastrointestinal, Liver and Pancreatic Diseases

Congenital Diseases

- Cleft palate
- Cleft lip

- Dental malposition
- Jaw anomalies
  - Prognatia superior/inferior
  - Brachygnatia superior/inferior
- Megaoesophagus
- Hiatic hernia
- Megacolon
- Portosystemic shunt
- Cricopharyngeal achalasia
- Oesophageal diverticuli
- Lymphangiectasia [Dog]
- Atresia ani/coli
- Rectovaginal fistula
- Hepatic cysts
- Pancreatic hypoplasia
- Copper storage disease [Dog]
- Glycogen storage disease

Acquired Diseases

- Infectious stomatitis
- Toxic stomatitis
- Persistent deciduous teeth
- Dental enamel defects
- Tonsillitis
- Foreign bodies
- Hiatic hernia
- Gastrointestinal invagination
- Infectious gastroenteritis
- Overeating
- Intestinal parasites
- Lactose intolerance
- Infectious hepatitis
- Hepatic abscesses
- Neonatal icterus [esp Cat]
- Juvenile diabetes mellitus
- Oral papilloma [Dog]
- Rectal prolapse

Urinary Tract Diseases

Congenital Diseases

- Renal amyloidosis
- Polycystic kidneys
- Ectopic ureters
- Renal dysplasia
- Renal agenesia
- Cystine tubular resorption disturbance (Cystine uroliths) [esp Dog]
- Dalmation urate defect (Urate uroliths) [Dog]
- Fanconi syndrome
- Nephroblastoma
- Persistent urachus

Acquired Diseases

- (Struvite) Urolithiasis
- Infectious cystitis
- FLUTD [Cat]
- Trauma
- Pyelonephritis

Muscular/Bone Diseases

Congenital Diseases

Bones
- Chondrodysplasia [esp Dog]
- Hip dysplasia (HD) [esp Dog]
- Congenital patellar luxation
- Shoulder joint dysplasia [esp Dog]
- Elbow dysplasia [esp Dog]
- Tibial dysplasia [esp Dog]
- Radial agenesia
- Juvenile bone cysts
- Dwarfism (STH deficiency [Dog])
- Acromegaly (STH excess)

- Mucopolysaccharidosis Type I, VI [Siamese cat]
- Osteogenesis imperfecta
- Osteopetrosis
- Polydactyly

Muscles
- Scotty Cramp [Dog]
- Golden Retriever myopathy [Dog]
- Labrador Retriever myopathy [Dog]
- Irish Terrier myopathy [Dog]
- Collie dermatomyositis [Dog]
- X-chromosomal muscular dystrophy [Dog]
- Congenital myotonia
- Glycogen storage disease
- Contraction of the infraspinous muscle [Dog]
- Contraction of the quadriceps muscle [Dog]

Neuromuscular

- Myasthenia gravis

Acquired Diseases

Bones
- Bone/Joint trauma
- Hypertrophic osteodystrophy [Dog]
- Osteochondrosis dissecans (OCD) [Dog]
- Isolated anconaeal process [Dog]
- Fragmented medial coronoid process [Dog]
- Premature distal ulnar growth plate closure [Dog]
- Premature distal radial growth plate closure [Dog]
- Panosteitis [Dog]

- Aseptic femoral head necrosis (Legg-Calvé-Perthes Disease) [Dog]
- Weakness of the flexor tendon (Hyperextension syndrome)
- Growth plate damage/premature closure
- Malnutrition
  - Vitamin A deficiency/overload
  - Ca:P imbalance
  - Protein overload
- Craniomandibular osteopathy [Dog]
- Hypervitaminosis A [Cat]

Muscles
- Feline hypokalaemia [Cat]
- Toxoplasma myositis
- Autoimmune myositis

Skin Diseases

Congenital Diseases

- Acanthosis nigricans [Dog]
- Collagenoses/Collagenopathies (Ehlers-Danlos syndrome)
- Epitheliogenesis imperfecta
- Canine ichthyosis [Dog]
- Epidermolysis bullosa
- Acrodermatitis
- Congenital seborrhoea
- Acromutilation syndrome
- Dermoid cyst [esp Dog]
- Chediak-Higashi syndrome [Persian cats]
- Canine colour mutant alopecia [Dog]
- Hypotrichosis
- Hairless dog/cat breeds
- Follicular dysplasia of the black hair [Dog]

- Pattern baldness [Dachshund]
- Alopecia [Yorkshire terrier]
- Tyrosinaemia [Dog]
- Zinc reactive dermatosis [Dog]
- Vitiligo [Rottweiler]
- Paw collagenosis [German Shepherd Dog]
- Digital hyperkeratosis [Irish Terrier]
- Epidermal dysplasia [West Highland White Terrier]
- Cyclic neutropenia [Grey Collie]
- Psoriasiform lichenoid dermatosis [Springer Spaniel]
- Mucinosis [Shar Pei]
- Hypophyseal dwarfism [German Shepherd Dog]
- Congenital hypothyroidism [Dog]

Acquired Diseases

- Viral dermatitis
- Bacterial dermatitis
- Mycotic dermatitis
- Parasitic dermatitis
- Allergic dermatitis
- Toxic dermatitis
- Diet related dermatoses
- Puppy/kitten pyodermia/ juvenile cellulitis
- Infantile pustulosis
- Feline eosinophilic granuloma [esp Cat]
- Traumatic skin diseases

Central Nervous Diseases

Congenital Diseases

- Hydrocephalus
- Cerebellar hypoplasia
- Epilepsy
- Congenital vestibular disturbances/deafness
- Lissencephaly
- Meningoencephalocele
- Narcolepsy/Cataplexy
- Dys-/Hypomyelinogenesis
- Lysosomal storage disease
- Cerebellar abiotrophies
- Neuroaxonal dystrophy [Dog]
- Cerebellar degeneration [Bull Mastiff]
- Leucoencephalomyelopathy [Rottweiler]
- White Dog Shaker syndrome [Dog]
- Necrotising encephalopathy [Yorkshire Terrier]

Acquired Diseases

- Parvoviral cerebellar hypoplasia
- Infectious encephalitis
- Meningoencephalitis
- Granulomatous meningoencephalitis (Reticulosis)
- Toxic encephalopathy
- Metabolic encephalopathy
- Head trauma

Spinal Diseases

Congenital Diseases

- Wobbler syndrome (atlantoaxial instability) [Dog]
- Atlantoaxial subluxation [Dog, Miniature breeds]
- Spina bifida
- Meningomyelocele

- Multiple cartilaginous exostoses (Osteochondromatosis)
- Fused/Hemivertebrae
- Lordosis/Kyphosis/Scoliosis
- Miniature poodle: Demyelopathy [Dog]
- Neuroaxonal dystrophy [Rottweiler]
- Hereditary ataxia
- [Jack Russell/Fox terrier]
- Myelomalacia [Afghan]
- Mucopolysaccharidosis [Siamese cats]
- Myelodysplasia [Weimaraner]
- Dermoid cysts [esp Dog]
- Feline sacrocaudal dysgenesis [Cat]
- Arachnoidal cysts
- Spinal stenosis

Acquired Diseases

- Infectious meningomyelitis
- Granulomatous meningoencephalomyelitis
- Discospondylitis/Osteomyelitis
- Feline hypervitaminosis A [Cat]
- Lymphosarcoma [esp Cat]
- Spinal trauma
Necrotising vasculitis

Ocular Diseases

Congenital Diseases

- Distichiasis
- Entropium/ectropium
- Symblepharon
- Corneal/conjunctival dermoid
- Nasolacrimal duct stenosis
- Congenital keratoconjunctivitis sicca [esp Dog]

- Congenital corneal opacity
- Progressive retinal atrophy
- Coloboma
- Retinal dysplasia
- Eye anomaly [Collie/Sheltie]
- Eyelid agenesia
- Microphthalmus
- Enophthalmos
- Strabismus
- Feline mucopolysaccharidosis [Cat]
- Gangliosiderosis
- Mannosiderosis
- Congenital glaucoma
- Congenital lens opacity (cataract)
- Juvenile cataract
- Hypo-/aplasia of the optical nerve
- Congenital xerophthalmia

Acquired Diseases

- Infectious keratoconjunctivitis
- Ulcerative keratitis
- Keratoconjunctivitis sicca
- Infectious uveitis
- Glaucoma
- Juvenile cataract

Infectious Diseases

Puppies

Viruses
- Distemper
  - Paramyxovirus
- Canine Parvovirosis
  - Parvovirus
- Canine Herpesvirosis
  - Herpes virus

- Canine Coronavirosis
  - Coronavirus
- Canine infectious tracheobronchitis (CAV-2) Canine parainfluenza virus
- (Rabies
  - Rabies virus)
- Pseudorabies/Aujeszky-Disease
  - Herpes virus suis
- Hepatitis contagiosa canis
  - CAV-1
- Tick borne encephalitis (TBE)
  - Flavivirus

Bacteria

- Coliform infections
  - E. coli, Enterobacter sp., Klebsiella sp., Proteus sp.
- Lyme Borreliosis
  - Borrelia burgdorferi
- Bordetellosis
  - Bordetella bronchiseptica
- Streptococcosis
  - Streptococcus spp. Serogroup G, C, B
- Staphylococcosis
  - Staphylococcus sp.
- Salmonellosis
  - Salmonella spp.
- Campylobacteriosis
  - Campylobacter jejuni
- Mycobacteriosis
  - Mycobacterium tuberculosis, M. bovis, M. avium
- Brucellosis
  - Brucella canis
- Tyzzer Disease
  - Bacillus piliformis
- Leptospirosis
  - Leptospira spp.

- Listeriosis
  - Listeria monocytogenes
- Clostridiosis
  - Clostridium difficile, Cl. perfringens
- Pasteurellosis
  - Pasteurella multocida
- Mycoplasmosis
  - Mycoplasma spp.
- Yersiniosis
  - Yersinia spp.
- Tularaemia
  - Francisella tularensis
- Actinomycosis
  - Actinomyces spp.
- Nocardiosis
  - Nocardia spp.
- L-phase infections
- Tetanus
  - Clostridium tetani
- Botulism
  - Clostridium botulinum
- Helicobacteriosis
  - Helicobacter pylori

Rickettsia

- Q Fever
  - Coxiella burnetti
- Ehrlichiosis
  - Ehrlichia canis
  - Anaplasma phagocytophilum
- Rocky Mountain Spotted Fever
  - Rickettsia rickettsii

Fungi

- Dermatomycosis
  - Microsporum sp., Trichophyton sp., Candida sp., Malassezia sp.
- Systemic mycosis
  - Cryptococcus sp., Blastomyces sp.,

Coccidioides sp.,
Histoplasma sp., Aspergillus
sp., Sporothrix sp.

Protozoa
- Giardiose
  - Giardia duodenalis
- Coccidiosis
  - Cystoisospora spp.,
    Toxoplasma sp.,
    Hammondia sp.,
    Sarcocystis sp.,
    Cryptosporidium sp.
- Babesiosis
  - Babesis canis
- Balantidiosis
  - Balantidium coli
- Pneumocystosis
  - Pneumocystis carinii
- Leishmaniosis
  - Leishmania donovani
- Amoebic dysentery
  - Entamoebia histolytica
- Hepatozoonosis
  - Hepatozoon canis
- Encephalitozoonosis
  - Encephalitozoon
    cuniculi

Trematodes
- Liver fluke infestation
  - Opisthorchis sp.
- Intestinal fluke infestation
  - Alaria sp., Nanophyeltus sp.,
    Heterophyes sp.
- Lung fluke
  - Paragonimus sp.

Tape worms (Cestodes)
- Dipylidiosis
  - Dipylidium caninum,
    Joyeuxiella spp.,
    Diplopylidium spp.
- Taeniose

- Taenia pisiformis, T. ovis,
  T. cervi, T. multi-ceps, T.
  hydatigena, T. serialis, T.
  crassiceps
- Mesocestoidosis
  - Mesocestoides lineatus, M.
    litteratus
- Echinococcosis
  - Echinococcus granulosus,
    (E. multilocularis)
- Diphyllobothriosis
  - Diphyllobothrium latum
- Spirometrosis
  - Spirometra spp.

Round Worms (Nematodes)
- Round worm infestation
  - Toxocara canis, Toxascaris
    leonina
- Hook worm infestation
  - Ancylostoma caninum,
    Uncinaria stenocephala
- Whip worm infestation
  - Trichuris vulpis
- Lung worm infestation
  - Capillaria aerophila,
    Filaroides osleri, Crenosoma
    vulpis, Angiostrongylus
    vasorum
- Strongyloidosis
  - Strongyloides stercoralis
- Trichinellosis
  - Trichinella spiralis
- Stomach worm infestation
  - Spirocerca lupi
- Giant kidney worm infestation
  - Dioctophyme renale,
    Capillaria plica
- Heart worm infestation
  - Dirofilaria immitis
- Tongue worm infestation
  - Linguatula serrata

Ticks
- Common wood tick infestation
  - Ixodes ricinus
- Brown dog tick infestation
  - Rhipicephalus sanguineus

Mites
- Mange
  - Demodex canis, Sarcoptes canis, Cheyletiella sp.
- Harvest mite infestation
  - Neotrombicula autumnalis
- Red mite infestation
  - Dermanyssus gallinae
- Ear mite infestation
  - Otodectes cynotis

Fleas
- Dog flea infestation
  - Ctenocephalides canis
- Infestation with other species
  - Pulex irritans, Ctenocephalides felis, Archaeopsylla erinacei, Ceratophyllus gallinae

Lice
- Dog louse infestation
  - Linognathus setosus

Biting lice
- Canine chewing louse infestation
  - Trichodectes canis

Kittens

Viruses
- Cat flu
  - Calici virus, Herpes virus, Reovirus, Parainfluenza virus
- Feline Leukaemia
  - FeLV
- Feline Immunodeficiency
  - FIV

- Feline Infectious peritonitis
  - FIP Coronavirus
- Parvovirosis/feline panleucopenia
  - Parvovirus
- (Rabies
  - Rabies virus)
- Pocks
  - Orthopoxvirus
- Feline Rotavirosis/feline astrovirosis
  - Rotavirus/Astrovirus
- Pseudorabies/Aujeszky-Disease
  - Herpes virus suis

Bacteria
- Streptococcosis
  - Streptococcus spp. Serogroup G, C, B
- Staphylococcosis
  - Staphylococcus spp.
- Chlamydiosis
  - Chlamydia psittaci
- Pasteurellosis
  - Pasteurella multocida
- Mycoplasmosis
  - Mycoplasma spp.
- Salmonellosis
  - Salmonella spp.
- Campylobacteriosis
  - Campylobacter jejuni
- Coliform infections
  - E. coli, Enterobacter sp., Klebsiella sp., Proteus sp.
- Mycobacteriosis
  - Mycobacterium tuberculosis, M. bovis, M. avium, M. lepraemurium
- Tyzzer Disease
  - Bacillus piliformis
- Lyme Borreliosis
  - Borrelia burgdorferi

- Listeriosis
  - Listeria monocytogenes
- Clostridiosis
  - Clostridium difficile
- Bordetellosis
  - Bordetella bronchiseptica
- Yersiniosis
  - Yersinia spp.
- Tularaemia
  - Francisella tularensis
- Actinomycosis
  - Actinomyces spp.
- Nocardiosis
  - Nocardia spp.
- L-phase infections
- Helicobacteriosis
  - Helicobacter pylori

Rickettsia

- Haemobartonellosis
  - Haemobartonella felis
- Ehrlichiosis
  - Ehrlichia canis
- Q Fever
  - Coxiella burnettii

Fungi

- Dermatomycosis
  - Microsporum sp., Trichophyton sp., Candida sp., Malassezia sp.
- Systemic mycosis
  - Cryptococcus sp., Blastomyces sp., Coccidioides sp., Histoplasma sp., Aspergillus sp., Sporothrix sp.

Protozoa

- Giardiosis
  - Giardia duodenalis
- Coccidiosis
  - Cystoisospora spp., Toxoplasma sp.,

Hammondia sp., Besnoitia sp., Sarcocystis sp., Cryptosporidium sp.
- Leishmaniosis
  - Leishmania donovani
- Pneumocystosis
  - Pneumocystis carinii
- Babesiosis
  - Babesia felis
- Cytauxzoonosis
  - Cytauxzoon felis

Trematodes

- Liver fluke infestation
  - Opisthorchis felineus, Heterophytes sp.

Tapeworms (Cestodes)

- Dipylidiosis
  - Dipylidium caninum, Joyeuxiella spp., Diplopylidium spp.
- Taeniosis
  - Taenia taeniaeformis
- Diphyllobothriosis
  - Diphyllobothrium latum
- (Echinococcosis)
  - Echinococcus multilocularis
- Mesocestoidosis
  - Mesocestoides lineatus, M. litteratus

Round Worms (Nematodes)

- Common round worm infestation
  - Toxocara cati, Toxascaris leonina
- Hook worm infestation
  - Ancylostoma tubaeforme, Uncinaria stenocephala
- Stomach worm infestation
  - Ollulanus tricuspis

- Giant kidney worm infestation
  - Dioctophyme renale, Capillaria plica
- Lung worm infestation
  - Capillaria aerophila, Crenosoma vulpis, Aelurostrongylus abstrusus
- Heart worm infestation
  - Dirofilaria immitis
- Tongue worm infestation
  - Linguatula serrata
- Trichinellosis
  - Trichinella spiralis

Ticks
- Common wood tick infestation
  - Ixodes ricinus
- Brown dog tick infestation
  - Rhipicephalus sanguineus

Mites
- Mange
  - Demodex cati, Sarcoptes spp., Cheyletiella sp., Notoedres cati
- Harvest mite infestation
  - Neotrombicula autumnalis
- Red mite infestation
  - Dermanyssus gallinae
- Ear mite infestation
  - Otodectes cynotis

Fleas
- Cat flea infestation
  - Ctenocephalides felis
- Infestation with other species
  - Pulex irritans, Ctenocephalides canis, Archaeopsylla erinacei, Ceratophyllus gallinae

Biting Lice
- Cat chewing louse
  - Felicola subrostratus

Metabolic Diseases
Congenital Diseases

- Enzyme deficiency diseases (Fructose-/lactose intolerance)
- Hypophyseal dwarfism [Dog]
- Congenital diabetes insipidus centralis/renalis [Dog]
- Congenital primary hyperparathyroidism
- Congenital hypothyroidism
- Glycogen storage disease

Acquired Diseases

- Juvenile diabetes mellitus
- Hypoglycaemia
- Hypophyseal dwarfism [Dog]
- Secondary parathyroidism (alimentary/renal causes)
- Hypocortisolism (Addison's disease) [Dog]

Diet-Related Diseases

- Hypertrophic osteodystrophy [Dog]
  - Calcium excess, phosphate deficiency, protein excess
- Feline hypokalaemia [Cat]
- Malnutrition
- Secondary parathyroidism (Calcium deficiency, Phosphate excess)
- Hypervitaminosis D
- Osteomalacia/Rachitis (Vitamin D deficiency)
- Thiamine deficiency/Vitamin B1 deficiency [Cat]
- Taurine deficiency [esp Cat]
- Carnitine deficiency [esp Dog]

- Hypervitaminosis A [Cat]
- Vitamin E deficiency [Cat]

Immune System Diseases
Congenital Immunosuppression

- X-chromosomal combined immune deficiency[Basset Hound]
- Cyclic neutropenia [Grey Collie]
- Thymal hypoplasia
- IgA deficiency [German Shepherd Dog, Beagle, Shar Pei]
- IgM deficiency [Dobermann]
- C3 deficiency [Brittany Spaniel]
- Chediak-Higashi syndrome [Persian cat]
- Mucopolysaccharidosis [Siamese cat, Short-haired cat]
- Leucocyte adhesion defect [Irish Setter]

Acquired Immunosuppression

- Malnutrition/ Colostrum deficiency
- Viral immunosuppression
  - FeLV/FIV [Cat]
  - Canine distemper virus [Dog]
  - Parvovirus
- Associated pathogens
  - Demodex sp.
  - Toxoplasma sp.
  - Microsporum sp.
  - Trichophyton sp.
  - Aspergillus sp.
  - Candida sp.
  - Cryptococcus sp.
  - Nocardia sp.
  - Pneumocystis sp.
  - Listeria sp.
  - Pseudomonas sp.
  - Staphylococcus sp.
  - (Ehrlichia sp.)
- Medical immunosuppression
  - Glucocorticoids
  - Cytostatics
- Other Causes
  - Splenectomy
  - Bone marrow damage
  - Bone tumours/malignant tumours

Allergic Diseases

- Neonatal isoerythrolysis [Cat]
- Atopy/Inhalation allergy
- Contact allergy
- Flea allergy
- Drug allergy
- Food allergy
- Insect bite/sting allergy
- Blood transfusion incompatibility

Coagulopathies
Congenital Diseases
Thrombocytopenia
- Cyclic neutropenia [Grey Collie]

Thrombocytopathy
- Von Willebrand syndrome [esp Dog]
- Canine thrombopathy [Dog]
- Thrombasthenia (Glanzmann) [Dog]

- Chediak-Higashi syndrome [Cat]
- Ehlers-Danlos syndrome

Plasmatic Coagulopathies

- Factor VIII deficiency (Haemophilia A)
- Factor IX deficiency (Haemophilia B)
- Von Willebrand syndrome [esp Dog]
- Factor VII deficiency [Dog]
- Factor X deficiency [Dog]
- Factor XI deficiency [Dog]
- Factor XI deficiency (Hagemann) [Cat]

Acquired Diseases

Thrombocytopenia

- Infectious thrombocytopenia
- Immunothrombocytopenia
- Disseminated intravasal coagulation (DIC)
- Bone marrow damage

Thrombocytopathy

- Drugs
- Hyperviscosity syndrome
- Organ failure

Plasmatic Coagulopathies

- Disseminated intravasal coagulation (DIC)
- Vitamin K deficiency/antagonism
- Drugs

15 Geriatrics

Geriatric Diseases

Important illnesses of advanced age

Common Causes	
Dog	Cat
+++ Hip joint arthrosis (Coxarthrosis)	+++ Diabetes mellitus
++ Dilated cardiomyopathy	++ Hyperthyroidism
++ Mitral valve fibrosis	++ Feline asthma
++ Diabetes mellitus	++ Hypertrophic/dilated cardiomyopathy
++ Tumour disease	++ Chronic renal failure
++ Prostatic disease	
++ Chronic gastroenteritis	++ Cholangiohepatitis
++ Hypercortisolism	++ Tumour disease

Common Causes	
Dog	Cat
++ Cardiac Arrhythmias (Cushing's disease)	++ Cardiac Arrhythmias
++ Lens opacity/cataract	
+ Hearing loss	

Cardiac Diseases

Acquired Diseases

- Primary cardiomyopathy
  - Dilated cardiomyopathy [esp Dog]
  - Hypertrophic cardiomyopathy [esp Cat]
  - Restrictive cardiomyopathy
- Secondary cardiomyopathy
  - Toxoplasmosis
  - Taurine/Carnitine deficiency
  - Cor pulmonale
  - Hyperthyroidism [Cat]
  - Hypothyroidism [Dog]
  - Hypo-/Hyperkalaemia
  - Hypo-/Hypercalcaemia
  - Diabetes mellitus
  - Hypercortisolism (Cushing's disease) [Dog]
  - Uraemia
  - Renal hypertension
  - Acromegaly
  - Glycogen storage disease
  - Infectious myocarditis
  - Allergic myocarditis
  - Toxic myocarditis
  - Traumatic myocarditis

- Heart valve diseases
  - Mitral valve fibrosis
  - Tricuspid valve fibrosis
  - Bacterial endocarditis
- Cardiac arrhythmias
- Feline aortic thrombosis [esp Cat]
- Pericardial diseases

Tumour Diseases

- Haemangiosarcoma [esp Dog]
- Heart base tumour (Chemodectoma [esp Dog])
- Thyroid carcinoma
- Mesothelioma
- Lymphosarcoma [esp Cat]
- Tumour metastasis

Respiratory Diseases

Acquired Diseases

- Tracheal collapse
- Infectious bronchopneumonia
- Allergic bronchopneumonia (feline asthma)
- Pulmonary oedema
- Pleuritis/Mediastinitis
- Chronic rhinitis/sinusitis

- Laryngeal paralysis
- Pulmonary thromboembolism

Tumour Diseases

Tumours of the Nasal Cavity
- Squamous cell carcinoma
- Adenocarcinoma
- Osteosarcoma
- Chondrosarcoma
- Fibrosarcoma
- Myxosarcoma
- Haemangioendothelioma
- Lymphosarcoma [esp Cat]
- Nasopharyngeal polyps [Cat]

Laryngeal Tumours
- Lymphosarcoma [esp Cat]
- Squamous cell carcinoma
- Adenocarcinoma

Tracheal Tumours
- Squamous cell carcinoma
- Adenocarcinoma

Primary Lung Tumours
- Squamous cell carcinoma
- Adenocarcinoma

Metastatic Lung Tumours
- Mammary carcinoma
- Prostatic carcinoma
- Thyroid carcinoma
- Lymphosarcoma [esp Cat]
- Malignant histiocytosis [Bernese Moutain Dog]
- Malignant melanoma
- Haemangioendothelioma

Mediastinal Tumours
- Heart base tumour (Chemodectoma) [esp Dog]
- Thyroid carcinoma
- Mesothelioma
- Lymphosarcoma [esp Cat]

Gastrointestinal Diseases

Acquired Diseases

- Periodontal Disease
  - Plaque/tartar
  - Feline odontoclastic resorptive lesions [Cat] (FORL)
  - Decay
  - Dental abscess
  - Dental fracture
  - Oronasal fistula
  - Periodontitis
- Stomatitis/Gingivitis/Glossitis
- Pharyngitis/Laryngitis
- Chronic gastroenteritis/ colitis
  - Pyloric stenosis [esp Dog]
  - Motility disturbances
  - Gastric-/intestinal ulcer
  - Infectious gastroenteritis
  - Allergic gastroenteritis
  - Toxic gastroenteritis
  - Lymphangiectasia [Dog]
  - Hyperthyroidism [Cat]
  - Organ failure
- Gastric dilation/volvulus [Dog]
- Constipation
- Anal sac impaction/abscess
- Perineal hernia
- Megaoesophagus
- Megacolon

Tumour Diseases

Tumours of the Oral Cavity

- Epulis [esp Dog]
- Papilloma [esp Dog]
- Squamous cell carcinoma
- Fibrosarcoma

- Melanoma
- Salivary gland adenoma/carcinoma

Pharyngeal Tumours
- Nasopharyngeal polyps [Cat]
- Squamous cell carcinoma
- Tonsillar carcinoma
- Lymphosarcoma

Oesophageal Tumours
- Squamous cell carcinoma

Gastric/Intestinal Tumours
- Adenocarcinoma
- Squamous cell carcinoma
- Lymphosarcoma [esp Cat]
- Leiomyoma
- Polyps

Perianal Tumours
- Hepatoid gland adenoma/carcinoma [Dog]
- Anal sac carcinoma

Hepatic/Exocrine Pancreatic Diseases

Acquired Diseases

- Liver cirrhosis
- Cholangitis/cholangiohepatitis [esp Dog]
- Secondary hepatopathy
  - Diabetes mellitus
  - Hypercortisolism (Cushing's disease) [Dog]
  - Right–sided heart failure
  - Lipidosis
  - Hyperthyroidism [Cat]
  - Acute pancreatitis
- Acute pancreatitis
- Exocrine pancreatic insufficiency
- Infectious hepatitis

- Toxic hepatitis
- Liver cysts/Bile duct cysts

Tumour Diseases

- Hepatocellular adenoma/carcinoma
- Cholangioadenoma/–carcinoma
- Haemangioma/Haemangiosarcoma
- Pancreatic adenoma/carcinoma
- Lymphosarcoma [esp Cat]
- Tumour metastasis

Urinary Tract Disease

Acquired Diseases

- Acute/chronic renal failure
- Cystitis
- Pyelonephritis
- Urolithiasis
- Feline lower urinary tract disease (FLUTD) [Cat]
- Urinary incontinence

Tumour Diseases

Renal Tumours
- Renal cell carcinoma
- Nephroblastoma
- Lymphosarcoma [esp Cat]
- Tumour metastasis

Urinary Bladder Tumours

- Transitional cell carcinoma
- Papilloma
- Lymphosarcoma [esp Cat]

Blood/Splenic Diseases

Acquired Diseases

- Anaemia
  - Haemolytic anaemia
  - Aplastic anaemia
  - Blood loss anaemia
- Splenic rupture
  [esp Dog]
- Coagulopathies
  - Thrombocytopenia
  - Thrombocytopathy
  - Plasmatic coagulopathy

Tumour Diseases

Lymphatic Tumours
- Lymphosarcoma/Leukaemia
  [esp Cat]
- Lymphatic leukaemia
  [esp Cat]
- Plasmocytoma/multiple
  myeloma [esp Dog]
- Thymoma

Myeloid Tumours
- Myeloid leukaemia
- Erythroid leukaemia
- Polycythaemia vera
- Megakaryocyte leukaemia
- Monocyte leukaemia

Splenic Tumours
- Haemangioendothelioma
  [esp Dog]
- Lymphosarcoma
  [esp Cat]

Other Tumours
- Mast cell tumour [esp Dog]
- Malignant histiocytosis
  [Bernese Mountain Dog]

Metabolic Diseases

Acquired Diseases

Primary Metabolic Diseases
- Diabetes mellitus
- Hyperthyroidism [Cat]
- Hypoglycaemia
  (Hyperinsulinism)
- Hypercortisolism (Cushing's
  disease) [Dog]
- Feline hypokalaemia [Cat]
- Obesity
- Diabetes insipidus (central/
  renal)
- Hypothyroidism [Dog]
- Secondary parathyroidism
  (alimentary/renal)
- Hypocortisolism (Addison's
  disease) [Dog]
- Glycogen storage disease

Diet-Related Diseases
- Hypervitaminosis A [Cat]
- Thiamine deficiency [Cat]
- Taurine deficiency
- Carnitine deficiency

Tumour Diseases

- Hypophyseal adenoma
- Thyroid adenoma/carcinoma
- Parathyroid adenoma
- Phaeochromocytoma (tumour
  of the adrenal medulla)
- Insulinoma
- Gastrinoma

Central Nervous Diseases

Acquired Diseases

- Metabolic encephalopathy

- Granulomatous meningoencephalitis/reticulosis
- Geriatric peripheral vestibular syndrome
- Gradual age-related hearing loss (Presbyacusis)
- Cerebral circulatory disorders
- Seizures
- Encephalomeningitis

Tumour Diseases

- Lymphosarcoma [esp Cat]
- Meningeoma [esp Cat]
- Ependymoma
- Astrocytoma
- Oligodendroglioma
- Medulloblastoma
- Vestibular Schwannoma

Spinal Diseases

Acquired Diseases

- Spondylosis deformans
- Degenerative discopathy
- Lumbosacral stenosis (Cauda equina syndrome)
- Degenerative myelopathy
- Dura mater ossification
- Discospondylitis/Osteomyelitis
- Fibrocartilaginous embolism
- Thromboembolism
- Spinal trauma

Tumour Diseases

- Lymphosarcoma [v. a. Cat]
- Osteosarcoma
- Osteochondrosarcoma
- Multiple myeloma [esp Dog]

Bone/Muscular Diseases

Acquired Diseases

- Arthrosis/Degenerative joint disease
  - Hip arthrosis (Coxarthrosis) [esp Dog]
  - Shoulder arthrosis [esp Dog]
  - Other Arthroses [esp Dog]
- Pathological fractures
  - Osteomyelitis
  - Senile osteoporosis
  - Bone tumours
- Cruciate ligament rupture (degenerative)
- Degenerative meniscal damage
- Hygroma [esp Dog]
- Senile osteoporosis
- Arthritis
  - Infectious arthritis
  - Immunoreactive arthritis (rheumatoid arthritis)
- Traumatic fractures
- Hypertrophic pulmonary osteopathy
- Patellar luxation
- Tendovaginitis/bursitis
- Polymyopathy
- Polyneuropathy

Tumour Diseases

Bone Tumours

- Osteoma/Osteosarcoma
- Chondroma/Chondrosarcoma
- Osteochondroma
- Fibrosarcoma
- Haemangiosarcoma
- Fibrosarcoma
- Synovial cell sarcoma

Muscle Tumours
- Rhabdomyoma/
  Rhabdomyosarcoma

Ocular Diseases

Acquired Diseases

- Glaucoma
- Lens opacity/cataract
- Progressive retinal atrophy
- Keratoconjunctivitis sicca
- Plasmacellular
  keratoconjunctivitis [Dog]
- Hypertension [esp Cat]
- Senile corneal degeneration
- Senile iridal atrophy
- Conjunctival granuloma
  [Collie]
- Lens luxation
- Uveitis anterior

Tumour Diseases

Eyelid Tumours
- Papilloma
- Adenoma/carcinoma of the
  Meibomian gland
- Squamous cell carcinoma
- Lymphosarcoma [esp Cat]
- Melanoma
- Mast cell tumour [esp Dog]
- Basalioma

Conjunctival Tumours
- Papilloma
- Squamous cell carcinoma
- Lymphosarcoma [esp Cat]
- Melanoma
- Haemangioma

Ocular Tumours
- Melanoma
- Papilloma

- Lymphosarcoma [esp Cat]
- Ciliary body adenoma/
  carcinoma
- Haemangioma/
  Haemangiosarcoma
- Retinoblastoma
- Medulloepithelioma
- Optic nerve glioma/
  meningioma

Orbital Tumours
- Fibrosarcoma
- Lymphosarcoma [esp Cat]
- Osteosarcoma
- Squamous cell carcinoma
- Adenocarcinoma

Reproductive Tract Diseases

Acquired Diseases

Female Genitalia
- Mastitis
- Pyometra endometritis
  complex
  - Chronic endometritis
  - Glandular cystic endometrial
    hyperplasia [Dog]
  - Pyometra
- Ovarian cysts

Male Genitalia
- Prostatic enlargement [Dog]
  - Prostatic hyperplasia
  - Prostatic cysts
  - Prostatitis/Prostatic abscess
  - Prostatic tumours
  - Paraprostatic cyst
- Balanoposthitis

Tumour Diseases

Female Genitalia
- Ovarian tumours

- – Granulosa cell tumour
- – Cystadenoma/carcinoma [Dog]
- Uterine tumours
  - – Leiomyoma
  - – Polyps
  - – Adenoma/Adenocarcinoma
  - – Fibrosarcoma
- Vaginal/vulval tumours
  - – Leiomyoma
  - – Fibroma/Fibrosarcoma
  - – Papilloma
  - – Squamous cell carcinoma
  - – Canine transmissible venereal tumour [Dog]
- Mammary tumours
  - – Feline fibroadenoma [Cat]
  - – Adenoma/Adenocarcinoma
  - – Benign/malignant mixed tumours

Male Genitalia

- Testicular tumours [esp Dog]
  - – Leydig cell tumour
  - – Sertoli cell tumour
  - – Seminoma
- Prostatic tumours [Dog]
  - – Adenocarcinoma
- Penile tumours [Dog]
  - – Canine transmissible venereal tumour
  - – Squamous cell carcinoma
  - – Papilloma
  - – Adenocarcinoma

Skin Diseases

Acquired Diseases

- Seborrhoea
- Infectious dermatitis
- Allergic dermatitis
- Autoimmune diseases

- Metabolic dermatosis
- Pigment disturbances
- Otitis externa

Tumour Diseases

- Atheroma
  - – Epidermoid cyst
  - – Sebaceous gland adenoma
  - – Sebaceous gland retention cyst
- Basal cell tumour
- Squamous cell carcinoma
- Mast cell tumour
- Histiocytoma [Dog]
- Fibroma/Fibrosarcoma
- Lipoma/Liposarcoma
- Melanoma
- Papilloma
- Cutaneous Lymphosarcoma [esp Cat]
- Hepatoid gland adenoma [esp Dog]
- Sweat gland adenoma
- Trichoepithelioma
- Haemangioma/ Haemangiopericytoma/ Haemangiosarcoma
- Intracutaneous keratinised epithelioma
- Anal sac carcinoma
- Dermal leukaemia
- Canine transmissible venereal tumour

Immunoreactive Diseases

Acquired Diseases

- Viral Immunosuppression
  - – FeLV/FIV [Cat]
  - – Canine distemper virus [Dog]
  - – Parvovirus

- Drug-related immuno-suppression
  - Glucocorticoids
  - Cytostatics
- Other Causes
  - Splenectomy
  - Bone marrow damage
  - Tumour disease
  - Diabetes mellitus
  - Hyperoestrogenism
  - Liver cirrhosis
  - Chronic renal failure

Allergic Diseases
- Atopy/Inhalation allergy
- Food allergy
- Contact allergy
- Flea allergy
- Drug allergy
- Blood transfusion
- incompatibility

- Insect sting/Insect bite allergy

Autoimmune Diseases
- Lupus erythematosus
  - Systemic lupus erythematosus
  - Discoid lupus erythematosus
- Pemphigus complex
  - Pemphigus vulgaris
  - Pemphigus foliaceus
  - Pemphigus erythematosus
  - Pemphigus vegetans
  - Bullous pemphigoid
- Autoimmune haemolytic anaemia
- Autoimmune thrombocytopenia
- Rheumatoid arthritis
- Polyarteritis nodosa
- Myasthenia gravis

16 Zoonoses

Zoonoses

Infectious diseases that are transmissible from animals to humans

Dog † Human

Viruses

- (Rabies virus [bite])

Bacteria

- Brucella canis [contact]
- Leptospira sp. [urine]
- Salmonella sp. [contact]
- Campylobacter jejuni [contact]
- Streptococcus sp. Group A [contact]
- Bordetella bronchiseptica [contact]
- Borrelia burgdorferi [ticks]
- Pasteurella multocida [bite]
- Francisella tularensis [ticks]
- Yersinia pestis [fleas, bite]
- Mycobacterium sp. [contact]

Rickettsia

- (Ehrlichia canis [ticks])

Fungi

- Microsporum canis [contact]
- Trichophyton mentagrophytes [contact]
- Malassezia pachydermatis [contact]
- Candida albicans [contact]
- Aspergillus fumigatus [contact]

Ectoparasites

- Fleas
  - Ctenocephalides canis/felis
  - Pulex irritans
  - Others
- Lice
  - Linognathus setosus

- Biting Lice
  - Trichodectes canis
- Mites
  - Sarcoptes sp.
  - Cheyletiella sp.
  - Neotrombicula autumnalis
  - Dermanyssus gallinae

Endoparasites

- Protozoa
  - Cryptosporidia sp. [contact]
  - Giardia duodenalis [contact]
  - (Leishmania sp. [sand flies])
  - (Entamoeba histolytica [contact])
- Round worms
  - Toxocara canis [contact]
  - Toxascaris leonina [contact]
  - Ancylostoma sp. [contact]
  - (Dirofilaria sp. [mosquitos])
- Tape worms
  - Dipylidium caninum [fleas, contact]
  - Taenia sp. [contact]
  - Echinococcus sp. [contact]

Cat † Human
Viruses

- Rabies Virus [Bite]
- Orthopoxvirus bovis [contact]

Bacteria

- Brucella sp. [contact]
- Salmonella sp. [contact]
- Campylobacter jejuni [contact]
- Listeria monocytogenes [contact]

- Bordetella bronchiseptica [contact]
- Borrelia burgdorferi [ticks]
- Pasteurella multocida [bite]
- Francisella tularensis [ticks]
- Yersinia pestis [fleas, bite]
- Mycobacterium sp. [contact]
- Afipia felis [bite/scratch]

Rickettsia/Chlamydia

- Chlamydia psittaci [contact]
- Bartonella henselae [bite/scratch]
- Coxiella burnetii [contact]

Fungi

- Microsporum canis [contact]
- Trichophyton mentagrophytes [contact]
- Cryptococcus neoformans [contact]
- Pneumocystis carinii [contact]
- Sporothrix schenckii [contact]

Ectoparasites

- Fleas
  - Ctenocephalides canis/felis
  - Pulex irritans
  - Others
- Biting lice
  - Felicola subrostratus
- Mites
  - Notoedres cati
  - Otodectes cynotis
  - Sarcoptes sp.
  - Cheyletiella sp.
  - Neotrombicula autumnalis
  - Dermanyssus gallinae

Endoparasites

- Protozoa
  - Toxoplasma sp. [contact]
  - Cryptosporidia sp. [contact]
  - Giardia duodenalis [contact]
- Roundworms
  - Toxocara cati [contact]
  - Toxascaris leonina [contact]
  - Ancylostoma sp. [contact]
- Tapeworms
  - Dipylidium caninum [fleas, contact]
  - (Echinococcus multilocularis) [contact]

Rodents † Human

Viruses

- Lymphocytic choriomeningitis [contact]

Bacteria

- Salmonella sp. [contact]
- Campylobacter jejuni [contact]
- Listeria monocytogenes [contact]
- Bordetella bronchiseptica [contact]
- Leptospira sp. [urine]
- Pasteurella multocida [bite]
- Francisella tularensis [ticks]
- Yersinia sp. [contact]
- Mycobacterium sp. [contact]
- Spirillum minus [rat bite]

Chlamydia

- Chlamydia psittaci [contact]

Fungi

- Microsporum canis [contact]
- Trichophyton mentagrophytes [contact]

Ectoparasites

- Fleas
- Biting lice
- Mites

Domestic Birds † Human

Viruses

- Influenza A Virus
- Avian influenza (Paramyxovirus)

Bacteria

- Salmonella sp. [contact]
- Campylobacter jejuni [contact]
- Pasteurella multocida [bite]
- Mycobacterium sp. [contact]

Chlamydia

- Chlamydia psittaci [contact]

Fungi

- Trichophyton mentagrophytes [contact]

Ectoparasites

- Fleas
- Biting lice
- Mites

Endoparasites

- Cryptosporidia sp. [contact]

17 Laboratory Findings

Haematology

Red Blood Cell Count

Haematocrit (Hct)

Reference Parameters

Dog: 44–52% (0,44–0,52 l/l)
Cat: 30–45% (0,30–0,45 l/l)

↑ **Parameters**
- Physiological
  - Greyhounds
  - Training
  - Excitement (splenic contraction)
- Dehydration
- Shock
- Congenital heart disease (Right-left shunt)
- Chronic pulmonary disease
- Hypercortisolism (Cushing's disease) [Dog]
- Hyperthyroidism [Cat]
- Renal tumours
- Altitude sickness
- Polycythaemia vera

↓ **Parameters**
- Physiological: puppies/ kittens, pregnancy, sedation/ anaesthesia
- Anaemia

Reference Parameters

Dog: 5,5–8,5 × 10^6 μl (× 10^{12} l)
Cat: 5,0–10,0 × 10^6 μl (× 10^{12} l)

↑ **Parameters**
- Physiological
  - Greyhounds
  - Training
  - Excitement (splenic contraction)
- Dehydration
- Shock
- Congenital heart disease (Right-left shunt)
- Chronic pulmonary disease
- Hypercortisolism (Cushing's disease) [Dog]
- Hyperthyroidism [Cat]
- Renal tumours
- Altitude sickness
- Polycythaemia vera

↓ **Parameters**
- Physiological: puppies/ kittens, pregnancy, sedation/ anaesthesia
- Anaemia

Haemoglobin (Hb)

Reference Parameters

Dog: 15,0–19,0 g/dl
(9,3–11,8 mmol/l)
Cat: 9,0–15,0 g/dl
(5,6–9,3 mmol/l)

↑ **Parameters**
- Physiological
  - Greyhounds
  - Training
  - Excitement (splenic contraction)
- Dehydration
- Shock

- Congenital heart disease
  (Right-left shunt)
- Chronic pulmonary
  disease
- Hypercortisolism
  (Cushing's disease) [Dog]
- Hyperthyroidism [Cat]
- Renal tumours
- Altitude sickness
- Polycythaemia vera

↓ **Parameters**
- Physiological: puppies/
  kittens, pregnancy,
  sedation/anaesthesia
- Anaemia

Mean Corpuscular Volume (MCV)

Calculation

$$\text{MCV (fl/\mu m}^3) = \frac{\text{Hct (\%)} \times 10}{\text{Erythrocyte number} (\times 10^6 /\mu l)}$$

Reference Parameters

Dog: 67–80 fl/μm^3
Cat: 40–55 fl/μm^3
↑ **Parameters**
- Physiological
  – Puppies/kittens
- Regenerative anaemia
  (reticulocytes, normoblasts)
- Folic acid deficiency anaemia
  – Malabsorption syndrome
  – Folic acid antagonism
    (Sulfonamides/
    Trimethoprim, Phenytoin)
- Erythroleukaemia
- Hyperthyroidism [Cat]
- Congenital macrocytosis

↓ **Parameters**
- Haemobartonella felis [Cat]
- Iron deficiency anaemia
- Vitamin B$_6$ deficiency

Mean Corpuscular Haemoglobin Concentration (MCHC)

Calculation

$$\text{MCHC (g/dl)} = \frac{\text{Hb (g/dl)} \times 100}{\text{Hct (\%)}}$$

Reference Parameters

Dog: 32–36 g/dl
Cat: 30–36 g/dl
↑ **Parameters**
- Measuring error
- Haemolysis
- Lipidaemia
- Heinz bodies [Cat]
↓ **Parameters**
- Regenerative anaemia
  (reticulocytes, normoblasts)
- Iron deficiency anaemia
- Vitamin B$_6$ deficiency anaemia
- Hypoalbuminaemia
- Congenital hypochromic
  anaemia

Reticulocyte Number

Method

Vital stain (Brillant cresyl blue)

Reference Parameters

Dog: 5–10/1000 Ery
Cat: 5–20/1000 Ery
↑ **Parameters**
- Regenerative anaemia
  – Haemolytic anaemia

- Blood loss anaemia
- Therapeutic success in non-regenerative anaemias
- Physiological
  - Pregnancy
  - Neonates/puppies/ kittens
- Chronic pulmonary disease
- Lead poisoning
- Congenital diseases
  - Cyclic neutropenia [Grey Collie]
  - Pyruvate kinase deficiency [Basenji, Beagle]
  - Porphyria [Siamese cat]
  - Stomatocytosis [Alaska Malamute]

↓ **Parameters**
- Non-regenerative anaemia
  - Aplastic anaemia/bone marrow insufficiency

Reticulocyte Index (RI)

Calculation

$$RI = \frac{\text{Reticulocyte number (\%)} \times \text{Hct (\%)}}{\text{Reticulocyte maturation time (days)} \times \text{normal Hct (\%)}}$$

Reticulocyte maturation time =
  with Hct 45%: 1 day
  with Hct 25%: 2 days
  with Hct 15%: 2,5 days
normal Hct = Dog: 45%
  Cat: 40%

↑ **Parameters**
- RI > 2 (regenerative anaemia)
- RI > 3 (haemolytic anaemia)

↓ **Parameters**
- RI < 2 (non-regenerative anaemia)

Distinguishing Features of Anaemia

Findings	Haemolytic Anaemia insufficiency	Acute Haemorrhage	Chronic Haemorrhage	Bone Marrow
Blood Laboratory				
Haematocrit	↓	↓	↓	↓
Erythrocytes	↓	↓	↓	↓

Findings	Haemolytic Anaemia insufficiency	Acute Haemorrhage	Chronic Haemorrhage	Bone Marrow
Haemoglobin (HB)	↓	↓	↓	↓
MCH	–	–	↓	–
MCV	–	–	–/↑	–
MCHC	–	–	↓	–
Protein (TP)	–	↓	↓	–
Bilirubin	↑	–	–	–
Coombs Test	(+)	–	–	–

LDH	↑	–	–	–
Serum iron	↑	–	↓	–
Blood Smear				
Reticulocyte Index	↑ > 2,5	–	↑ > 2,5	↑ > 2,5
Blood parasites	(+)	–	–	–
Autoagglutination	(+)	–	–	–
Spherocytes	+	–	–	–
Macrocytosis	–	–	–	+
Microcytosis	+	–	+	–
Anisocytosis	(+)	–	(+)	–
Heinz bodies	(+)	–	–	(+)
Urinalysis				
Haemoglobin/ Bilirubinuria	+	–	–	–
Bone marrow smear	active	–	active	Low in cell

White Blood Cell Count

Leucocyte Number

Reference Parameters

Dog: 6000–12000 /µl
Cat: 6000–11000 /µl

↑ **Parameters (Leucocytosis)**
- Bacterial infectious diseases
- Lymphatic leukaemia/ lymphosarcoma
- Physiological
  - Excitement (stress-leucogram)
  - Pregnancy
- Glucocorticoids
  - Chronic stress
  - Glucocorticoid/ACTH Therapy
  - Hypercortisolism (Cushing's disease) [esp Dog]
- Non-infectious inflammations
- Hyperthyroidism [Cat]
- FIP [Cat]

↓ **Parameters (Leucopenia)**
- Viral infectious diseases
- Septicaemia/Endotoxaemia
- Anaphylaxis
- Bone marrow insufficiency/ infiltration
- Parasitic infectious diseases
  - Toxoplasma sp.
  - (Leishmania sp.)

Neutrophil Granulocytes

Reference Parameters

Dog: banded: 0–4%
  segmented: 50–75%

Cat: banded: 0–4%
  segmented: 60–75%

↑ **Parameters (Neutrophilia)**
- Infectious diseases
  (esp bacterial)
- Regenerative anaemia
  - Haemolytic anaemia
  - Blood loss anaemia
- Leukaemia
  - Myeloid leukaemia
- Physiological
  - Excitement (stress
    leucogram)
  - Pregnancy
- Glucocorticoids
  - Chronic stress
  - Glucocorticoid/ACTH
    Therapy
  - Hypercortisolism
    (Cushing's disease) [esp Dog]
- Other medicines
  - Anabolics
  - Oestrogen
- Hyperthyroidism [Cat]
- Lupus erythematosus
- Non-infectious inflammation
  - Burns
  - Acute pancreatitis
  - Necrosis
  - Tumours
  - Uraemia
  - Diabetic ketoacidosis

Left Shift (↑banded)
- Acute infectious diseases
  (esp bacterial)
- Regenerative anaemias
- Non-infectious inflammation
- Viral infectious diseases
  (Recovery phase)

**Right Shift
(Hypersegmentation)**

- Glucocorticoids
- Old stale blood sample
- Folic acid deficiency

↓ **Parameters (Neutropenia)**
- Septicaemia/Endotoxaemia
- Infectious diseases
  (esp viral, Toxoplasma
  sp., Ehrlichia sp.)
- Anaphylaxis
- Lupus erythematosus
- Toxic causes
  - Uraemia
  - Medicines
  - Poisoning
  - Oestrogens
    (Testicular tumours)
  - Radiation
- Bone marrow insufficiency
- Cyclic neutropenia
  [Grey Collie]

Eosinophil Granulocytes

Reference Parameters

Dog: 0–4%
Cat: 0–4%

↑ **Parameters (Eosinophilia)**
- Allergy
  - Atopy/Inhalation allergy
  - Food allergy
  - Contact allergy
  - Hormone allergy
  - Parasitic allergy
    (Ectoparasites, Larva
    migrans)
  - Bacterial/fungal allergy
- Eosinophilic granuloma
  complex
- Eosinophilic pneumonia/feline
  asthma
- Eosinophilic gastroenteritis

- Hypocortisolism (Addison's disease) [Dog]
- Eosinophilic myositis [Dog]
- Panosteitis [Dog]
- Medicines (esp Methimazole, Carbimazole) [Cat]
- Breed predisposition in the German Shepherd Dog

↓ **Parameters (Eosinopenia)**

- Glucocorticoids
  - Chronic stress
  - Glucocorticoid/ACTH Therapy
  - Hypercortisolism (Cushing's disease) [esp Dog]
- Acute stress (Adrenalin)
- Acute infectious diseases

Basophil Granulocytes

Reference Parameters

Dog: 0–1%
Cat: 0–1%

↑ **Parameters (Basophilia)**

- (Dirofilaria immitis [Dog])
- Basophilic leukaemia
- Allergy
- Hyperlipidaemia
- Abscess
- Basenji puppies
- Differentiation: Mast cells

Lymphocytes

Reference Parameters

Dog: 13–30%
Cat: 15–30%

↑ **Parameters (Lymphocytosis)**

- Physiological
  - Puppies/kittens

  - Excitement
- Lymphatic leukaemia
- Chronic inflammation
  - Chronic infectious diseases
  - Chronic allergy
  - Autoimmune diseases
  - Vaccination reactions
- Hypocortisolism (Addison's disease) [Dog]
- Medicines (esp Methimazole, Carbimazole) [Cat]

↓ **Parameters (Lymphopenia)**

- Glucocorticoids
  - Chronic stress
  - Glucocorticoid/ACTH Therapy
  - Hypercortisolism (Cushing's disease) [esp Dog]
- Acute infectious diseases (esp viral)
- Cytostatics
- Septicaemia/Endotoxaemia
- Radiation
- Exposure to the heat/cold
- Primary/secondary immunodeficiency
- Chronic renal failure
- Lymphatic congestion

Monocytes

Reference Parameters

Dog: 0–4%
Cat: 0–4%

↑ **Parameters (Monocytosis)**

- Physiological [old dogs]
- Glucocorticoids
  - Chronic stress
  - Glucocorticoid/ACTH therapy

- Hypercortisolism (Cushing's disease) [esp Dog]
- Chronic infectious diseases
- Necrosis
  - Trauma
  - Tumours
  - Haemolysis
  - Haemorrhage

- Acute stress (Adrenalin)
- Monocytic leukaemia
- Autoimmunohaemolytic anaemia
- Relative monocytosis with neutropenia
- Granulomatous diseases

Further Examination Parameters

Blood Sedimentation Rate (BSR)

Material

0,4 ml Sodium citrate (3,8%) per 2 ml full blood

Method

Westergren method (vertical) [Dog]
DeHag method (vertical) [Cat]

Reference Parameters

Dog: after 1 h: 0–2 mm after 2 h: 1–4 mm
Cat: after 1 h: 0–2 mm after 2 h: 2–10 mm

↑ **Parameters**
- Physiological (Pregnancy)
- Infectious diseases (esp pyometra)
- Tumour diseases (esp leukaemia, plasmocytoma)
- Trauma
- Rheumatoid arthritis

↓ **Parameters**
- Dehydration
- Polycythaemia vera
- Heart failure (hypoxia)
- Chronic lung disease (hypoxia)
- Allergy

Blood Parasites (Direct Detection)

Buffy Coat

- Microfilaria
  - (Dirofilaria immitis [esp Dog])
  - (Dirofilaria repens [esp Dog])
  - (Dipetalonema reconditum [esp Dog])
  - (Dipetalonema dracunculoides [esp Dog])
  - (Dipetalonema grassi [esp Dog])
  - (Brugia phahangi [esp Dog])
  - (Wuchereria bancrofti) [esp Dog]
- (Trypanosoma spp. [esp Dog])

Erythrocytes

- Haemobartonella felis [Cat]
- Babesia spp.
- Haemobartonella canis [Dog]
- (Cytauxzoon felis [Cat])

Leucocytes

- (Ehrlichia canis in lymphocytes, monocytes [Dog])
- (Hepatozoon canis in monocytes [Dog])
- (Leishmania donovani infantum very rare in monocytes [esp Dog])

Blood Chemistry

Proteins

Total Protein (TP)

Reference Parameters

Dog: 6,0–8,0 g/dl (60–80 g/l)
Cat: 6,0–8,0 g/dl (60–80 g/l)

↑ **Parameters (Hyperproteinaemia)**

- with ↑ Haematocrit:
  - Dehydration with normal or ↓ Haematocrit:
  - Masked anaemia + dehydration (hyperalbuminaemia)
  - Hyperglobulinaemia
  - Hyperfibrinogenaemia

↓ **Parameters (Hypoproteinaemia)**

- With ↓ haematocrit
  - overinfusion
  - haemorrhage
- Physiological: puppies/kittens
- ↓ Protein synthesis
  - Cachexia
  - Malabsorption syndrome
  - Liver cirrhosis/ portosystemic shunt
  - Congestive heart failure
- ↑ Protein loss
  - Burns
  - Blood loss
  - Protein-losing enteropathy
  - Protein-losing nephropathy
  - Septicamia/endotoxaemia
  - Peritonitis

Albumin

Reference Parameters

Dog: 2,5–4,0 g/dl (25–40 g/l)
Cat: 2,5–4,0 g/dl (25–40 g/l)

↑ **Parameters (Hyperalbuminaemia)**

- Dehydration
- Anabolic agents therapy

↓ **Parameters (Hypoalbuminaemia)**

- Physiological (puppies)
- ↓ Protein synthesis
  - Cachexia
  - Malabsorption syndrome
  - Liver cirrhosis/ portosystemic shunt
  - Congestive heart failure
- ↑ Protein loss
  - Burns
  - Blood loss
  - Protein-losing enteropathy
  - Protein-losing nephropathy

- Septicaemia/Endotoxaemia
- Peritonitis
- Dwarfism (STH deficiency) [Dog]

Globulin

Reference Parameters

Dog: 2,4–4,5 mg/dl (24–45 mg/l)
Cat: 2,8–5,5 mg/dl (28–55 mg/l)

↑ **Parameters (Hyperglobulinaemia)**
- Physiological (neonates)
- Acute inflammation (α-Globulins)
- Chronic inflammation (γ-Globulins)
- Liver diseases
  - Acute hepatitis (α-Globulins)
  - Chronic hepatitis (β_2-Globulins)
  - Liver cirrhosis (γ-Globulins)
  - Liver tumours (β_1-Globulins)
- Tumours
  - esp lymphatic leukaemia/ lymphosarcoma
  - Multiple myeloma/ plasmocytoma (monoclonal hypergammaglobulinaemia)
- Infectious diseases
  - FIP (γ-Globulins) [Cat] Canine Distemper virus (α_2-, γ-Globulins) [Dog]
  - FeLV/FIV (γ-Globulins) [Cat]
  - Ectoparasites (γ-Globulins)
  - (Leishmania sp. [γ-Globulins]) [esp Dog]
  - (Ehrlichia sp. [α_2-, β-, γ-Globulins]) [Dog]
  - (Dirofilaria sp. [γ-Globulins]) [esp Dog]
  - (Systemic mycoses [γ-Globulins])
- Immunoreactive diseases
  - Lymphocytic cholangitis [Cat]
  - Lupus erythematosus
  - Renal amyloidosis
  - Glomerulonephritis
  - Rheumatoid arthritis

↓ **Parameters (Hypoglobulinaemia)**
- Primary/secondary immune deficiency
- Blood loss
- Protein-losing enteropathy
- Protein-losing nephropathy

A/G Ratio

Reference Parameters

Dog: 0,6–1,1
Cat: 0,6–1,2

↑ **Parameters**
- Hypoglobulinaemia
- Primary/secondary immune deficiency

↓ **Parameters**
- Hyperglobulinaemia (< 0,5 FIP suspicion)
- Hypoalbuminaemia

C-reactive Protein (CRP)

Reference Parameters

Dog: < 10 µg/ml

↑ **Parameters**
- Acute inflammatory process

- Bacterial infection
- Autoimmune disease
- Tumour disease
- Encephalitis
- Myocarditis

Haptoglobin

Reference Parameters

Dog: 0,3–0,5 mg/dl

Blood Glucose (BG)

Reference Parameters

Dog: 70–120 mg/dl
(3,9–6,7 mmol/l)
Cat: 70–150 mg/dl
(3,9–8,3 mmol/l)

↑ **Parameters**
(Hyperglycaemia)

- Physiological
  - Stress [esp Cat]
  - Postprandial
- Diabetes mellitus
- Hypercortisolism
  (Cushing's disease) [esp Dog]
- Hyperthyroidism [Cat]
- Progesterone (Dioestrus) [Bitch]
- Medicines
  - Glucocorticoids
  - Adrenalin
  - Xylazine
  - Ketamine
  - Alphaxolon/Alphadolon
    (Saffan®)
  - Thiazides
  - Insulin overdose (Somogyi
    effect)

↑ **Parameters**
- acute inflammatory process
  - Bacterial infection
  - Autoimmune disease
  - Tumour disease
  - Encephalitis
  - Myocarditis

- Seizures
- Acromegaly (STH excess)
- Acute Pancreatitis [esp Dog]
- Phaeochromocytoma
- Measuring error (Dextrose
  DTI, Lipidaemia, Haemolysis)

↓ **Parameters**
(Hypoglycaemia)

- Septicaemia/Endotoxaemia
- Hyperinsulinism (Insulinoma,
  Insulin therapy)
- Liver failure (cirrhosis/
  portosystemic shunt)
- Malabsorption syndrome
- Cachexia
- Glycogen storage disease
- Hypocortisolism (Addison's
  disease) [Dog]
- Idiopathic in puppies and small
  dog breeds
- Seizures (Status epilepticus)
- Polycythaemia
- Ethylene glycol poisoning
- Measuring error (stale blood
  sample)

Fructosamine

Reference Parameters

Dog: up to 340 μmol/l
Cat: up to 340 μmol/l
↑ **Parameters (with Hyperglycaemia)**

- Longer duration of hyperglycaemia (2–3 weeks) (Diabetes mellitus therapeutic control)

↓ **Parameters (with Hyperglycaemia)**

- Stress hyperglycaemia [esp Cat]

Liver Parameters

Glutamate Pyruvate Transaminase (GPT)/Alanine Aminotransferase (ALT)

Reference Parameters

Dog: up to 55 U/l
Cat: up to 70 U/l
↑ **Parameters**

- Hepatitis
  - Infectious hepatitis
  - Leptospira sp. [Dog]
  - FIP Coronavirus [Cat]
  - FeLV/FIV [Cat]
  - CAV-1 (Hepatitis c. c.) [Dog]
  - Toxoplasma sp.
  - Toxic hepatitis
  - Lymphocytic cholangitis [esp Cat]
  - Feline cholangiohepatitis [Cat]
- Hepatosis
  - Congested liver (Right sided heart failure)
  - Feline hepatic lipidosis [Cat]
  - Liver amyloidosis
  - Glycogen storage disease
  - Copper storage disease [Dog]
  - Diabetes mellitus
    - Hyperthyroidism [esp Cat]
    - Hypercortisolism (Cushing's disease) [esp Dog]
- Liver tumours/Liver cysts
- Bile duct obstruction
  - Intrahepatic cholestasis
  - Extrahepatic cholestasis (stones, tumours)
- Acute pancreatitis [esp Dog]
- Shock
- Fever
- Myocarditis
- Medicines
  - Glucocorticoids
  - Phenobarbital
  - Primidone
  - Mebendazole

Alkaline Phosphatase (AP)

Reference Parameters

Adult Dog: up to 110 U/l; Adult Cat: up to 140 U/l; Puppies/kittens: up to 6 times elevated
↑ **Parameters**

- Physiological (growth, training)
- Liver disease
- Liver regeneration
- Bile duct obstruction
- Bone disease

- Bone regeneration (healing fracture)
- Hypercortisolism (Cushing's disease) [esp Dog]
- Septicaemia/endotoxaemia
- Cachexia
- Pregnancy [esp Cat]
- Hyperthyroidism [Cat]
- Diabetes mellitus
- Medicines
  - Glucocorticoids
  - Phenobarbital
  - Primidone
  - Mebendazole

Bilirubin (Total Bilirubin)

Reference Parameters

Dog: up to 0,2 mg/dl (3,4 μmol/l)
Cat: up to 0,2 mg/dl (3,4 μmol/l)
↑ **Parameters (Hyperbilirubinaemia)**

Predominantly indirect (nonconjugated) Bilirubin:

- Acute haemolysis
- Full blood transfusion
- Internal haemorrhage/ haematoma

Predominantly direct (conjugated) Bilirubin:

- Hepatitis
  - Infectious hepatitis
  - Leptospira sp. [Dog]
  - FIP Coronavirus [Cat]
  - FeLV/FIV [Cat]
  - CAV-1 (Hepatitis c. c.) [Dog]
  - Toxoplasma sp.
  - Toxic hepatitis

- Lymphocytic cholangitis [esp Cat]
- Feline cholangiohepatitis [Cat]
- Hepatosis
  - Congested liver (Right sided heart failure)
  - Feline hepatic lipidosis [Cat]
  - Liver amyloidosis
  - Glycogen storage disease
  - Copper storage disease [Dog]
  - Diabetes mellitus
  - Hyperthyroidism [esp Cat]
  - Hypercortisolism (Cushing's disease) [esp Dog]
  - Liver cirrhosis
- Liver tumours/liver cysts
- Bile duct obstruction
  - Intrahepatic cholestasis
  - Extrahepatic cholestasis (stones, tumours)
- Medicines
  - Glucocorticoids
  - Phenobarbital
  - Primidone
  - Mebendazole

Ammonium

Reference Parameters

Dog: up to 100 μg/dl (up to 59 μmol/l); Cat: up to 100 μg/dl (up to 59 μmol/l)
↑ **Parameters**

- Portosystemic shunt
- Liver cirrhosis
- Acute hepatitis
- Extreme uraemia
- Congenital disorders of the urea cycle [Dog]

- Arginine deficiency [Cat]
- Extensive physical strain
- Ammonium poisoning
- Measuring error (stale blood samples

Glutamate Oxaloacetate Transaminase (GOT)/Aspartate Aminotransferase (AST)
Reference Parameters

Dog: up to 25 U/l
Cat: up to 30 U/l
↑ **Parameters**
- Liver disease
- Skeletal muscle disease
- Myocardial disease (esp myositis, myocardial infarction, aortic thrombosis)
- Extensive physical strain
- Measuring error (haemolysis)

Gamma Glutamyl Transferase (GGT)
Reference Parameters

Dog: up to 6 U/l
Cat: up to 6 U/l
↑ **Parameters**
- Chronic liver disease
- Bile duct obstruction

Lactate Dehydrogenase (LDH)
Reference Parameters

Dog: up to 130 U/l
Cat: up to 200 U/l
↑ **Parameters**
- Physiological (oriental cat breeds)

- Skeletal muscle disease
- Myocardial disease
- Liver disease
- Malignant tumours
- Measuring error (haemolysis)

Bile Acids
Reference Parameters

Dog: up to 20 μmol/l
(12 h fasting value)
Cat: up to 20 μmol/l
(12 h fasting value)
↑ **Parameters**
- Physiological (postprandial)
- Hepatitis
  - Infectious hepatitis
  - Leptospira sp. [Dog]
  - FIP Coronavirus [Cat]
  - FeLV/FIV [Cat]
  - CAV-1 (Hepatitis c. c.) [Dog]
  - Toxoplasma sp.
  - Toxic hepatitis
  - Lymphocytic cholangitis [esp Cat]
  - Feline cholangiohepatitis [Cat]
- Bile duct obstruction
  - Intrahepatic cholestasis
  - Extrahepatic cholestasis (stones, tumours)
- Hypercortisolism (Cushing's disease) [esp Dog]
- Glucocorticoid therapy
- Hyperthyroidism [esp Cat]
- Diabetes mellitus
- Portosystemic shunt/liver cirrhosis

Triglycerides

Reference Parameters

Dog: 50–100 mg/dl
(0,6–1,2 mmol/l)
Cat: 50–100 mg/dl
(0,6–1,2 mmol/l)

↑ **Parameters**

- Physiological (postprandial)
- Diabetes mellitus
- Hypothyroidism [Dog]
- Acute pancreatitis [esp Dog]
- Hypercortisolism (Cushing's disease) [esp Dog]
- Glucocorticoid therapy
- Bile duct obstruction
- Starvation (with obesity)
- Idiopathic hyperlipidaemia [Miniature Schnauzer]
- Protein-losing nephropathy

Cholesterol

Reference Parameters

Dog: 100–300 mg/dl
(2,5–8,0 mmol/l)
Cat: 75–150 mg/dl
(2,0–4,0 mmol/l)

↑ **Parameters**

- Physiological (postprandial)
- Diabetes mellitus
- hypothyroidism [esp Cat]
- Acute pancreatitis [esp Dog]
- Hypercortisolism (Cushing's disease) [esp Dog]
- Glucocorticoid therapy
- Bile duct obstruction
- Starvation (with obesity)
- Idiopathic hyperlipidaemia (Miniature Schnauzer)
- Protein-losing nephropathy

Cholinesterase

Reference Parameters

Dog: 1,5–3,0 kU/l
Cat: 1,0–3,0 kU/l

↓ **Parameters**

- Organophosphate poisoning
- Acute/chronic liver disease

Beta Hydroxybutyrate(β-HB)

Reference Parameters

Dog/Cat: laboratory dependent

↑ **Parameters**

- Diabetic ketoacidosis
- Starvation

Gastrointestinal Parameters

Gastrin

Reference Parameters

Dog: 25–110 ng/l

↑ **Parameters**
(Hypergastrinaemia)

- Gastrinoma (Zollinger-Ellison syndrome) [esp Dog]
- Pyloric stenosis [esp Dog]
- Duodenal ulcer
- Renal failure
- Hyperparathyroidism

- Atrophic gastritis
- Short bowel syndrome
(Billroth II) [Dog]

Folic Acid

Reference Parameters

Dog: 3,5–11,0 ng/ml
Cat: 3,2–34,0 ng/ml
↑ **Parameters**
- Intestinal bacterial overgrowth
- Exocrine pancreatic insufficiency
↓ **Parameters**
- Malabsorption syndrome
- Folic acid antagonism
  - Sulfonamides/Trimethoprim
  - Phenytoin

Cobalamin (Vitamin B$_{12}$)

Reference Parameters

Dog: 300–800 pg/ml
Cat: 120–1200 pg/ml
↑ **Parameters**
- Vitamin B$_{12}$ supplementation
- Antibiotic therapy
↓ **Parameters**
- Intestinal bacterial overgrowth
- Intestinal parasites (esp tape worms)
- Malabsorption syndrome
- Exocrine pancreatic insufficiency

Pancreatic Parameters

Amylase

Reference Parameters

Dog: up to 1700 U/l
Cat: up to 1800 U/l
↑ **Parameters (2–3 times)**
- Acute pancreatitis [esp Dog]
- Pancreatic necrosis
- Pancreatic tumours
- Renal failure
- Gastric/intestinal perforation
- Glucocorticoid therapy

Lipase

Reference Parameters

Dog: up to 300 U/l

Cat: up to 280 U/l
↑ **Parameters (2–3 times increased)**
- Acute pancreatitis [esp Dog]
- Pancreatic necrosis
- Pancreatic tumours
- Renal failure
- Liver disease (esp Liver tumours)
- Glucocorticoid therapy

Trypsin-like Immunoreactivity (TLI) Test

Reference Parameters

Dog: 5–35 µg/l
Cat: 17–48 µg/l

↑ **Parameters**
- Acute pancreatitis
- Renal failure
- Prerenal azotaemia
- Malnutrition

↓ **Parameters**
- Exocrine pancreatic insufficiency

Pancreas Specific Lipase (cPL, fPL)

Reference Parameters

Dog: < 200 µg/l (cPL)
Cat: < 3,5 µg/l (fPL)

↑ **Parameters**
- (Acute) pancreatitis

Renal Parameters

Urea

Reference Parameters

Dog: 20–50 mg/dl
(3,3–8,3 mmol/l)
Cat: 30–65 mg/dl
(5,0–11,0 mmol/l)
Urea (mg/dl) =
Urea-N/BUN (mg/dl) × 2,14

↑ **Parameters (Azotaemia)**

Prerenal Azotaemia
- Dehydration
- Shock
- Blood loss
- Congestive heart failure
- Hypocortisolism (Addison's disease) [Dog]
- Hypoalbuminaemia
- Hyperthyroidism [esp Cat]
- Fever
- Diet (Carbohydrate deficiency + Protein excess)
- Extensive physical strain

Renal Azotaemia
- Acute renal Failure
  - Trauma
  - Renal infarction
  - Interstitial nephritis
  - Toxic nephritis
  - Glomerulonephritis
  - Pyelonephritis
- Chronic renal failure
  - Interstitial nephritis
  - Glomerulonephritis
  - Pyelonephritis
  - Renal fibrosis
  - Renal amyloidosis
  - Kidney stone (Nephrolithiasis)
  - Renal tumours
  - Renal cysts [esp Cat]

Postrenal Azotaemia
- Urinary tract obstruction
  - Urolithiasis
  - FLUTD [Cat]
  - Urinary tract tumours
  - Prostatic enlargement [Dog]
  - Pelvic fracture

- Ruptured bladder /torn ureter/urethra
↓ **Parameters**
- Liver failure (cirrhosis/ portosystemic shunt)
- Polyuria/Polydipsia (esp hypercortisolism, Diabetes insipidus)

Creatinine

Reference Parameters

Dog: up to 1,5 mg/dl (up to 130 μmol/l)
Cat: up to 2,0 mg/dl (up to 170 μmol/l)
↑ **Parameters (Azotaemia)**
Prerenal Azotaemia
- Dehydration
- Shock
- Blood loss
- Congestive heart failure
- Hypocortisolism (Addison's disease) [Dog]
- Hypoalbuminaemia
- Hyperthyroidism [esp Cat]
- Fever
- Catabolism
- Diet (Carbohydrate deficiency + Protein excess)
- Extensive physical strain

Renal Azotaemia
- Acute renal failure
  - Trauma
  - Renal infarction

  - Interstitial nephritis
  - Toxic nephritis
  - Glomerulonephritis
  - Pyelonephritis
- Chronic renal failure
  - Interstitial nephritis
  - Glomerulonephritis
  - Pyelonephritis
  - Renal fibrosis
  - Renal amyloidosis
  - Kidney stones (Nephrolithiasis)
  - Renal tumours
  - Renal cysts [esp Cat]

Postrenal Azotaemia
- Urinary tract obstruction
  - Urolithiasis
  - FLUTD [Cat]
  - Urinary tract tumours
  - Prostatic enlargement [Dog]
  - Pelvic fracture
- Ruptured bladder/ torn ureter/urethra
- Measuring error (Cephalosporin therapy, diabetic ketoacidosis)

Cystatin C

Reference Parameters

Dog: 0,3–1,3 mg/l
Cat: < 1,0 mg/l
↑ **Parameters**
- Early detection parameter of renal failure

Distinguishing Features of Azotaemia

Findings	Prerenal Causes	Acute Renal Failure	Chronic Renal Failure	Postrenal Causes
Clinical findings				
Fever	(+)	(+)	N	N
Uraemic breath	+	+	+	+
Polydipsia/ Polyuria	N	N	+	N
Oliguria/Anuria	+	+	(+) final stage	+
Renal size	N	↑	↓	(↑)
Pain on renal palpation	N	+	N	+
Ultrasound	N	Structural change	Structural change	Obstructive causes
Bladder size	N	N	N	Full bladder
Blood pressure	N	N	(≠)	N
Excretion urography	N	↓	↓	N
Blood laboratory				
Urea	↑	↑	↑	↑
Creatinine	↑	↑	↑	↑
Haematocrit	(↑)	N	(↓)	(↑)
Erythrocytes	(↑)	N	(↓)	(↑)
Reticulocytes	N	N	(↓)	N
Potassium	N	↑	↓(↑ final stage)	↑
Phosphorus	N	↑	↑	↑
Blood gas analysis	(metabolic acidosis)	metabolic acidosis	(metabolic acidosis)	metabolic acidosis
Urinalysis				
Specific gravity	> 1,034 [Cat] > 1,029 [Dog]	< 1,034 [Cat] < 1,029 [Dog]	< 1,012 [Cat] < 1,008 [Dog]	irrelevant
Protein	N	+	(+)	irrelevant
Urine sediment	N	active	active	active

Muscle Parameters

Creatine Kinase (CK)

Reference Parameters

Dog: up to 90 U/l
Cat: up to 130 U/l
↑ **Parameters**
• Skeletal muscle diseases
  (Rhabdomyolysis)
  – Muscle trauma
  – Spinal diseases
  – Seizures
  – Myositis
  – Myopathy
  – Extensive physical strain
• Myocardial damage (only
  CK-MB)

α-Hydroxybutyrate Dehydrogenase (α-HBDH)

Reference Parameters

Dog: up to 50 U/l
Cat: up to 97 U/l

↑ **Parameters**
• Myocardial disease

Troponin

Reference Parameters

Dog: up to 0,6 ng/ml
Cat: up to 0,5 ng/ml
↑ Parameters
• Myocardial disease

Brain Natriuretic Peptide (BNP/ Nt-proBNP) [Previously: Atrial Natriuretic Peptide (ANP)]

Reference Parameters

Dog: < 900 pmol/l
Cat: < 50 pmol/l
↑ **Parameters**
• Myocardial disease
• false-positive parameters with
  renal failure

Hormones

Thyroxin (T_4)
Free Thyroxin (fT_4)

Reference Parameters

T4: Dog: 1,3–3,6 µg/dl
       (17–46 nmol/l)
     Cat: 0,9–4,0 µg/dl
       (12–52 nmol/l)
fT_4: Dog: 0,6–3,7 ng/dl
     Cat: 0,5–2,6 ng/dl
↑ **Parameters**

• Hyperthyroidism
  – Thyroid adenoma/
    carcinoma
  – Thyroiditis/abscess
• Physiological (puppies/kittens)
• Hyperoestrogenism
  – Ovarian cysts
  – Ovarian tumours
  – Oestrogen therapy
  – Oestrus [Dog]
• Hyperprogesteronism

- Pregnancy
- Progestagen therapy
- Hyperinsulinism
  - Insulinoma
  - Insulin therapy

↓ **Parameters**
- Primary hypothyroidism
  - Lymphocytic thyroiditis
  - Chronic thyroiditis
  - Follicular atrophy
  - Thyroid carcinoma
  - Iodine deficiency
  - Bilateral thyroidectomy
- Secondary hypothyroidism
  - TSH deficiency
    (Hypophyseal lesion)
  - Autoimmune
    hypothyroidism
- Congenital hypothyroidism
  (dwarfism)
- Euthyroid systemic disease
- Medicines
  - Glucocorticoids
  - Anticonvulsants
  - Methimazole/Carbimazole
  - Propylthiouracil
  - Testosterone

Insulin

Reference Parameters

Dog: 9–32 mU/l (Fasting value)
Cat: 4–20 mU/l (Fasting value)
↑ **Parameters
(Hyperinsulinism)
Hyperinsulinism +
Hypoglycaemia**
- Physiological (postprandial)
- Insulinoma
  - β-Islet cell tumour

- Extrapancreatic tumour
  (paraneoplastic syndrome)

**Hyperinsulinism +
Hyperglycaemia**
- Diabetes mellitus
  (Type 2: Insulin resistance)
  - Obesity
  - Hypersomatotropism
    (STH)
  - Hyperprogesteronism
  - Hyperthyroidism
  - Glucocorticoid therapy
  - Hypercortisolism
    (Cushing's disease)

↓ **Parameters
(Hypoinsulinism)
Hypoinsulinism +
Hyperglycaemia**
- Diabetes mellitus
  (Insulin deficiency)
- Insulin antagonism
  - esp Adrenalin/
    Noradrenalin
  - Glucocorticoid therapy
  - Hypercortisolism
    (Cushing's disease)
  - Xylazine

Insulin-Glucose Ratio

Reference Parameters

Dog: up to 0,3 (Insulin (mU/l):
  Glucose (mg/dl)
Cat: up to 0,3
↑ **Parameters**
- Physiological (postprandial)
- Insulinoma
  - β-Islet cell tumour
  - Extrapancreatic tumour
    (Paraneoplastic syndrome)

Beta-Oestradiol (17β-)
Reference Parameters

Dog: cycle dependent
Cat: cycle dependent
↑ **Parameters (Hyperoestrogenism)**
- Ovarian cysts
- Ovarian tumours
- Testicular tumours

Progesterone
Reference Parameters

Dog: cycle dependent
Cat: cycle dependent
↑ **Parameters (> 2 ng/ml = 3 mmol/l)**
- Corpus luteum function (from oestrus for about 60 days)
- LH Peak
  - Ideal mating date about 4 days post LH Peak (Progesterone check every 2 days from day 9 of heat)
↓ **Parameters (< 2 ng/ml = 3 mmol/l)**
- Anoestrus
- Luteolysis

Relaxin
Reference Parameters

Dog/Cat: < 20 %
↑ **Parameters**
- Pregnancy diagnosis from day 28 in the Dog

Canine Prostate-Specific Arginine Esterase (CPSE)
Reference Parameters

Dog: < 70 ng/ml
↑ **Parameters**
- Early detection of prostatic hyperplasia in the dog

Erythropoetin
Reference Parameters

Dog: 0–6 mU/ml (Dog/Cat)
↑ **Parameters**
- Polycythaemia
↓ **Parameters**
- non-regenerative anaemia in renal failure

Insulin-like Growth Factor (IGF-1)
Reference Parameters

Dog/Cat: 50–500 ng/ml
↑ **Parameters**
- Acromegaly
↓ **Parameters**
- Dwarfism

Further Hormones

- ADH (Vasopressin)
- Parathormone
- Gastrin
- Luteinising hormone (LH)
- Testosterone
- T_3, fT_3
- ACTH
- Cortisol

Medications/Toxicology

Digoxin

Therapeutic Plasma Concentration

Dog/Cat: 0,5–2,0 µg/l
↑ **Parameters**
- Digitalis intoxication
- Renal failure

↓ **Parameters**
- Subtherapeutic blood level

Potassium Bromide

Therapeutic Plasma Concentration

Dog/Cat: 1000–3000 mg/l
↑ **Parameters**
- Potassium bromide intoxication

↓ **Parameters**
- Subtherapeutic blood level

Phenobarbital

Therapeutic Plasma Concentration

Dog: 15–40 mg/l
Cat: 10–30 mg/l
↑ **Parameters**
- Phenobarbital intoxication

↓ **Parameters**
- Subtherapeutic blood level

Cyclosporin

Therapeutic Plasma Concentration

Dog: 100–500 ng/ml
Cat: 250–1000 ng/ml

Further Medicines

- Phenytoin
- Primidon
- Valproic acid
- Benzodiazepines

Toxicology

- Thallium
- Lead
- Arsenic
- Cadmium
- Chrome
- Cobalt
- Dicoumarols (Rat poisons)
- Mercury
- Nickel
- Organophosphates (see Cholinesterase)
- Methaemoglobin
- Slug pellets/Carbamate

Electrolytes

Sodium (Na)

Reference Parameters

Dog: 140–155 mmol/l
Cat: 145–158 mmol/l

↑ **Parameters (Hypernatriaemia)**

- ↑ Water loss
  - Diarrhoea
  - Hyperthermia
  - Fever
  - Panting
  - Diabetes mellitus (insulin therapy)
  - Diabetes inspidus (polyuria)
  - Polyuria without polydipsia (ie pyometra)
  - Hypercortisolism (Cushing's disease)
- ↑ Sodium intake
  - Salty food/water
  - Infusions with hypertonic saline solutions
  - Infusions of sodium bicarbonate solutions
- Primary Hyperaldosteronism

↓ **Parameters (Hyponatriaemia)**

- ↑ Sodium loss
  - Vomitus/Diarrhoea
  - Chronic renal failure (Polyuria)
  - Acute renal failure (polyuric phase)
  - Hypocortisolism (Addison's disease)
  - Diuretics

- Diluting effect
  - Psychogenic polydipsia
  - Infusions of hypotonic solutions
  - Increased ADH secretion (SIADH)
  - Congestive heart failure (hypertension)
  - Hyperlipidaemia

Potassium (K)

Reference Parameters

Dog: 3,5–5,1 mmol/l
Cat: 3,0–4,8 mmol/l

↑ **Parameters (Hyperkalaemia)**

- ↓ Potassium excretion
  - Acute renal failure (Anuria/Oliguria)
  - Urinary tract obstruction (FLUTD, urolithiasis)
  - Bladder rupture
  - Potassium sparing diuretics (spironolactone)
  - ACE inhibitors
  - NSAID
  - Hypocortisolism (Addison's disease)
- ↑ Potassium intake
  - Oral/intravenous potassium substitution
- Potassium shift into extracellular space
  - Metabolic acidosis
  - Diabetic ketoacidosis
  - Muscle trauma

- Hyperosmolarity
  (Hypertonic infusion
  solution, mannitol,
  Diabetes mellitus)
- Digitalis intoxication
- Succinylcholine
- Arginine
- Haemolysis (Akita)
- Old stale blood sample
  (Leucocytes, thrombocytes)

↓ Parameters (Hypokalaemia)
- ↑ Potassium excretion
  - Chronic renal failure
    (polyuria)
  - Postobstructive diuresis
  - Diuretics
  - Infusion of saline solutions
  - Mineralocorticoids
  - Primary hyperaldosteronism
  - Glucocorticoids (Polyuria)
  - Hypercortisolism (Cushing's
    disease) (Polyuria)
  - Chronic vomitus/
    diarrheoa
- ↓ Potassium intake
  - Potassium poor diet
  - Parenteral nutrition
- Potassium shift into
  intracellular space
  - Insulin (+ Glucose)
  - Metabolic/respiratory
    alkalosis
  - Sodium bicarbonate

Chloride (Cl)

Reference Parameters

Dog: 96–113 mmol/l
Cat: 110–130 mmol/l

**↑ Parameters
(Hyperchloraemia)**
- Metabolic acidosis
  - Diarrhoea
  - Shock
  - Renal failure
  - Diabetic ketoacidosis
  - Lactic acidosis (muscle ache)
  - Ethylene glycol poisoning
    (anti freeze)
  - Metaldehyde poisoning
    (slug pellets)
  - Carboanhydrase inhibitor
- Same causes as
  hypernatriaemia

**↓ Parameters
(Hypochloraemia)**
- Metabolic alkalosis
  - Acute vomitus (gastric
    acid)
- Diuretics
- Same causes as hyponatriaemia

Calcium (Ca)

Reference Parameters

Dog: 2,3–3,0 mmol/l
Cat: 2,3–3,0 mmol/l

**↑ Parameters
(Hypercalcaemia)**
- Malignant tumours
  - Lymphosarcoma
  - Adenocarcinoma
  - Multiple myeloma
- Primary hyperparathyroidism
  (parathyroid adenoma)
- Osteolysis
  - Bone tumours
  - Osteomyelitis

- Osteoporosis (inactivity osteoporosis)
- Hypocortisolism (Addisonian crisis)
- Seizures (status epilepticus)
- Hypervitaminosis D
  - Calciferol poisoning (Rodenticides)
  - Calcium rich diet/ supplementation
  - Toxic plants (esp jasmine) (Cestrum sp.)
- Chronic renal failure
- Hyperalbuminaemia
- Hypothermia
- ↓ **Parameters (Hypocalcaemia)**
- Eclampsia (peripartal tetany)
- Hypoparathyroidism
  - Autoimmune disease
  - Parathyroidectomy (bilateral thyroidectomy)
  - (Para)thyroid tumour
  - Canine distemper virus
- Secondary parathyroidism
  - Alimentary (calcium deficiency, phosphate excess, malabsorption syndrome)
  - Renal (chronic renal failure)
- Acute renal failure (Hyperphosphataemia)
- Ethylene glycol poisoning (antifreeze)
- Acute pancreatitis
- Hypoalbuminaemia

- Phosphate containing enema [esp Cat]
- Hypercalcitoninaemia (C-cell thyroid adenoma)
- Gastrinoma (Zollinger-Ellison syndrome) [Dog]
- Urinary tract obstruction (hyperphosphataemia)
- Measuring error (EDTA plasma, haemolysis)

Phosphate (P)

Reference Parameters

Young dogs < 1 Year: 1,6–3,2 mmol/l
Adult dogs: 0,8–1,6 mmol/l
  Cat: 0,8–1,9 mmol/l
↑ **Parameters (Hyperphosphataemia)**
- Phosphate rich diet
- Renal failure (acute/chronic)
- Urinary tract obstruction (FLUTD, Urolithiasis)
- Ruptured bladder
- Osteolytic bone tumours
  - Mammary carcinoma
  - Prostatic carcinoma
  - Squamous cell carcinoma
  - Fibrosarcoma
  - Lymphosarcoma
  - Multiple myeloma
  - Osteosarcoma
  - Hypervitaminosis D
  - Calciferol poisoning (Rodenticides)
  - Calcium rich diet/ supplementation

- Toxic plants (esp jasmin, Cestrum sp.)
- Hypoparathyroidism
  - Autoimmune disease
  - Parathyroidectomy (bilateral thyroidectomy)
  - Thyroid/parathyroid tumours
  - Canine distemper virus
- Hyperthyroidism [Cat]
- Hypocortisolism (Addison's disease)
- Acromegaly [bitch]
- Measuring error (haemolysis)

↓ **Parameters (Hypophosphataemia)**

- Antacids (Aluminium hydroxide)
- Malignant tumours
- Diabetic ketoacidosis
- Primary hyper-parathyroidism [Dog]
- Diuretics
- Glucocorticoid therapy
- Hypercortisolism (Cushing's disease) [esp Dog]
- Hypovitaminosis D/ Rachitis/Osteomalacia
- Liver cirrhosis
- Dwarfism (STH deficiency)
- Respiratory alkalosis (Hyperventilation)

Magnesium (Mg)

Reference Parameters

Dog: 0,6–1,3 mmol/l
Cat: 0,6–1,3 mmol/l

↑ **Parameters (Hypermagnesiaemia)**

- Acute renal failure (oliguria/ anuria)
- Antacids (magnesium aluminium hydroxide)
- Oral magnesium supplementation
- Hypocortisolism (Addison's disease)

↓ **Parameters (Hypomagnesiaemia)**

- Malabsorption syndrome
- Parenteral nutrition
- Diuretics
- Diarrhoea
- Vomitus
- Pancreatitis
- Hypoparathyroidism
- Medications
  - Cisplatin
  - Aminoglycosides
  - Amphetamins
  - Insulin

Trace Elements

- Iron
- Zinc
- Copper
- Selenium

Blood Gas Analysis (BGA)

Reference Parameters (arterial)

	Dog	Cat
pH	7,36–7,44	7,36–7,44
pCO_2	4,8–5,3 kPa	3,7–4,3 kPa
pO_2	11,3–12,7 kPa	11,3–12,7 kPa
Standard bicarbonate:	22–26 mmol/l	22–26 mmol/l
BE (StBicarbonate-24):	+2,5 to –2,5	+2,5 to –2,5
Anion gap $Na^+ - (Cl^- + HCO_3^-)$	8–12 mmol/l	8–12 mmol/l

Evaluation

pH	pCO_2	Standard bicarbonate	BE	Evaluation
↓	↓ (compensation)	↓	↓ (–)	Metabolic acidosis
↓	↑	↑ (renal compensation)	↑ (+) (compensation)	Respiratory acidosis
↑	↑ (compensation)	↑	↑ (+)	Metabolic alkalosis
↑	↓	↓ (compensation)	↓ (–) (compensation)	Respiratory alkalosis

Metabolic acidosis

↑ **Anion Gap (normochloraemic acidosis)**
- Diabetic ketoacidosis
- Lactacidosis
  - Heart failure (hypoxia)
  - Respiratory disease (hypoxia)
  - Muscular strain (status epilepticus, dog racing)
  - Liver failure
  - Renal failure (uraemia)
  - Tumour disease
  - Medicines (Acetylsalicylic acid, Paracetamol, Ethylene glycol poisoning, Alcohols)

Normal Anion Gap (hyperchloraemic acidosis)
- Diarrhoea
- Renal tubular acidosis
- Hypocortisolism (Addison's disease)

- Medicines (ammonium chloride, calcium chloride, Carboanhydrase inhibitor)
- Parenteral nutrition (Arginine, Lysine, Histidine)

Respiratory Acidosis
- Respiratory obstructive diseases
- Disturbance of the respiratory centre
  - CNS lesion
  - Poisoning (endogenous/ exogenous)
  - Hypokalaemia
  - Anaesthesia
- Neuromuscular causes
  - Myasthenia gravis
  - Botulismus
  - Tetanus
  - Hypokalaemia
  - Tick paralysis
  - Phrenic paralysis
  - Poisoning

Metabolic Alkalosis
- Acid loss
  - Chronic vomitus (gastric content)
  - Diuretics
- Potassium deficiency

- Chronic renal failures
- Urinary tract obstruction
- Primary hyperaldosteronism
- Hypercortisolism (Cushing's disease)
- Glucocorticoid therapy
- Alkaline intake
  - Sodium bicarbonate

Respiratory Alkalosis
- Central nervous excitement (Hyperventilation in case of fear, pain)
- Hypoxia
  - Pulmonary disease
  - Congestive heart failure
  - Anaemia
- Disturbance of the respiratory centre
  - CNS lesion
  - Septicaemia/endotoxaemia
  - Hepatic encephalopathy (Liver cirrhosis, portosystemic shunt)
  - Heat stroke
  - Anaesthesia (respiration)
  - Medicines (acetylsalicylic acid, aminophyllines)

Serum Electrophoresis

Reference Parameters

	Dog	Cat
Albumin (g/dl)	2,2–4,4 (47–59%)	2,6–5,6 (45–60%)
α_1-Globulin (g/dl)	0,2–0,5 (4–7%)	0,2–1,3 (4–14%)
α_2-Globulin (g/dl)	0,3–0,9 (5–12%)	0,4–1,1 (7–12%)
β_1-Globulin (g/dl)	0,5–1,4 (11–20%)	1,1–1,4 (11–15%)
γ-Globulin (g/dl)	0,4–1,4 (8–18%)	0,6–2,6 (10–28%)

↑ **α₁-Globulin**
- Physiological: Neonates
- Acute/chronic inflammation
- Tumour disease
- Rheumatoid arthritis

↓ **α₁-Globulin**
- Liver cirrhosis

↑ **α₂-Globulin**
- Chronic inflammation
- Systemic mycosis
- Tumour disease

↓ **α₂-Globulin**
- Liver cirrhosis
- Chronic inflammation
- Systemic mycosis
- Protein-losing nephropathy
- Haemolytic anaemia
- Canine distemper [Dog]
- FIP [Cat]
- Rheumatoid arthritis

↑ **β₁-Globulin**
- Protein-losing nephropathy

↓ **β₁-Globulin**
- Autoimmune disease
- Haemolytic anaemia

↑ **β₂-Globulin**
- Acute inflammation
- Protein-losing enteropathy
- Systemic mycosis
- Liver cirrhosis
- Tumour disease
- FIP [Cat]

↑ **γ-Globulin**

Monoclonal Gammaglobulinaemia

- Multiple myeloma/plasmacytoma [esp Dog]
- Lymphatic leukaemia/Lymphosarcoma
- (Ehrlichia sp. [Dog])

Polyclonal Gammaglobulinaemia

- Infectious diseases
  - FIP [Cat]
  - CAV-1 (Hepatitis c. c.) [Dog]
  - Brucella sp. [Dog]
  - Ectoparasitosis
  - (Leishmania sp. [esp Dog])
  - (Ehrlichia sp. [Dog])
  - (Rickettsia sp. [Dog])
  - (Dirofilaria sp. [esp Dog])
- Chronic inflammation
  - Pyometra
  - Feline Cholangiohepatitis [Cat]
  - Pyoderma
- Autoimmune disease
  - Systemic lupus erythematosus
  - Pemphigus complex
  - Rheumatoid arthritis
  - Autoimmune haemolytic anaemia
- Tumour diseases

↓ **γ-Globulin**
- Primary/secondary immune deficiency
- Neonates (colostrum deficiency)
- Immunosuppression

Immunoserology

ANA Test (Antinuclear Antibodies)

Reference Parameters

Dog/Cat: negative

Positive

- Systemic lupus erythematosus
- Discoid lupus erythematosus
- Pemphigus complex
- Infectious disease
  - Demodex sp.
  - FeLV/FIV [Cat]
  - FIP [Cat]
- Flea allergy
- Immune haemolytic anaemia
- Immune thrombocytopenia
- Rheumatoid arthritis
- Bacterial endocarditis
- Feline cholangiohepatitis [Cat]
- Lymphocytic thyroiditis
- Tumour disease
- False positive
  - Griseofulvin
  - Hydralazine
  - Procainamide
  - Sulfonamide
  - Tetracyclins
  - Propylthiouracil
  - Methimazole/Carbimazole

False Negative

- Glucocorticoids
- Cytostatics

Coombs Test (Direct)

Reference Parameters

Dog/Cat: negative
(no agglutination)

Positive (Erythrocyte Agglutination)

- Immune haemolytic anaemia
- Blood parasites

Rheumatoid Factor (Rose-Waaler Test)

Reference Parameters

Dog/Cat: negative

Positive

- Rheumatoid arthritis
- Systemic lupus erythematosus

Blood Types

Dog

- DEA 1,1
- DEA 1,2
- DEA 3
- DEA 4
- DEA 5
- DEA 6
- DEA 7
- DEA 8 Incompatibility reactions with DEA-1,1-positive donors and DEA-1, 1-negative recipients

Cat

- Blood type A (96% of all cats)
- Blood type B (esp British Shorthair, Devon Rex)
- Blood type AB

Incompatibility reactions with Blood type A donors and blood type B recipients

Neonatal isoerythrolysis in kittens of blood type A fathers and blood type B mothers

Acetylcholine Receptor Antibody Test

Reference Parameters

Dog/Cat: negative
Positive
• Myasthenia gravis

Microscope Slide Agglutination Test

Test Proceedings

1. Centrifugation of an EDTA blood sample
2. Pipette the plasma off, add same amount of saline and mix
3. Repeat this 3 × times
4. Produce a microscope slide preparation with a cover slide

Positive (Erythrocyte Agglutination)
• Immune haemolytic anaemia

Thyroglobulin Antibody Test

Reference Parameters

Dog/Cat: negative
Positive
• Autoimmune hypothyroidism

(Anti-)Thrombocyte Antibody Test

Reference Parameters

Dog/Cat: negative
Positive
• Autoimmune thrombocytopenia
• Secondary after Ehrlichiosis/ Anaplasmosis

Insulin Antibodies

Reference Parameters

Dog/Cat: negative
Positive
• Insulin resistance with Diabetes mellitus

Further Immunological Tests

• Allergy test (monoclonal antibody test)
• Immune electrophoresis

Microbial Serology

Microbe	Species	Test	Material
Viruses			
Adenovirus I + II	Dog	Antibody Antigen (PCR)	Serum/Plasma EDTA blood, smear

Canine Parainfluenza virus (CPIV)	Dog	Antibody Antigen (PCR)	Serum/Plasma Smear
Coronavirus (CCoV, FECV, FIPV)	Dog/Cat	Antibody Antigen (PCR)	Serum/Plasma Faeces/Smear/ Effusion
Feline Calici virus (FCV)	Cat	Antibody Antigen (PCR)	Serum/Plasma Smear/ EDTA blood
FeLV	Cat	Antigen (ELISA) Antigen (PCR)	Serum/Plasma EDTA blood, Saliva
FIV	Cat	Antigen (ELISA) Antigen (PCR)	Serum/Plasma EDTA blood
FSME	Dog	Antibody Antigen (PCR)	Serum/Plasma Liquor/Serum/ Tick
Herpes virus (CHV, FHV)	Dog/Cat	Antibody Antigen (PCR)	Serum/Plasma EDTA blood, Smear
Influenza A	Dog/Cat	Antigen (PCR)	Smear
Viruses			
Feline cow pox (Orthopoxvirus)	Cat	Antigen (PCR)	Biopsy/Skin scrape
Papilloma virus	Dog	Antigen (PCR)	Biopsy/Skin scrape
Parvovirus (CPV, FPV)	Dog/Cat	Antibody Antigen (PCR)	Serum EDTA blood/Faeces
Rotavirus	Cat	Antigen	Faeces Serum/Plasma
Distemper virus	Dog	Antibody Antigen (PCR)	Liquor/Smear
Bacteria			
Anaplasma spp.	Dog/Cat	Antibody Antigen(PCR)	Serum/Plasma EDTA blood,Tick
Bartonella sp.	Cat	Antigen (PCR)	Serum/Plasma
Bordetella sp.	Dog/Cat	Antigen (PCR)	EDTA blood, Smear
Borrelia spp.	Dog	Antibody Antigen (PCR)	Smear Serum/Plasma
Brucella sp.	Dog	Antibody Antigen (PCR)	Synovia/Liquor, Skin biopsy, Tick
Campylobacter sp.	Dog/Cat	Antibody Antigen (PCR)	Serum/Plasma
Chlamydia/ Chlamydophila spp.	esp Cat/ Dog	Antibody Antigen (PCR)	Faeces Serum/Plasma

Coxiella spp.	Dog/Cat	Antibody	Conjunctival Smear
		Antigen (PCR)	Serum/Plasma
Ehrlichia spp.	Dog/Cat	Antibody	Smear
		Antigen (PCR)	Serum/Plasma
			EDT

Bacteria

Helicobacter spp.	Dog/Cat	Antibody	Serum/Plasma
		Antigen	Faeces, Smear, Vomit
Leptospira spp.	Dog	Antibody	Serum/Plasma
		Antigen (PCR)	Smear, Urine
MRSA	Dog/Cat	Antigen (PCR)	Faeces/Smear
Mycoplasma spp.	Dog/Cat	Antigen (PCR)	EDTA blood
Rickettsia spp.	Dog	Antibody	Serum/Plasma
Salmonella spp.	Dog	Antibody	Serum/Plasma
		Antigen (PCR)	Faeces
Staphylococcus spp.	Dog/Cat	Antibody	Serum
Yersinia spp.	Dog/Cat	Antibody	Serum
		Antigen (PCR)	Faeces

Parasites

Babesia spp.	Dog/Cat	Antibody Antigen (PCR)	Serum/Plasma
Cryptosporidia spp.	Dog/Cat	Antigen (PCR)	EDTA blood, Tick
Dirofilaria sp. (adult)	Dog/Cat	Antigen (ELISA)	Faeces Serum/Plasma
Hepatozoon sp.	Dog	Antigen (PCR)	EDTA blood, Smear, Tick
Leishmania sp.	Dog	Antibody Antigen (PCR)	Serum Biopsy
Neospora sp.	Dog	Antibody Antigen (PCR)	Serum/Plasma Liquor/Faeces
Sarcoptes sp.	Dog	Antibody	Serum
Toxoplasma sp.	Dog/Cat	Antibody Antigen (PCR)	Serum Liquor/Faeces
Tritrichomonas sp.	Cat	Antigen (PCR)	Faeces

Fungi

| Aspergillus sp. | Dog/Cat | Antibody | Serum/Plasma |
| Microsporum sp./ Trichophyton sp. | Dog/Cat | Antigen (PCR) | Hair/Skin Smear |

Moleculargenetic Examinations

Detection	Species/Breed
Pedigree Certification	Dog/Cat (oral mucosal smear)
Alaskan Malamute Polyneuropathy	Alaskan Malamute
Arrhythmogenic right ventricular Cardiomyopathy (ARVC)	Boxer
Brachyuria	Australian Shepherd et al
Canine Leucocyte Adhesion Deficiency (CLAD)	Irish Setter
Collie Eye Anomalie (CEA)	Collie, Australian Shepherd et al
Congenital Hypothyroidism (CGH)	Spanish Water Dog
Cystinuria	Newfoundland, Landseer
Degenerative Myelopathy (DM)	German Shepherd Dog et al
Dry Eye Curly Coat Syndrome	Cavalier King Charles Spaniel
Episodic Falling (EF)	Cavalier King Charles Spaniel
Hereditary Necrotising Myelopathy (ENM)	Dutch Kooikerhondje
Exercise Induced Collapse (EIC)	Labrador, Retriever, German Wirehaired, Pembroke Welsh Corgie et al
Factor VII Deficiency	Alaskan Klee Kai, Airedale Terrier, Beagle, Giant Schnauzer, Scottish Deerhound
Familiary Nephropathy	English Cocker Spaniel, English Springer Spaniel, Samoyed
Coat colour/colour variations/Hair length	Dog/Cat
Fucosidosis	English Springer Spaniel
Brittle Bone Disease (Osteogenesis imperfecta)	Short and Wire Haired Dachshund
Gangliosiderosis (GM1, GM2)	Husky, Portugese Water Dog, Siamese Cat, Burma, Korat, Oriental Shorthair
Globoid cell leucodystrophy (Krabbe disease)	West Highland White Terrier, Cairn Terrier
Glycogen Storage Disease (GSDII, GSDIIIa)	Finnish Lapphund, Swedish Lapphund, Lapp Reindeer Dog, Curly Coated Retriever, Norwegian Forest Cat

Gray Collie Syndrome (Canine Cyclic Neutropenia)	Collie
Haemophilia A (Factor VIII)	Havanese
Haemophilia B (Factor IX)	Rhodesian Ridgeback
Hereditary cataract (HSF4)	Australian Shepherd, Wäller
Hereditary Nasal Parakeratosis (HNPK)	Labrador Retriever
Hereditary Neuropathy	Greyhound
Hypertrophic Cardiomyopathy	Maine Coon, Ragdoll
Hyperuricosuria and Hyperuricaemia (SLC)	Dog
Proof of Identity	Dog/Cat
Imerslund–Gräsbeck Syndrome (IGS)	Beagle, Border Collie
Junctional Epidermolysis Bullosa (JEB)	German Short Hair
Juvenile Epilepsy	Lagotto Romagnolo
Juvenile Dilative Cardiomyopathy (JDCM)	Portuguese Water Dog
Copper Storage Disease	Bedlington Terrier
L2-Hydroxyglutaricaciduria (L2-HGA)	Staffordshire Terrier
Late onset Ataxia (LOA)	Parson Jack Russell Terrier
Malignant Hyperthermia	Dog
MDR1 Genetic defect (Ivermectin oversensitivity)	Australian Shepherd, Bobtail, Border Collie, German Shepherd Dog, Elo, Short and Long Haired Collie, Long Haired Whippet, McNab, Shetland Sheepdog, Silken Windhound, Wäller, White Swiss Shepherd Dog
Mucopolysaccharidosis VII	German Shepherd Dog, Brasilian Terrier
Muscular dystrophy (MD)	Cavalier King Charles Spaniel, Golden Retriever
Musladin–Lueke Syndrome (MLS)	Beagle Myostatin
Mutation	Whippet
Myotonia congenita	Miniature Schnauzer
Night blindness (CSNB)	Briard
Narcolepsy	Dobermann, Labrador Retriever
Necrotising Meningoencephalitis (NME)	Pug
Neonatal Cortical Cerebellar Abiotrophy (NCCD)	Beagle

Detection	Species/Breed
Neonatal Encephalopathy With Seizures (NEWS)	Standard Poodle
Neuronal Ceroid Lipofuscinosis (NCL)	American Staffordshire Terrier, American Bulldog, Australian Shepherd, Border Collie, Dachshund, English Setter, Tibetan Terrier
Phosphofructokinase deficiency	American Cocker Spaniel, German Spaniel, English Springer Spaniel, Whippet

Proof	Species
Polycystic Kidney Disease (PKD)	Bull Terrier, Persian, Siamese, Himalayan, European Shorthair, British Shorthair, American Shorthair et al
Primary Ciliary Dyskinesia (PCD)	Bobtail
Primary Lens luxation (PLL)	Dogs
Primary Open Angle Glaucoma (POAG)	Beagle
Progressive Retinal Atrophy (PRA)	Irish Setter, Collie, Welsh Corgi, Bullmastiff, Sloughi, Somali, Abessinier et al
Protein-Losing Nephropathy (PLN)	Soft-Coated Wheaten Terrier
Pyruvate Dehydrogenase Phosphatase-1 Deficiency (PDP1)	Clumber and Sussex Spaniel
Pyruvatekinase Deficiency	Basenji, Caim Terrier, West Highland White Terrier, Somali, Abyssinian
Retinal Dysplasia/Oculoskeletal Dysplasia (OSD)	Labrador Retriever, Samoyed
Spinal Muscular Atrophy (SMA)	Maine Coon
Startle Disease	Irish Wolfhound
Neutrophilic Syndrome (TNS)	Border Collie
Von Willebrand Disease (vWD1, vWD2, vWD3)	Bernese Mountain Dog, German Pinscher, Dobermann, German Wired Hair, German Short Hair, Dutch Kooiker, Scottish Terrier, Shetland Sheepdog et al

Proof	Species
X-Severe Combined Immunodeficiency (X-SCID)	Basset Hound, Welsh Corgie
Dwarfism	German Shepherd Dog, Saarloos Wolfhound, Czechoslovakian Wolfhound, Labrador Retriever

Examination material: EDTA blood/Oral mucosal smear

Coagulation

Thrombocyte Number

Reference Parameters

Dog: 150–500 × 10^9/l
Cat: 180–550 × 10^9/l

↑ **Parameters (Thrombocytosis)**
- Physiological
  - Excitement
  - Physical strain
  - Pregnancy
- Acute/chronic haemorrhage
- Acute/chronic inflammation
- Tumour disease
- Splenectomy
- Medicines
  - Vincristine
  - Adrenalin
  - Glucocorticoids

↓ **Parameters (Thrombocytopenia)**

↓ **Production (Bone marrow damage)**
- Infectious causes
  - FeLV/FIV [Cat]
  - FIP Coronavirus [Cat]
  - Parvovirus
  - (Ehrlichia sp. [Dog])

- Toxic Causes
  - Phenylbutazone
  - Metamizole/Carbimazole
  - Chloramphenicol
  - Phenobarbital
  - Sulfonamides
  - Tetracyclines
  - Cytostatics
  - Radiation
  - Heavy metal poisoning
  - Oestrogen (endogenous/ exogenous)
  - Levamisol
  - Acetylsalicylic acid
  - Paracetamol
  - Penicillin
  - Streptomycin
  - Diuretics
  - Acetazolamide
  - Propylthiouracil
  - Gold preparations
  - Uraemia
  - Endotoxins/Mycotoxins
- Immunoreactive Causes
  - Infection
  - Medicines
  - Autoimmune disease
- Bone marrow tumours
  - Multiple myeloma

- – Lymphatic leukaemia
- – Myeloid leukaemia
- Other Causes
  - – Myelofibrosis/Osteofibrosis
  - – Radiation
  - – Iron deficiency anaemia
  - – Hypocortisolism (Addison's disease)

↑ **Consumption**

- DIC
  - – Septicaemia/endotoxaemia
  - – Gastric dilation/volvulus
  - – Pyometra
  - – Urinary tract infection
  - – Haemorrhagic enteritis
  - – Splenic torsion
  - – Acute pancreatitis
  - – Shock
  - – Heart failure
  - – Liver failure
  - – Haemolysis
  - – Snake venom
  - – Heat stroke
  - – Electric accident
  - – Burns
  - – FIP [Cat]
  - – Tumour diseases
  - – (Dirofilaria sp. [Dog])
- Immunoreactive Causes
  - – Infection
  - – Medicines
  - – Autoimmune thrombocytopenia
  - – Systemic lupus erythematosus
- Infectious Causes
  - – FeLV/FIV [Cat]
  - – FIP Coronavirus [Cat]
  - – Parvovirus
  - – Canine distemper virus [Dog]
  - – CAV-1 (Hepatitis c.c.) [Dog]
  - – Canine Herpes virus [Dog]
  - – Leptospira sp. [Dog]
  - – Salmonella sp.
  - – Haemobartonella sp. [Cat]
  - – Babesia sp. [Dog]
  - – (Histoplasma sp.)
  - – (Ehrlichia sp. [Dog])
- Splenomegaly
- Chronic haemorrhage
- Feline aortic thrombosis [Cat]

Prothrombin Time (PT)

Indication

Measure for the **exogenous (extrinsic) system** + final common pathway of coagulation

Reference Parameters

Dog: 7–10 s
Cat: 7–12 s

↑ **Parameters (Prolonged Prothrombin Time)**

- Vitamin-K deficiency/ Antagonism
  - – Liver failure
  - – Malabsorption syndrome
  - – Feline Cholangiohepatitis [Cat]
  - – Obstructive jaundice
  - – Damage to the intestinal flora (Antibiosis)
  - – Dicoumarol poisoning (Rodenticides)
- Liver failure

- Factor VII deficiency [esp Beagle)
- Factor X deficiency [esp Cocker]
- DIC
- Systemic lupus erythematosus

Thromboplastin Time (Quick)

Indication

Measure for the **exogenous (extrinsic) system** + final common pathway of coagulation

Reference Parameters

Dog: 75–130%
Cat: 60–150%
↓ **Parameters (Prolonged Thromboplastin Time)**
- Vitamin K deficiency/ antagonism
  - Liver failure
  - Malabsorption syndrome
  - Feline cholangiohepatitis [Cat]
  - Obstructive jaundice
  - Damage to the intestinal flora (Antibiosis)
  - Dicoumarol poisoning (Rodenticides)
- Liver failure
- Factor VII deficiency [esp Beagle)
- Factor X deficiency [esp Cocker]
- DIC
- Systemic lupus erythematosus

(Activated) Partial Thromboplastin Time (PTT/aPTT)

Indication

Measure for the **endogenous (intrinsic) system** + final common pathway of coagulation

Reference Parameters

Dog: < 24 s; Cat: < 22 s
↑ **Parameters (Prolonged PTT/aPTT) with Normal PT/Quick**
- Haemophilia A (Factor VIII deficiency) (♂Dog/Cat)
- Haemophilia B (Factor IX deficiency) (♂ Dog/Cat)
- Factor XI deficiency (Dog)
- Factor XII deficiency (Hagemann) (Cat)
- Heparin therapy
↑ **PT/↓ Quick**
- Factor deficiency II, V, X
- Fibrinogen deficiency
- Vitamin K deficiency/ antagonism
- Fibrinolysis therapy
- Heparin therapy
- DIC
- Hyperfibrinolysis

Fibrin Degradation Products (FDP)

Indication

DIC/Suspicion of hyperfibrinolysis

Reference Parameters

Laboratory dependent
↑ **Parameters**
• DIC
    – Septicaemia/endotoxaemia
    – Gastric dilation/volvulus
    – Pyometra
    – Urinary tract obstruction
    – Haemorrhagic enteritis
    – Splenic torsion
    – Acute pancreatitis
    – Shock
    – Heart failure
    – Liver failure
    – Haemolysis
    – Snake venom
    – Heat stroke
    – Electric accident
    – Burns
    – FIP [Cat]
    – Tumour disease
    – (Dirofilaria sp. [Dog])
• Thromboembolism
    – Feline aortic
      thromboembolism [Cat]
    – Pulmonary
      thromboembolism
    – Therapeutic success in non-
      regenerative anaemia
• Hyperfibrinolysis
• Fibrinolysis therapy

Bleeding Time

Indication

Global coagulation test

Test Procedure

Measurement of the bleeding
time after ear laceration or
claw clipping (filter paper)

Reference Parameters

Dog: < 6 min Cat: < 3 min
↑ **Parameters (Prolonged
Bleeding Time)**
• Thrombocytopenia
• Thrombocytopathy
• Vitamin K deficiency/
  Antagonism
• DIC
• Von Willebrand syndrome

Factor Determination

• Von Willebrand factor
• Factor VIII
• Factor IX

Assessment of Coagulation Tests

Disease	Bleeding Time	PT/Quick	PTT/aPTT	Fibrin Degradation Products	Thrombocytes
Vit. K deficiency/ Dicoumarol poisoning	N	↑	N/↑	N	N
DIC	↑	N/↑	N/↑	↑	↓
Thrombocytopenia	↑	N	N	N	↓
Thrombocytopathy	↑	N	N	N	N
Von Willebrand syndrome	↑	N	N/↑	N	N
Haemophilia A (Factor VIII deficiency)	N	N	↑	N	N
Haemophilia B (Factor IX deficiency)	N	N	↑	N	N
Factor XI deficiency	N	N	↑	N	N
Factor XII deficiency	N	N	↑	N	N
Factor VII deficiency	N	↑	N	N	N
Factor X deficiency	N	↑	↑	N	N

Urinalysis

Urinary Output/Volume

Reference Parameters

Dog: 1–2 ml/kg KG/h
(20–40 ml/kg KG/d)
Cat: 1–2 ml/kg KG/h
(20–30 ml/kg KG/d)

↑ **Parameters (Polyuria)**
- See principal symptom:
  Polydipsia/Polyuria

↓ **Parameters (Oliguria/ Anuria)**
- See princical symptom:
  Oliguria/Anuria

Specific Gravity

Reference Parameters

Dog: >1,015
Cat: >1,015

↑ **Parameters (Hypersthenuria)**
- Dehydration
- Blood loss
- Shock
- Congestive heart failure
- Fever
- Renal infarction
- Proteinuria
- Glucosuria
- Medicines
  - Dextranes
- Oliguria (sometimes in acute renal failure)

↓ **Parameters (Hyposthenuria) Polyuria**
- Medicines
  - Glucocorticoids
  - Anticonvulsants
  - Diuretics
  - Continuous intravenous drip infusion
- Hypercortisolism (Cushing's disease) [esp Dog]
- Diabetes mellitus
- Hyperthyroidism [Cat]
- Hypokalaemia [esp Cat]
- Chronic renal failure

Urine Colour

Reference Parameters

Dog/Cat: pale to intense yellow

Light/Colourless
- Polyuria

Yellow–Orange
- Urine concentration
- Bilirubin
- Medicines
  - Nitrofurantoin
  - Sulfasalazine
  - Riboflavin
  - Fluorescein

Red
- Haematuria
- Haemoglobinuria
- Myoglobinuria
- Porphyria [Cat]
- Beetroot
- Medicines
  - Phenytoin
  - Bromsulphthalein (BSP)
  - Chronic lead poisoning
  - Chronic mercury poisoning
- Stale urine sample

Green–Brown
- Bilirubin/Biliverdin
- Myoglobin
- Pseudomonas infection
- Phenols

Blue
- Methylene blue

Milky
- Pyuria (pus)
- Lipiduria

Urine Chemistry

Reference Parameters

Dog/Cat:
pH: 5,5–7,0
Total Protein: 60–530 mg/l
Creatinine: < 1,06 g/l
Protein-Creatinine
Ratio: < 0,5
Glucose: negative
Ketones: negative
Bilirubin: Dog: up to (+)
                          Cat: negative
Haemoglobin: negative
Myoglobin: negative

↑ pH Alkaline
- Stale urine sample
- Postprandial
- Bacterial cystitis
- Diet (protein poor)
- Respiratory alkalosis (Hyperventilation)
- Vomitus (Stomach contents esp with pyloric stenosis)
- Urinary tract obstruction
- Medicines
  - Sodium bicarbonate
  - Lactate
  - Acetazolamide

↓ pH acid
- Diabetic ketoacidosis
- Azotaemia
- Diarrhoea
- Vomitus (small intestinal content/bile)
- Respiratory acidosis
- Hypoxia
  - Obstructive respiratory tract disease
  - Cardiac disease (esp right-left shunt)
- Shock
- Protein degradation
  - Protein rich diet
  - Cachexia
- Medicines
  - Methionin
  - Ammonium chloride
  - Vitamin C
  - Furosemide
  - NaCl
  - Acidifying dietary food (stone prophylaxis)

↑ Protein (Proteinuria)
- Physiological (oestrus)
- Urinary tract infection/ tumours/ Urolithiasis
- Infection of the reproductive organs/tumours (esp pyometra, prostatitis, ejaculation)
- Haematuria
- Haemoglobinuria
- Myoglobinuria
- Hyperproteinaemia
- Acute/chronic renal failure

↑ Protein/Creatinine Ratio
- Glomerulonephritis
- Amyloidosis

- Bense-Jones Proteinuria

↑ **Glucose (Glucosuria)**

With ↑ Blood glucose (Hyperglycaemia)

- Physiological
  - Stress [esp Cat]
  - Postprandial
- Diabetes mellitus
- Hypercortisolism (Cushing's disease) [esp Dog]
- Hyperthyroidism [Cat]
- Progesterone (Dioestrus, bitch)
- Medicines
  - Glucocorticoids
  - Progestagen therapy
  - Adrenalin
  - Xylazine
  - Ketamine
  - Alphaxolon/Alphadolon (Saffan®)
  - Thiazides
  - Insulin overdose (Somogyi effect)
- Acromegaly (STH excess)
- Acute pancreatitis [esp Dog]
- Phaeochromocytoma

With Normal Blood Glucose

- Fanconi syndrome (primary renal glucosuria)
- Acute/chronic renal failure

↑ **Ketones (Ketonuria)**

- Diabetic ketoacidosis
- Hypoglycaemia (Insulinoma)
- Trauma (Lipolysis)
- Fasting esp with obesity (lipolysis)
- Diet food (fat rich + poor in carbohydrates)

↑ **Bilirubin (Bilirubinuria)**

- Haemolysis
  - Intravasal (haemolytic anaemia)
  - Extravasal (haematuria)
- Hepatitis
- Hepatosis
- Liver tumours/cysts
- Bile duct obstruction

↑ **Haemoglobin (Haemoglobinuria)**
  - Urine sediment: Erythrocytes
  - Serum CK: normal
- Haemolysis
  - Intravasal (haemolytic anaemia)
  - Extravasal (Haematuria)
- Hypoglycaemia

↑ **Myoglobin (Myoglobinuria)**
  - Urine sediment: without erythrocytes
  - Serum CK: ↑
- Muscle trauma
- Seizures
- Myositis

Urine sediment

↑ **Erythrocytes (Haematuria)**

- See principal symptom: Urine, bloody

↑ **Leucocytes (Pyuria)**

- Pyelonephritis
- Cystitis/Urethritis
- Endometritis/Pyometra
- Prostatitis/Balanoposthitis

Bacteria

- Rods (gram negative)
  - E. coli
  - Klebsiella sp.
  - Enterobacter sp.

- Proteus sp.
- Pseudomonas sp.
- Corynebacterium sp.
- Cocci (gram positive)
  - Staphylococcus sp.
  - Streptococcus sp.
- Spirochaetes
  - Leptospira sp. [Dog]

Fungi

- Candida sp.

Parasites

- Capillaria sp.
- (Dioctophyma sp.)
- (Dirofilaria Microfilaria [esp Dog])

Epithelial Cells

- Renal tubular epithelium (nephritis)
- Transitional epithelium (Cystitis/Pyelonephritis)
- Squamous epithelium
- Tumour cells

Casts

- Hyaline casts
  - Proteinuria
- Epithelial casts → Granular casts → Wax casts
  - Tubular nephropathy
  - Interstitial nephritis
  - Amyloidosis (Wax cylinder)
- Fatty casts
  - Tubular nephropathy [esp Cat]
- Erythrocyte casts
  - Renal haemorrhage (nephritis, trauma, tumours)
- Leucocyte casts
  - Acute nephritis/ pyelonephritis

- Haemoglobin casts
  - Haemolysis

Crystals

pH alkaline

- Struvite (shape: coffin lid)
- Ca Carbonate (shape: spheres, discs)
- Ca Phosphate (shape: long prisms)
- Ammonium urate (shape: thornapple)
  - Dalmatians
  - Liver disease (portosystemic shunt)

pH Acidic

- Oxalate (Monohydrate. shape: dumbbell) (Dihydrate. shape: envelope)
- Cystine (shape: flat hexagonal sheets)
- Urate (shape: prisms)

Rare Crystals

- Ethylene glycol poisoning (Ca Oxalate)
- Allopurinol
- Sulfonamides (shape: needles)
- Bilirubin (shape: brown needles)
- Cholesterol (shape: colourless flat sheets)
- Leucin (shape: spheres, discs)
- Tyrosin (shape: yellow needles)

Further Urine Examinations

- Bence-Jones Proteins
  - Multiple myeloma/ plasmocytoma

- Cortisol/Creatinine ratio
  - Adrenal gland function test
- Bacterial culture
- SDS Gel electrophoresis
- Poisonings

- Thallium
- Arsenic
- Cadmium/mercury
- Organophosphates
- p-Nitrophenyl

Faecal Examination

Faecel Examination

Parasites

Direct Faecal Examination (Microscope Slide)
  - Obligatory preliminary investigation

Flotation
- Protozoa
  - Cryptosporidium sp.
  - Giardia sp.
  - Isospora sp.
  - Toxoplasma sp. [Cat]
  - Pneumocystis sp.
  - Sarcocystis sp.
  - Balantidium sp. [Dog]
  - (Entamoeba sp.)
- Tape worms (Cestodes) (Oocysts)
  - Dipylidium sp.
  - Joyeuxiella sp.
  - Diplopylidium sp.
  - Spirometra sp.
  - Echinococcus sp.
  - Taenia sp.
  - Mesocestoides sp.
- Round worms (Nematodes) (Oocysts)
  - Toxocara sp.
  - Toxascaris sp.
  - Ancylostoma sp.
  - Uncinaria sp.

- Trichuris sp. [Dog]
- Capillaria sp.
- (Spirocerca sp. [Dog])

Sedimentation
- Tape worms (Oocyts)
  - Diphyllobothrium sp. [Dog]

Baermann–Wetzel Method
- Lung worms (Larvae)
  - Strongyloides sp. [esp Dog]
  - Filaroides sp. (rare) [Dog]
  - (Aleurostrongylus sp. [Cat])
  - (Angiostrongylus sp. [Dog])
  - (Crenosoma sp. [esp Dog])

Sticky Tape Preparation
- Trichuris sp. [Dog]

Viruses
- Parvovirus antigen
- Coronavirus antigen

Bacteria
- Bacterial culture
  - Salmonella sp.
  - Campylobacter sp.
  - Yersinia sp.
  - E. coli
  - Clostridium sp.
- Bacterial toxins
  - Clostridium toxin

Fungi
- Fungal culture

Digestion products
↑ **Muscle Fibres and/or**

↑ **Starch**

• Exocrine pancreatic insufficiency

↑ **Fat**

• Malabsorption syndrome
• Maldigestion syndrome

↑ **Lysozyme/PMN Elastase**

• Colitis
• Colonic carcinoma

↑ **Lactic Acid**

• Lactase deficiency

↑ **Plasma Proteins**

• Protein-losing enteropathy

↓ **Chymotrypsin**

• Exocrine pancreatic insufficiency

↓ **Elastase**

• Exocrine pancreatic insufficiency

Blood/(Occult Blood)

• See principal symptoms: Faeces, bloody

Analysis of Body Cavity Effusions

Thoracic Effusion

Causes

Transudate

• Congestive heart failure (Right sided heart failure)
• Hypoalbuminaemia

Modified Transudate

• Congestive heart failure
• Tumours
• Diaphragmatic hernia
• Pancreatitis
• Autoimmune diseases
• Liver cirrhosis

Exudate

• Pus (Pyothorax)
  – Actinomyces sp.
  – Nocardia sp.
  – Pasteurella sp.
  – Bacteroides sp.
  – Fusobacterium sp.
  – Pneumonia
  – Foreign body perforation
  – Oesophageal perforation
  – Tumour necrosis

  – Thoracocentesis
• Blood
  – Lung lobe torsion
  – Coagulopathies
  – Trauma
  – Tumours
• Chyle
  – Congestive heart failure
  – Trauma
  – Tumour
  – Lymphangiectasia [Dog]
  – Diaphragmatic hernia
  – Lung lobe torsion
  – (Dirofilaria sp. [esp Dog])
• Other causes
  – FIP Coronavirus [Cat]
  – Tumours
  – Diaphragmatic hernia
  – Lung lobe torsion

Abdominal Effusion

Causes

Transudate

• Hypoalbuminaemia

- Protein-losing enteropathy
- Protein-losing nephropathy
- Liver cirrhosis/ portosystemic shunt
- Feline cholangiohepatitis [Cat]
- Cachexia
- Burns
- Tumour
- Lymph vessel obstruction
- Liver cirrhosis

Modified Transudate
- Right sided heart failure
- Pericardial disease
- Tumours

Exudate
- Pus
  - Penetrating wound
  - Ruptured pyometra
  - Intestinal perforation
  - Intestinal obstruction (Ileus)
  - Septicaemia/ruptured abscess
  - Peritonitis
- Blood
  - Traumatic organ/ blood vessel rupture
  - Coagulopathy
  - Splenic rupture/ Haemangiosarcoma [Dog]
- Chyle
  - Lymph vessel obstruction/ rupture
  - Retroperitoneal haematoma
  - Lymphangiectasia [Dog]
  - Liver cirrhosis
  - Heart disease
  - Intestinal obstruction (Ileus)

- Acute pancreatitis
- Tumour
- Pseudochyle
  - Tumour
  - Chronic inflammation
- Urine
  - Ruptured bladder/torn ureter/urethra
- Bile
  - Gall bladder rupture
  - Liver rupture
- Other Causes
  - Intestinal torsion/volvulus
  - Testicular torsion/ cryptorchism
  - Gastric/intestinal rupture
  - Pancreatic rupture
  - Acute pancreatitis
  - Tumours
  - FIP [Cat]
  - Diaphragmatic hernia
  - Vena cava syndrome (Dirofilaria sp. [Dog])

Pericardial Effusion

Causes

Modified Transudate
- Congestive heart failure
- Uraemia
- Hypoalbuminaemia
- Cardiac arrhythmias
- Pericardio-diaphragmatic hernia

Exudate
- Pus (Pericarditis)
  - Canine distemper virus [Dog]
  - FIP Coronavirus [Cat]
  - Leptospira sp. [Dog]

- Actinomyces sp.
- Nocardia sp.
- Mycobacterium sp.
- Toxoplasma sp.
- Pasteurella sp.
- Streptococcus spp.
- Staphylococcus spp.
- E. coli
- Cryptococcus sp. [Cat]
- Tumours
- Blood
  - Atrial rupture
  - Foreign body
  - Haemangiosarcoma [esp Dog]
  - Coagulopathy
  - Pericarditis

Cytological Malignancy Criteria

Changes in Cell Shape

- Cell pleomorphism (Variable cell shape)
  - Atypical
  - Loss of differentiation
  - Heterotypical

Nuclear Changes

- Polynuclear cells
- Macrocaryosis
  - ↑ nucleus
  - ↑ nucleus cytoplasm ratio
- Anisocaryosis (nuclei of variable size/shape)
- Hyperchromasia of the nuclear wall
- Polyploidy
- Atypical mitoses

Changes of the Nucleoli

- ↑ Nucleoli number
- Macronucleosis (↑ Nucleoli size)
- Anisonucleosis (Nucleoli of variable size/shape)

Cytoplasmatic Changes

- Atypical size
  - expansion
  - shape
  - contents
  - staining

Distinguishing Features of Body Cavity Effusion

Test	Transudate	Mod. Transudate	Exudate	Blood	Chyle
Colour	clear	cloudy	cloudy yellow/brown (FIP/bile)	bloody	milky
Erythrocytes	(-)	(-/+)	(+)	+	(+)
Thrombocytes	(-)	(-)	(-)	+	(-)
Leucocytes/µl	↓ (< 1000) (Lymph)	↑ (< 7000) (Lymph/Neutro)	↑ (> 7000) (Neutro) ↓ (< 5000) (FIP)	Like blood	↓ (< 1000) (Mono/Lymph)
Tumour cells	(-)	(-/+)	(-/+)	(-/+)	(-)
Bacterial culture	(-)	(-)	(+)	(-)	(-)
Specific gravity	< 1,018	1,018–1,025	↑ (> 1,025)	↑ (> 1,025)	↑ (> 1,025)
Protein (g/dl) (relevant only wih thoracic effusion)	↓ (< 2,5)	2,5–5,0	↑ (> 2,5)	↑ (> 2,5)	↑ (> 2,5)
A/G Ratio	↑ (> 0,6)	↑ (> 0,6)	↓ (< 0,6) (FIP)	↑ (> 0,6)	↑ (> 0,6)
Rivalta test (Cat)	(-)	(-)	(+) (FIP)	(-)	(-)
LDH (U/l)	↓ (< 200)	↓ (< 200) (Heart disease) ↑ (> 200) (Neoplasia)	↑ (> 1600) (FIP)	↑/↓	↓ (< 200)

Bilirubin	< Serum	< Serum	↑ (> Serum) (Gall bladder rupture)	↑/↓	< Serum
Creatinine	< Serum	< Serum	↑ (> Serum) (Urinary tract rupture)	< Serum	< Serum
Amylase/Lipase	< Serum	< Serum	↑ (> Serum) (Pancreatic rupture /Pancreatitis)	< Serum	< Serum
Cholesterol	< Serum	< Serum	↑ (> Serum) (Pseudochyle)	< Serum	< Serum
Triglycerides	< Serum	< Serum	< Serum	< Serum	↑ (> Serum)
Ether clearance test	not relevant	not relevant	(-)	not relevant	(+) (clearance)

Liquor Analysis

Causes	Colour	Pressure	Cells(/µl)	Protein (g/dl)	Globulin (Pandy/ Nonne–Apelt)	Glucose (% Serum)
Normal	clear	5–15 cm H₂O	< 5	< 1	(–)	< 60
Acute trauma/ haemorrhage	clear/bloody	N/↑	↑ (Ery)	N/↑	(+)	N
Viral Meningoencephalitis	clear/ cloudy (FIP)	N/↑	↑ (Lymph, Neutro)	N/↑(FIP)	(–/+) (FIP)	N/↓
Bacterial Meningoencephalitis	cloudy	↑	↑ (Neutro)	↑	++	↓
Rickettsial Meningoencephalitis	clear	↑	↑ (Ery, Lymph, Mono)	↑	(+)	↓
Mycotic Meningoencephalitis	clear/cloudy	↑	↑ (Ery, Neutro)	↑	(+)	↓
Parasitic Meningoencephalitis	clear/bloody	↑	↑ (Ery, Eos, Neutro)	↑	(+)	↓
Granulomatous Meningoencephalitis	clear/bloody	↑	↑ (Ery, Eos, Lympho)	↑	++	N
Brain tumours	clear	N/↑	N/↑ (Lymph)	N/↑	(–/+)	N/↓
Degenerative Diseases	clear	N	N	N/↑	(–/+)	N

Synovial Analysis

Causes	Colour	Viscosity	Mucin clot test	Spontaneous clotting	Leucocytes (/μl)	Glucose (% Serum)	Culture	Rheuma factor
Normal	clear/light yellow	↑	fast	(–)	< 200	> 90	(–)	(–)
Degenerative Arthrosis	clear/cloudy yellow	↑	solid	(–/+)	< 5000	N	(–)	(–)
Immuneractive Arthritis	clear/cloudy yellow/red	↓	friable	(+)	↑ (> 5000)	N	(–)	(–/+)
Septic Arthritis	clear/cloudy yellow/red	↓	friable	(+)	↑ (> 100 000)	↓ (< 50)	(+)	(–)
Trauma	clear/cloudy red	↓	solid	(–)	< 5000	N	(–)	(–)

Further examination parameters: Tumour cytology, electrophoresis, Lupus erythematosus cytology, synovial biopsy, Lyme Borrelia antigen (PCR)

Analysis of Tracheobronchial Secretion (TBS)

Cytology	Culture	Evaluation
Physiological cell count		
• Low in cells – ciliated epithelium – goblet cells • ↓ Mucous	Physiological flora	Physiological
Mucoid cell count		
• Rich in cells – ciliated epithelium – goblet cells • ↑ Mucous	Physiological flora	Tracheal collapse Tracheal hypoplasia Respiratory tract tumours Chronic dry cough Aspiration pneumonia
Mucopurulent cytology		
• Rich in cells – cell debris – Neutrophil granulocytes • ↑ Mucous • Bacteria	Bordetella bronchiseptica E. coli Pseudomonas spp. Further facultative pathogenic microbes	Bacterial tracheobronchitis/Pneumonia Foreign body

Haemorrhagic cell count

- Rich in cells
  - Erythrocytes
- ↓ Mucous

Physiological flora
Mycobacterium spp.

Lung contusion
Chronic dry cough
Foreign body
Coagulopathy
Tuberculosis

Eosinophilic cell count

- Rich in cells
  - Eosinophilic granulocytes
- Parasitic larvae
  - Filaroides sp. [Dog]
  - Capillaria sp.
  - (Crenosoma sp. [Dog])
  - Aelurostrongylus sp. [Cat]
  - (Angiostrongylus sp. [Dog])
  - (Dirofilaria sp. [esp Dog])
- ↑ Mucous

Physiological flora
Bacterial secondary infection
Mycoses
  - Cryptococcus sp.

Allergic bronchopneumonia
Parasitic bronchopneumonia
Mycotic bronchopneumonia
  - (Histoplasma sp.)
  - (Blastomyces sp.)
  - (Coccidioidomyces sp.)
  - Secondary mycoses

Analysis of Tracheobronchial Secretion (TBS) (Contd)

Cytology	Culture	Evaluation
Mixed cell count		
• Rich in cells – ciliated epithelium – Lymphocytes – Neutrophil granulocytes – Macrophages • ↑ Mucous	Physiological flora Bacterial secondary infection	Congestive heart failure Viral tracheobronchitis/pneumonia
Tumourous cell count		
• Rich in cells – esp bronchial carcinoma – Lymphatic leukaemia [Cat] • ↑ Mucous • Bacteria	Physiological flora Bacterial secondary infection	Bronchial carcinoma Lymphatic leukaemia [Cat]

Vaginal Cytology (Physiological Cycle of the Bitch)

Cycle	Cycle length	Vulva	Secretion	Cytology
Proestrus	7–9 Days	swelling	bloody	• Erythrocytes • Epithelial cells – Basophil intermedial cells

Oestrus	4–8 Days	swelling	Serosanguineous	• Epithelial cells
				  – Acidophil superficial cells
				  – Anuclear superficial cells
				  – Intermediate cells

Metoestrus	4–6 Weeks	reduced swelling	cloudy mucous	• Erythrocytes
				• Neutrophil granulocytes
				• Epithelial cells
				  – Basophil intermediate cells
				  – Basophil parabasal cells

Anoestrus	3–5 Months	normal	normal	• Epithelial cells
				  – Basophil basal cells
				  – Basophil parabasal cells
				  – Basophil intermediate cells

Endocrine Function Tests

Adrenal Gland Function

Dexamethasone Suppression Test (Low Dose Screening Test)

Indication
- Polydipsia/Polyuria with suspicion of hypercortisolism (Cushing's disease) [esp Dog]

Test Procedure in the Dog
1. Base cortisol level (Plasma/Serum)
2. Dexamethasone 0,01 mg/kg BW i. v.
3. Cortisol suppression level after 4hrs (plasma/serum)
4. Cortisol suppression level after 8hrs (plasma/serum)

Test Procedure in the Cat
1. Base cortisol level (plasma/serum)
2. Dexamethasone 0,1 mg/kg BW i. v.
3. Cortisol suppression level after 8hrs (plasma/serum)

Evaluation
(see table below)

Base level	Suppression level (4 h)	Suppression level (8 h)	Evaluation
N/↑	N/↑ (< 50%)	↑ (> 10 nmol/l or ng/ml)	Cushing's disease (adrenal or pituitary)
N/↑	↓ (50%, < 10 nmol/l or ng/ml)	↑ (> 10 nmol/l or ng/ml)	Pituitary Cushing's disease Physiological
N/↓	↓ (50%, < 10 nmol/l or ng/ml)	↓ (< 10 nmol/l or ng/ml)	Iatrogenic Cushing's disease

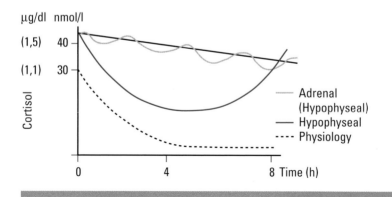

Dexamethasone Suppression Test (High Dose Screening Test)

Indication
- Differentiation between adrenal and pituitary hypercortisolism (Cushing's disease) in the dog

Test Procedure
1. Base cortisol level (plasma/serum)
2. Dexamethasone 0,1 mg/kg BW i. v./i. m.
3. Cortisol suppression level after 3 h/4 h (plasma/serum)
4. Cortisol suppression level after 8 h (plasma/serum)

Evaluation
(see table below)

Base level	Suppression level (4 h)	Suppression level (8 h)	Evaluation
N/↑	↑ (< 50%)	↑ (< 50%)	Cushing's disease (esp adrenal/[pituitary])
N/↑	↓ (> 50%)	↑	Pituitary Cushing's disease
N/↑	↑	↓ (> 50%)	Pituitary Cushing's disease
N/↑	↓ (> 50%)	↓ (> 50%)	Pituitary Cushing's disease

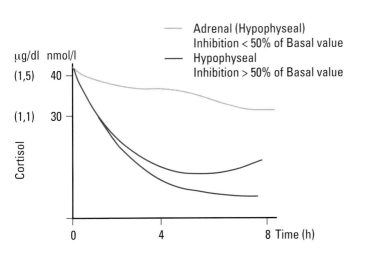

ACTH Stimulation Test

Indication
- Differentiation between spontaneous and iatrogenic hypercortisolism (Cushing's disease)
- Hypocortisolism (Addison's disease) suspicion
- Therapeutic control with hypercortisolism (Cushing's disease)

Test Procedure
1. Base cortisol level (plasma/serum)
2. Dog: ACTH (Synacten®) 0,25 mg/Dog (25 IU) i. v./i. m. Cat: ACTH (Synacten®) 0,125 mg/Cat (12,5 IU) i. v./i. m.
3. Cortisol stimulation level after 60 min (plasma/serum)

Evaluation
Cushing's disease: Stimulation value > 150 nmol/l or ng/ml or > 3 times the base parameters

Trilostan therapeutic control: 15–55 nmol/l or ng/ml (see table below)

Base level	Stimulation level (90 min)	Evaluation
N/↑	↑ (> × 5)	Spontaneous Cushing's disease
N/↓		Iatrogenic Cushing's disease
N/↓	↓	
N/↑/↓	↑ (< × 5)	Hypocortisolism (Addison's disease)

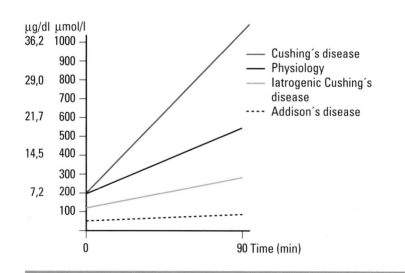

Cortisol/Creatinine Ratio

Indication
- Suspicion of hypercortisolism (Cushing's disease)
- Differentiation between adrenal Cushing's disease and pituitary Cushing's disease

Calculation
- Urine Cortisol (μmol/l)
  - Urine Creatinine (μmol/l)

Test Procedure
1. Cortisol/Creatinine base level (morning urine on the 1st day)
2. Cortisol/Creatinine base level (Morning urine on the 2nd day)
3. Dexamethasone 0,1 mg/ kg BW p. o. 3 × in 8 hour intervals (2nd day)
4. Cortisol/Creatinine Suppression level (morning urine on the 3rd day)

Evaluation
(see table below)

Base level 1st day	Base level 2nd day	Suppression level 3rd day	Evaluation
N/↑	↑		Cushing's disease (adrenal or pituitary)
N/↑	↑	↑	Cushing's disease (adrenal/ [pituitary])
N/↑	↑	↓ (< 50%)	Pituitary Cushing's disease

Thyroid Function

K Value

Indication
- Hypothyroidism

Calculation (12h Fasted Parameters)
$k = 0{,}7 \times fT_4$ (pmol/l)
- Cholesterol (mmol/l)

Evaluation
$K < -4$ = Hypothyroidism

TRH Stimulation Test

Indication
- Suspicion of hypothyroidism [Dog]

Test Procedure
1. T_4/fT_4 base level (plasma/serum)
2. TRH (Thyreoliberin®) 200 μg/animal i. v.

3. T_4/fT_4 stimulation level (90 min) (plasma/serum)
4. T_4/fT_4 stimulation level (3 h)

Evaluation
(see table below)

Base level	Suppression level (3 h)	Evaluation
N/↓	↑ (< 50%)	Hypothyroidism
N/↓	↑ (> 50%)	Physiological

TSH Stimulation Test

Indication
• Suspicion of hypothyroidism [Dog]
• Reagent currently unavailable

Test Procedure
1. T_4 base level (plasma/serum)
2. TSH 0,1 IE/kg BW i. v.
3. T_4 stimulation level (4 h/6 h) (plasma/serum)

Evaluation
(see table below)

Base level	Stimulation level (4 h/6 h)	Evaluation
N/↓	↑ (< 3 µg/dl = 35 nmol/l)	Hypothyroidism
N/↓	↑ (> 3 µg/dl)	Physiological

T_3 Suppression test

Indication
• Suspicion of hyperthyroidism [Cat]

Test Procedure
1. T_4/fT_4 base level (plasma/serum)
2. T_3 (Thybon®) 25 µg/Cat p. o. 6 times in 8hr intervals
3. T_4/fT_4 suppression level ca. 2–4 h after final T_3 administration (plasma/serum)

Evaluation
(see table below)

Base level	Suppression level (4 h)	Evaluation
N/↑	↓ (> 50%)	Physiological
N/↑	N /↓ (< 50%)	Hyperthyroidism

Gonade Function

HCG Stimulation Test

Indication
- Evidence of hormone producing gonades (ie retained ovarian tissue after incomplete removal, cryptorchism)

Test Procedure
1. Testosterone or Oestradiol Base value (Serum)
2. HCG (Ovogest®) 500 I.E. i. v.
3. Stimulation level after 60 min

Evaluation
- Male dog: Testosterone stimulation level > 1 ng/ml with cryptorchism
- Bitch: Oestradiol stimulation level > 15 ng/ml with retained ovarian tissue

GnRH Stimulation Test

Indication
- Evidence of hormone producing gonades (ie retained ovarian tissue after incomplete removal, cryptorchism)

Test Procedure
1. Testosterone or Oestradiol base level (serum)
2. Buserelin (Receptal®) 0,32 µg/ animal i. v.
3. Stimulation level after 1hr in the male dog and 3 hours in the bitch

Evaluation
- Male dog: Testosterone stimulation level > 1 ng/ml with cryptorchism
- Bitch: Oestradiol stimulation level > 15 ng/ml with retained ovarian tissue

Further Function Tests

STH Stimulation Test

Indication
- Suspected STH Deficiency [Dog]
  - Diabetes mellitus (Type II)
  - Hypophyseal dwarfism
  - Dermatosis

Test Procedure
1. STH base level (serum)
2. Xylazine 100 µg (0,01 mg)/kg BW i. v. or Clonidin 10–30 µg (0,001–0,003 mg)/kg BW
3. STH stimulation parameters (30–60–90 min) (freeze serum after sampling)

Evaluation
(see table below)

Base level	Stimulation Parameters	Evaluation
N /↓	N /↓	STH deficiency Physiological
N /↓	↑	

Diabetes Insipidus Fluid Deprivation Test

Indication
- Polydipsia/Polyuria with suspected Diabetes insipidus

Test Procedure

1. Specific gravity/ osmolality (urine)
2. 24 h fluid deprivation
3. Specific gravity/ osmolality (urine)
   - Termination in case of dehydration > 5 % body weight or azotaemia

Evaluation
(see table below) (Extreme simplification)

Base level	Final level (Specific gravity)	Final level (Urine osmolality)	Evaluation
↓	↑ > 1,030	> 3 × Serum	Physiological
	↓ < 1,030	< 3 × Serum	Diabetes insipidus

Bile Acid Stimulation Test

Indication
- esp portosystemic shunt

Test Procedure
1. Bile acid fasting level (serum)
2. Feed 100 g meat + 5 g fat/ 10 kg BW postprandial bile acid level after 2 h

Evaluation
- Postprandial bile acid level > 50 µmol/l with portosystemic shunt

18 Appendix: Normal Laboratory Values

Normal Haematological Values

Parameter	Unit	Dog	Cat
Haematocrit (Hct)	% (l/l)	44–52 (0,44–0,52)	30–45 (0,30–0,45)
Erythrocyte number	× 10^6/µl	5,5–8,5	5,0–10,0
Haemoglobin (Hb)	g/dl (mmol/l)	15,0–19,0 (9,3–11,8)	9,0–15,0 (5,6–9,3)
Mean corpuscular volume (MCV)	fl/µm³	67–80	40–55
Mean corpuscular haemoglobin concentration (MCHC)	g/dl	32–36	30–36
Reticulocyte number	/1000	5–10	5–20
Reticulocyte Index (RI)	%	45	40
Leucocyte number	/µl	6000–12 000	6000–11 000
Neutrophil granulocytes, banded	%	0–4	0–4
Neutrophil granulocytes, segmented	%	50–75	60–75
Eosinophil granulocytes	%	0–4	0–4
Lymphocytes	%	13–30	15–30
Monocytes	%	0–4	0–4
Basophil granulocytes	%	0–1	0–1
Lymphocytes	%	13–30	15–30
Monocytes	%	0–4	0–4

Normal Haematological Values (Contd)

Parameter	Unit	Dog	Cat
Blood Sedimentation Rate (BSR) Wester-Gren Method (vertical)	mm	0–2 (1 h) 1–4 (2 h)	0–2 (1 h)
DeHag Method (vertical)			2–10 (2 h)

Normal Blood Chemistry Values

Parameter	Unit	Dog	Cat
Total Protein (TP)	g/dl (g/l)	6,0–8,0 (60–80)	6,0–8,0 (60–80)
Albumin	g/dl (g/l)	2,5–4,0 (25–40)	2,5–4,0 (25–40)
Globulin	mg/dl (mg/l)	2,4–4,5 (24–45)	2,8–5,5 (28–55)
A/G Ratio		0,6–1,1	0,6–1,2
Blood glucose	mg/dl (mmol/l)	70–120 (3,9–6,7)	70–150 (3,9–8,3)
Fructosamine	μmol/l	up to 340	up to 340
Glutamate Pyruvate Transaminase (GPT)/ Alanine Amino-transferase (ALT)	U/l	up to 55	up to 70
Alkaline Phosphatase (AP)	U/l	Adult up to 110	Adult up to 140
Bilirubin (total bilirubin)	mg/dl (μmol/l)	0,2 (3,4)	0,2 (3,4)
Ammonium	μg/dl (μmol/l)	up to 100 (up to 59)	up to 100 (up to 59)
Glutamate Oxalo-acetate Transaminase (GOT)/Asparate Amino-transferase (AST)	U/l	up to 25	up to 30

Normal Blood Chemistry Values (Contd)

Parameter	Unit	Dog	Cat
Gamma Glutamyl Transferase (GGT)	U/l	up to 6	up to 6
Lactate Dehydrogenase (LDH)	U/l	up to 130	up to 200
Bile Acids	μmol/l	up to 20 (Fasting value)	up to 20 (Fasting value)
Triglycerides	mg/dl (mmol/l)	50–100 (0,6–1,2)	50–100 (0,6–1,2)
Cholesterol	mg/dl (mmol/l)	100–300 (2,5–8,0)	75–150 (2,0–4,0)
Acetylcholinesterase	kU/l	1,5–3,0	1,0–3,0
Gastrin	ng/l	25–110	–
Folic acid	ng/ml	3,5–11,0	3,2–34,0
Cobalamin (Vitamin B12)	pg/ml	300–800	120–1200
Amylase	U/l	up to 1700	up to 1800
Lipase	U/l	up to 300	up to 280
TLI Test	μg/l	5–35	17–48
Urea	mg/dl (mmol/l)	20–50 (3,3–8,3)	30–65 (5,0–11,0)
Creatinine (Crea)	mg/dl (μmol/l)	up to 1,5 (up to 130)	up to 2,0 (up to 170)
Creatine Kinase (CK)	U/l	up to 90	up to 130
Thyroxin (T$_4$)	μg/dl (nmol/l)	1,3–3,6 (17–46)	0,9–4,0 (12–52)
Free Thyroxin (fT$_4$)	ng/dl	0,6–3,7	0,5–2,6
Insulin	mU/l	9–32 (Fasting value)	4–20 (Fasting value)
Insulin/Glucose Ratio	Insulin (mU/l): Glucose (mg/dl)	Up to 0,3	Up to 0,3

Electrolytes, Normal Values

Parameter	Unit	Dog	Cat
Sodium (Na)	mmol/l	140–155	145–158
Potassium (K)	mmol/l	3,5–5,1	3,0–4,8
Chloride (Cl)	mmol/l	96–113	110–130
Calcium (Ca)	mmol/l	2,3–3,0	2,3–3,0
Phosphate (P)	mmol/l	Adult 0,8–1,6	Adult 0,8–1,9
Magnesium (Mg)	mmol/l	0,6–1,3	0,6–1,3

Blood Gas Analysis (BGA), Normal Values

Parameter	Unit	Dog	Cat
pH		7,36–7,44	7,36–7,44
pCO_2	kPa	4,8–5,3	3,7–4,3
pO_2	kPa	11,3–12,7	11,3–12,7
Standard bicarbonate	mmol/l	22–26 +2,5	22–26 +2,5
BE (StBicarbonate–24)		to –2,5	to –2,5
Anion gap	mmol/l	8–12	8–12

Serum Electrophoresis, Normal Values

Parameter	Unit	Dog	Cat
Albumin	g/dl (%)	2,2–4,4 (47–59)	2,6–5,6 (45–60)
α_1-Globulin	g/dl (%)	0,2–0,5 (4–7)	0,2–1,3 (4–14)
α2-Globulin	g/dl (%)	0,3–0,9 (5–12)	0,4–1,1 (7–12)
β_1-Globulin	g/dl (%)	0,5–1,4 (11–20)	1,1–1,4 (11–15)
γ-Globulin	g/dl (%)	0,4–1,4 (8–18)	0,6–2,6 (10–28)

Coagulation, Normal Values

Parameter	Unit	Dog	Cat
Thrombocyte number	× 10⁹/l	150–500	180–550
Prothrombin time (PT)	s	7–10	7–12
Thromboplastin time (Quick)	%	75–130	60–150
(Activated) partial Thromboplastin time (PTT/aPTT)	s	Up to 24	Up to 22
Fibrin Degradation Products (FDP)	Laboratory dependent	Laboratory dependent	Laboratory dependent
Bleeding time	min	up to 6	up to 3

Urinalysis, Normal Values

Parameter	Unit	Dog	Cat
Urinary output/volume	ml/kg BW/h (ml/kg BW/d)	1–2 (20–40)	1–2 (20–30)
Specific gravity		>1,015	>1,015
Urine colour		pale to yellow	pale to strong yellow
pH		5,5–7,0	5,5–7,0
Protein	mg/dl	negative to 30	negative to 30
Glucose		negative	negative
Ketones		negative	negative
Bilirubin		up to (+)	negative
Haemoglobin/Myoglobin		negative	negative
Urine sediment		occasional epithelial cells	occasional epithelial cells

Index

abdominal girth, increased 12–17
    abdominal effusion/ascites 15–16
    organ enlargement 12–15
abdominal pain 8–11
    caudal 9–10
    cranial 9
    diffuse 10
    dorsal 11
anaemia 5–8
    blood loss 6–7
    bone marrow failure 7
    haemolysis 5–6
aural discharge 250–2
    ceruminal 250–1
    purulent 251

behavioural disorders 285–7
    aggression 285
    allotriophagia (compulsive ingestion of
        foreign bodies) 285–6
    automutilation 286
    barking, continuous 286
    fearfulness 286
    hypersexuality/nymphomania 287
    infanticide (killing/ingestion of puppies/
        kittens) 287
    micturition problems 287
    personality change 287
bite wounds 17
bleed, tendency to 17–21
    plasmatic coagulopathy 19–20
    thrombocytopathy 19
    thrombocytopenia 18–19

cardiovascular symptoms 47–70
    cardiac arrhythmias 52–6
        fast and irregular 54–5
        fast and regular 54
        slow and irregular 53–4
        slow and regular 52–3
    cardiac/respiratory arrest 47–9

        primary cardiac causes 48
        primary neurological causes 49
        primary respiratory causes 48
    cardiomegaly 58–61
        aorta 60
        left atrium 58–9
        left ventricle 59
        pulmonary segment 59–60
        right atrium 59
        right ventricle 59
        spherical heart 60
    cyanosis 68–70
        caudal body part 69
        central 68–9
        peripheral 69
    heart murmurs 49–52
        continuous murmur (machinery
          murmur) 51
        diastolic 50–1
        systolic 50
    heart sounds, pathological 56–8
        midsystolic clicks 57
    hypertension, arterial 61–2
    pulse alterations 63–4
        absent femoral pulse 63
        deficit 63
        jugular venous pressure 63
        strong 63
        weak 63
    syncope 64–8
        cardiovascular 64–6
        neurological 66
        other causes 66–7

dermatological symptoms 253–65
    dermal efflorescences 257–61
        primary 257, 258–9
        secondary 257–8, 259–61
    hair loss 253–7
        with pruritus 253–5
        without pruritus 255–6